Art of Illness

There is a long history of inventing illness, such as pretending to be sick for attention or accusing others of being ill. This volume explores the art of illness, and the deceptions and truths around health and bodies, from a multiplicity of angles from antiquity to the present.

The chapters, which are based on primary-source evidence ranging from antiquity to the late twentieth century, are divided into three parts. The first part explores how the idea of faking illness was understood and conceptualized across multiple fields, locations, and time periods. The second part uses case studies to emphasize the human element of those at the center of these narratives and how their behavior was shaped by societal attitudes. The third part investigates the development of regulations and laws governing malingering and malingerers. Altogether, they paint a picture of humans doing human actions—cheating, lying, stealing, but also hiding, surviving, working.

This book's careful, accessible scholarship is a valuable resource for academics, scientists, and the sophisticated undergraduate audience interested in malingering narratives throughout history.

Wendy J. Turner is Professor of History in the Department of History, Anthropology, and Philosophy at Augusta University, where she also holds affiliate professorships in the Center for Bioethics and Health Policy in the Institute for Public and Preventative Health and The Graduate School.

Routledge Advances in the History of Bioethics

Series Editors: Chris Mounsey, Stan Booth, and Madeleine Mant

Routledge Advances in the History of Bioethics aims to act as a nexus for debates typically in collections of diverse but explicitly interrelated essays about the histories and literatures of bioethical debates from a wide spectrum of disciplines, methodologies, periods and geographical contexts. This series champions conversations from within interdisciplinary collision spaces, considering the effects of physical and metaphysical environments upon factual and fictional spaces.

The History and Bioethics of Medical Education
"You've Got to Be Carefully Taught"
Edited by Madeleine Mant and Chris Mounsey

Reconsidering Extinction in Terms of the History of Global Bioethics
Edited by Stan Booth and Chris Mounsey

Stewardship and the Future of the Planet
Promise and Paradox
Edited by Rachel Carnell and Chris Mounsey

Coastal Environments in Popular Song
Lost Horizons
Edited by Glenn Fosbraey

Art of Illness
Malingering and Inventing Health Conditions
Edited by Wendy J. Turner

For more information about this series, please visit: https://www.routledge.com/Routledge-Advances-in-the-History-of-Bioethics/book-series/RAITHOB

Art of Illness

Malingering and Inventing
Health Conditions

Edited by Wendy J. Turner

Routledge
Taylor & Francis Group

NEW YORK AND LONDON

First published 2024
by Routledge
605 Third Avenue, New York, NY 10158

and by Routledge
4 Park Square, Milton Park, Abingdon, Oxon, OX14 4RN

Routledge is an imprint of the Taylor & Francis Group, an informa business

Library of Congress Cataloging-in-Publication Data
Names: Turner, Wendy J. (Wendy Jo), 1961– editor.
Title: Art of illness : malingering and inventing health conditions / edited by Wendy J. Turner.
Description: New York, NY : Routledge, 2024. | Series: Routledge advances in the history of bioethics | Includes bibliographical references and index.
Identifiers: LCCN 2023033464 (print) | LCCN 2023033465 (ebook) | ISBN 9781032589619 (hardback) | ISBN 9781032589626 (paperback) | ISBN 9781003452324 (ebook) | ISBN 9781003814375 (adobe pdf) | ISBN 9781003814382 (epub)
Subjects: LCSH: Malingering—History. | Malingering—Case studies. | Malingering—Law and legislation.
Classification: LCC RA1146 .A78 2024 (print) | LCC RA1146 (ebook) | DDC 616.8—dc23/eng/20230824
LC record available at https://lccn.loc.gov/2023033464
LC ebook record available at https://lccn.loc.gov/2023033465

ISBN: 978-1-032-58961-9 (hbk)
ISBN: 978-1-032-58962-6 (pbk)
ISBN: 978-1-003-45232-4 (ebk)

DOI: 10.4324/9781003452324

Typeset in Sabon
by Apex CoVantage, LLC

For Nathan Yanasak
My friend, champion, and husband

Contents

Abbreviations

ASB:	Archivio di Stato di Bologna, the State Archive of Bologna, Italy.
ASLu:	Archivio di Stato di Lucca, the State Archive of Lucca, Italy.
BAR:	British Archaeological Reports.
CIA:	Central Intelligence Agency, U.S. Intelligence Community.
COVID:	Shortened form of COVID-19, which is the abbreviation for "Coronavirus Identified in 2019".
CFS:	Chronic fatigue syndrome is a complicated disorder that causes extreme fatigue that continues for six months or more.
CSPD:	Calendar of State Papers: Domestic Series, Edward VI, Mary, and Elizabeth, 1547–1580, ed. Robert Lemon (London: Longman, etc. for HMPRO, 1856)
DSM:	(Sometimes DSM-I) American Psychiatric Association, *Diagnostic and Statistical Manual: Mental Disorders*. Washington, DC: Mental Hospital Service, 1952.
DSM-II:	American Psychiatric Association. *Diagnostic and Statistical Manual of Mental Disorders*, second edition. Washington, DC: American Psychiatric Association, 1968.
DSM-III:	American Psychiatric Association. *Diagnostic and Statistical Manual of Mental Disorders*, third edition. Washington, DC: American Psychiatric Association, 1980.
DSM-IV:	American Psychiatric Association. *Diagnostic and Statistical Manual of Mental Disorders*, fourth edition. Washington, DC: American Psychiatric Association, 1994.
DSM-5:	American Psychological Association, *Diagnostic and Statistical Manual of Mental Disorders*, fifth edition. Washington, DC: American Psychological Association, 2013.
EETS:	Early English Text Society.
FD:	"Factitious disorder".

HMPRO: His Majesty's Public Record Office. After about 1910, only called the Public Record Office (PRO), it has become a branch of The National Archive (TNA).

HMSO: His Majesty's Stationery Office.

IBS: Irritable bowel syndrome.

ICD: International Classification of Diseases, WHO. The current version is ICD-11 (2022). ICD-9 was used from 1979 to 1994. ICD-10 was in use from 1994 to 2021.

ME: Myalgic encephalomyelitis, commonly called chronic fatigue syndrome.

MED: *Middle English Dictionary,* second edition, edited by Robert E. Lewis, Ann Arbor: University of Michigan Press, 2007.

MISAS: "Medically insignificant signs in the absence of symptoms", see Chapter 4.

MRI: Magnetic resonance imaging.

MUS: "Medically unexplained symptoms".

OED: *Oxford English Dictionary,* Oxford: Oxford University Press, 2023, online: https://www.oed.com/.

PET: Positron emission tomography scan, used to reveal the metabolic or biochemical function of the tissue.

POTS: Postural orthostatic tachycardia syndrome, which causes the heart to race, dizziness, and fatigue when the patient moves from lying down to standing.

PRO: see below—TNA.

PTSD: Post-traumatic stress disorder.

s.v.: A Latin expression of sub verbo or sub voce, meaning "under the heading".

TB: Tuberculosis.

TNA: The National Archive. Located in Kew, London, this archival collection of records and other ephemera holds most of the royal, legal, and governmental records of England from the earliest history, even before the various kingdoms were united as England, until today with some records also pertaining to Ireland, Scotland, Wales, Sicily, Spain, France, and other locations globally.

WHO: World Health Organization.

Foreword

In the summer of 1249, Robert Malingre(s) and his wife, Maroie, transferred a Vermandois house and property to Emmeline le Poure, under the aegis of Adam le Conte. From the little documentation that exists, the transfer, from couple to individual, was without complication or challenge, easily escaping historian's notice.[1] For at least one etymologic authority, however, Robert's name suggested the origin of the term, 'malinger'.[2] Those who use medieval tax records to answer social historical questions are familiar with unpacking the meaning of names in those lists, with both profit and caution.[3] More typically, the roots of 'malinger' are seen in some association between *mal-* 'bad' via 'illness' and *haingre*, 'weak, thin', ultimately perhaps from Latin or German, with hypothetical medieval connections 'malgengos' (1225) and 'malengous' (1278).[4] Its more robust attestations, though, are of the late eighteenth and nineteenth centuries.[5]

While a true, etymologic linkage to Robert and his wife is dubious, the notion that 'malinger' might originate with a particular person signifies the *individuality* inherent in the word. The re'birth' of the individual in Western culture roughly in the eleventh to twelfth centuries (hotly debated by historians as it is) makes it possible to study malingering in Europe and beyond from the Middle Ages to now. But beyond individuality, that a certain person's baseline attributes are then overridden by fabrication to imitate another's, in order to change a bureaucratic categorization (whether governmental, religious, economic, cultural, or other)[6] is only possible if four elements exist: (a) that identification of an individual (and their attributes) can occur, (b) that the ability (and desire) to feign someone else's status for gain is possible, (c) that an institutional need to label those attributes (with functional consequences) is asserted, and (d) that the institution then recognizes that (b) can occur and wants to prevent it, using both individual and aggregate comparisons.[7] Thus, the components making up those elements, from institutions to individuals, from dissimulation to bureaucratic labeling, become analytic fixtures depending on and undergirding 'malingering'. Put in concrete terms, individual, neurotypical beggars in fourteenth-century Paris recognized that they could make more money from charitable giving if they feigned a disability (motor or sensory) and did so;[8] the French crown then promulgated laws to enjoin such dissimulation.[9] Malingering, in the form of avoiding a duty (work, military service, education, etc.), also developed a legal foothold and response; a number of English and French customaries from the twelfth century forward allowed for *essoin(e)*, a validated excuse for being a witness or other legally binding role due to illness or other accepted cause; faking *essoin(e)* was strongly discouraged.[10] Predating Talcott Parsons's sick role, the *essoin(e)* was much debated on both sides of the Channel.[11] All of these facets and more are fair game for study because of malingering's framework.

***

To some degree, the previous points explain the 'how' of assembling this book and its expert authors. But they also begin to suggest the 'why' as to malingering's value as analytic lens. Malingering is so valuable to investigate precisely because of its mediating influence in a wide variety of topics that affect the social contract, including, among many: identity, illness, disability, health, truth, verifiability, governmental categorization, sick roles, and social supports (and cohesion). Regarding the latter, Pierre Rosanvallon stressed that governmental means testing for social benefits can become socially divisive, not only because of the action itself, but because of the fractured levels of understanding policy in which,

> individuals do not evaluate the justice of the system ["la justice dans ses principes"] (according to the principle ["règle"] and its intention), but rather its practical and individualized effects ["du système"]. It is never the quantity ["condition"] of resources in general that is discussed, but the fact that someone knows such and such a family whose situation seems comparatively 'abnormally' favorable or unfavorable.[12]

The (dis)simulation need not only be intentionally fraudulent on the individual's part, but it can also be unintentionally errant on a bureaucracy's part. Malingering thus impacts cultural heuristics from the contested semiotics of psychology[13] (vide Freud's 'all neurotics are malingerers; they simulate without knowing it, and this is their sickness')[14] to the social roles of protest,[15] from the meaning of slavery[16] to the justification of pacifism,[17] while still evoking the power of countercultural farce[18] even to the boundaries of myth-making.[19] In contemporary policy, malingering impacts the interpretation of the U.S. Constitution's Fourth Amendment,[20] immigration processing,[21] and, of course, military service,[22] while pushing up against developmentalism.[23] And each of these dimensions has a sociocultural history that we need to understand in order to better address our current predicaments. The efforts of this volume's scholars (and their inevitable successors) are thus critical.

In 1897, the Franco-American physician and promoter of electricity, Dr Cornelius Herz (1845–98), traveled to England while resisting proceedings against him for a suspected crime. A Knight-Commander of the Légion d'Honneur, Herz was embroiled in a scandal that also involved President Georges Clémenceau, Thomas Edison, the Rothschilds, Jean-Martin Charcot, and the Panama Canal. He arrived in England and sought to avoid extradition on the grounds of a severe illness, necessitating evaluation by physicians. In particular, the consultants were charged with evaluating whether he was feigning illness, malingering. The artist H.S. Robert painted a skein of images of these encounters, reflecting not only the concern for fraud but also contemporary antisemitism.[24] A wealth of potential insights at a myriad of sociocultural levels remains to be learned from this story. And to this day, it is difficult to ascertain which luminaries of two premier medical establishments, French and English, were 'right' and which 'wrong' in characterizing the veracity or lack thereof in Herz's illness. Abundantly clear, however, is that his case casts an enormous range of topics and 'analysands' into relief—all because of the subject of malingering.

In guiding us a long way from thirteenth-century Vermandois, our Vergil, 'malingering', points out a wondrous path of riches before us. While it may not be that Robert and Maroie's property transfer led to the birth of 'to malinger', there is no doubt that the authors' knowledge and wisdom in the following pages will transfer to the reader with great profit and no dissimulation.

Walton O. Schalick, III, MD, PhD

Notes

1 Fernand Le Proux, "Chartes françaises du Vermandois de 1218 à 1250", *Bibliothèque de l'École des Chartes* 35 (1874): 437–77 at p. 466.

2 Alain Rey, éd., *Dictionnaire historique de la langue Française*, Nouvelle éd. (Paris: LeRobert, 2010), 1256.

3 See, among others, Sharon Farmer, *The Silk Industries of Medieval Paris* (Philadelphia: University of Pennsylvania Press, 2017), pp. 8ff & variously, and Walton O. Schalick, III, "Add One Part Pharmacy to One Part Surgery and One Part Medicine: Jean de Saint-Amand and the Development of Medical Pharmacology in Paris, c. 1230–1303" (Ph.D. diss., The Johns Hopkins University, 1997), 158–70.

4 The etymology is essentially unchanged from the 70s (*Shorter Oxford English Dictionary* (Oxford: Oxford University Press, 1973), vol. I, 1266), although the online *OED* entry from March 2022 suggests "back-formation" from "linger". See also Rey, *Dictionnaire*, 1256.

5 Christian Kay et al., eds., *Historical Thesaurus of the Oxford English Dictionary* (Oxford: Oxford University Press, 2009), vol. I at p. 67 and online OED from March 2022 "malinger" and "malingerer".

6 Williamson, for example, highlighted the differential transaction costs between the medieval and modern periods, including the impact of malingering (Oliver E. Williamson, *The Economic Institutions of Capitalism* (New York: Free Press, 1985), 223–26). See also Richard T. Lindholm, "Why Were Renaissance Florentine Wool Industry Companies So Small?" in *Quantitative Studies of the Renaissance Florentine Economy and Society* (London: Anthem Press, 2017), 235–62.

7 Frederick Schauer, "The Relevance of the Past to the Present", in his *The Proof: The Uses of Evidence in Law, Politics, and Everything Else* (Cambridge: Belknap/Harvard University Press, 2022), 203–25, at pp. 222–23.

8 Walton O. Schalick, III, "Neurology in the Middle Ages", in *Handbook of Clinical Neurology*, eds. Stanley Finger, François Boller, and Kenneth Tyler (Edinburgh, UK: Elsevier, 2010), 79–90.

9 Nineteenth-century echoic interpretations of medieval malingering resonated with modernist notions of disability and of work-avoidance (see, e.g., Kylee-Anne Hingston, "Grotesque Bodies: Hybridity and Focalization in Victor Hugo's Notre-Dame de Paris", in *Articulating Bodies: The Narrative Form of Disability and Illness in Victorian Fiction* (Liverpool: Liverpool University Press, 2019), 19–48).

10 Ron (F.R.P.) Akehurst, *The Establissements de Saint Louis: Thirteenth-Century Law Texts from Tours, Orléans, and Paris* (Philadelphia: University of Pennsylvania Press, 1996), 68 ff.

11 Talcott Parsons, "The Sick Role and the Role of the Physician Reconsidered", *Millbank Memorial Fund Quarterly* 53, no. 3 (1975): 257–78.

12 Pierre Rosanvallon, *The New Social Question: Rethinking the Welfare State*, transl. Barbara Harshaw (Princeton: Princeton University Press, 2000), 47–48 and his *La nouvelle question sociale: Repenser l'État-providence* (Paris: Éditions du Seuil, 1995), 91; I include the bracketed French original, as I believe the translations, otherwise excellent, miss a slight nuance that Rosanvallon intended in the original.

13 Eric Y. Drogin, " 'When I Said That I Was Lying, I Might Have Been Lying': The Phenomenon of Psychological Malingering", *Mental and Physical Disability Law Reporter* 25, no. 5 (2001): 711–15.

14 Thomas Szasz, "Malingering," in *Psychiatry: The Science of Lies* (Syracuse: Syracuse University Press, 2008), 17–32 at p. 17. For a creative riff on this resonant point, see Douglas Waxman, "The Dream: Freud & Szasz in Conversation", *Review of Disability Studies: An International Journal* 16, no. 1 (2020): 1–12.

15 William Urban, "Review of Prussian Society and the German Order: An Aristocratic Corporation in Crisis, c. 1410–1466, by M. Burleigh", *Journal of Baltic Studies* 15, no. 4 (1984): 308–10.

16 Dea H. Boster, " 'I Made Up My Mind to Act Both Deaf and Dumb': Displays of Disability and Slave Resistance in the Antebellum American South", in *Disability and Passing: Blurring the Lines of Identity*, eds. Jeffrey A. Brune and Daniel J. Wilson (Philadelphia: Temple University Press, 2013), 71–98.

17 Yücel Yanikdag, "From Cowardice to Illness: Diagnosing Malingering in the Ottoman Great War", *Middle Eastern Studies* 48, no. 2 (2012): 205–25.

18 Robert Brightman, "Traditions of Subversion and the Subversion of Tradition: Cultural Criticism in Maidu Clown Performances", *American Anthropologist* 101, no. 2 (1999): 272–87.

19 Edward Yelin, "The Myth of Malingering: Why Individuals Withdraw From Work in the Presence of Illness," *The Milbank Quarterly* 64, no. 4 (1986): 622–49.
20 Jamelia Morgan, "Disability's Fourth Amendment", *Columbia Law Review* 122, no. 2 (2022): 489–581, at p. 526.
21 Sarah C. Bishop, *Emotional Labor: A Story to Save Your Life* (New York: Columbia University Press, 2022), 60–87; Shauer, "The Relevance of the Past to the Present", 203–25.
22 Matthew Stibbe, "(Dis)entangling the Local, the National, and the International Civilian Internment in Germany and in German-Occupied France and Belgium in Global Context", in *Out of Line, Out of Place*, eds. Rotem Kowner and Iris Rachamimov (Ithaca, NY: Cornell University Press, 2022), 25–51.
23 Sandra W. Russ and Alexis W. Lee, "Assessing Disordered Thinking and Perception in Children and Adolescents", in *Psychological Assessment of Disordered Thinking and Perception*, eds. Irving B. Weiner and James H. Kleiger (Washington, DC: American Psychological Association, 2021), 271–86.
24 For a contemporary account on the British side, see "The Case of Dr. Cornelius Herz", *British Medical Journal* 2, no. 1711 (1893): 858–59. For a broader view, see Jean-Yves Mollier, *Le scandale de Panama* (Paris: Fayard, 1991), variously, and David G. McCullough extremely influential *The Path Between the Seas: The Creation of the Panama Canal, 1870–1914* (New York: Simon and Schuster, 1977), 98–99 and 213–38 variously.

Reference List

Akehurst, Ron (F.R.P.). *The Establissements de Saint Louis: Thirteenth-Century Law Texts from Tours, Orléans, and Paris*. Philadelphia: University of Pennsylvania Press, 1996.

Bishop, Sarah C. *Emotional Labor: A Story to Save Your Life*. New York: Columbia University Press, 2022.

Boster, Dea H. "'I Made Up My Mind to Act Both Deaf and Dumb': Displays of Disability and Slave Resistance in the Antebellum American South." In *Disability and Passing: Blurring the Lines of Identity*, edited by Jeffrey A. Brune and Daniel J. Wilson. Philadelphia: Temple University Press, 2013.

Brightman, Robert. "Traditions of Subversion and the Subversion of Tradition: Cultural Criticism in Maidu Clown Performances." *American Anthropologist* 101, no. 2 (1999): 272–87.

"The Case of Dr. Cornelius Herz." *British Medical Journal* 2, no. 1711 (1893): 858–59.

Drogin, Eric Y. "'When I Said That I Was Lying, I Might Have Been Lying': The Phenomenon of Psychological Malingering." *Mental and Physical Disability Law Reporter* 25, no. 5 (2001): 711–15.

Farmer, Sharon. *The Silk Industries of Medieval Paris*. Philadelphia: University of Pennsylvania Press, 2017.

Hingston, Kylee-Anne. "Grotesque Bodies: Hybridity and Focalization in Victor Hugo's Notre-Dame de Paris." In *Articulating Bodies: The Narrative Form of Disability and Illness in Victorian Fiction*. Liverpool: Liverpool University Press, 2019.

Kay, Christian, et al., eds. *Historical Thesaurus of the Oxford English Dictionary*. Vol. I. Oxford: Oxford University Press, 2009.

Le Proux, Fernand. "Chartes françaises du Vermandois de 1218 à 1250." *Bibliothèque de l'École des Chartes* 35 (1874): 437–77.

Lindholm, Richard T. "Why Were Renaissance Florentine Wool Industry Companies So Small?" In *Quantitative Studies of the Renaissance Florentine Economy and Society*. London: Anthem Press, 2017.

Little, William, (Henry) H. W. Fowler, and Jessie Coulson. *Shorter Oxford English Dictionary*. Vol. I. Oxford: Oxford University Press, 1973.

McCullough, David G. *The Path Between the Seas: The Creation of the Panama Canal, 1870–1914*. New York: Simon and Schuster, 1977.

Mollier, Jean-Yves. *Le scandale de Panama*. Paris: Fayard, 1991.

Morgan, Jamelia. "Disability's Fourth Amendment." *Columbia Law Review* 122, no. 2 (2022): 489–581.

Parsons, Talcott. "The Sick Role and the Role of the Physician Reconsidered." *Millbank Memorial Fund Quarterly* 53, no. 3 (1975): 257–78.

Rey, Alain, éd. *Dictionnaire historique de la langue Française*. Nouvelle ed. Paris: LeRobert, 2010.

Rosanvallon, Pierre. *La nouvelle question sociale: Repenser l'État-providence*. Paris: Éditions du Seuil, 1995.

———. *The New Social Question: Rethinking the Welfare State*. Translated by Barbara Harshaw. Princeton: Princeton University Press, 2000.

Russ, Sandra W., and Alexis W. Lee. "Assessing Disordered Thinking and Perception in Children and Adolescents." In *Psychological Assessment of Disordered Thinking and Perception*, edited by Irving B. Weiner and James H. Kleiger. Washington, DC: American Psychological Association, 2021.

Schalick, Walton O., III. "Add One Part Pharmacy to One Part Surgery and One Part Medicine: Jean de Saint-Amand and the Development of Medical Pharmacology in Paris, c. 1230–1303." Ph.D. diss., The Johns Hopkins University, 1997.

———, "Neurology in the Middle Ages." In *Handbook of Clinical Neurology*, edited by Stanley Finger, François Boller, and Kenneth Tyler. Edinburgh, UK: Elsevier, 2010.

Schauer, Frederick. "The Relevance of the Past to the Present." In *The Proof: The Uses of Evidence in Law, Politics, and Everything Else*. Cambridge: Belknap/Harvard University Press, 2022.

Stibbe, Matthew. "(Dis)entangling the Local, the National, and the International Civilian Internment in Germany and in German-Occupied France and Belgium in Global Context." In *Out of Line, Out of Place*, edited by Rotem Kowner and Iris Rachamimov. Ithaca, NY: Cornell University Press, 2022.

Szasz, Thomas. "Malingering," In *Psychiatry: The Science of Lies*. Syracuse: Syracuse University Press, 2008.

Urban, William. "Review of Prussian Society and the German Order: An Aristocratic Corporation in Crisis, c. 1410–1466, by M. Burleigh." *Journal of Baltic Studies* 15, no. 4 (1984): 308–10.

Waxman, Douglas. "The Dream: Freud & Szasz In Conversation." *Review of Disability Studies: An International Journal* 16, no. 1 (2020): 1–12.

Williamson, Oliver E. *The Economic Institutions of Capitalism*. New York: Free Press, 1985.

Yanikdag, Yücel. "From Cowardice to Illness: Diagnosing Malingering in the Ottoman Great War." *Middle Eastern Studies* 48, no. 2 (2012): 205–25.

Yelin, Edward. "The Myth of Malingering: Why Individuals Withdraw From Work in the Presence of Illness." *The Milbank Quarterly* 64, no. 4 (1986): 622–49.

Introduction

The Bioethics of Malingering, Misrepresentation of Health, and Forensics of Illness

Wendy J. Turner

There is a long history of people faking medical conditions from women claiming pregnancy to avoid the death penalty (if for only a few weeks), to members of the military feigning health conditions or infirmity to leave service. The performative aspects of health conditions can lend themselves to being reproduced: Individuals pretend to be "leprous" beggars with painted-on sores or to be lame with a bandaged leg and crutches. When those elements are not correct, when the lame man can limp away without crutches, the public may doubt the person is ill, impaired, or in need of assistance. In contemporary society, there are some locations where those who might be critical of others are told through signage: "Remember, not all disabilities are visible". People do abuse the "system" and/or the charity of others, for instance, those who use their grandmother's disabled parking decal to get a premium parking space at school and the local shopping center. Most of these individuals do not bother to hide the fact that they are cheating for selfish reasons.

There are also examples of unscrupulous family members that accuse healthy people of being unhealthy for gain. They might point to a family member who is a weak thinker and claim they are mentally disabled, or state that an aging individual is not being capable of managing affairs, or suggest that a person in the prime of life with any number of health-related conditions is too afflicted to manage on her own. These accusations permit the accuser to assume power over the weaker person (whether aging or disabled or having health issues) and their resources. These accusations can cause doubt in the mind of a jury, and every accusation needs to be investigated, true or not, causing delays that might advantage the accuser.

Complicating this situation is the role of physicians, who began serving as expert witnesses in trials in the Middle Ages. Although expected to be truthful and dispassionate—they began to be paid for this service because their time at court took away from the time they could spend in their clinic. In the United States and other places with accelerating economies, those payments became large, and the right "truth" could be purchased—real,

DOI: 10.4324/9781003452324-1

ethical, or not. In contemporary societies, there are often safeguards, but not always and not many; it depends on the stakes, where we are, and if the physician on the stand takes her oath of "do no harm" seriously or not. Even under the best and most ethical circumstances, sometimes at the trial, there is no clear answer and whatever the interpretation, it makes no difference to the health of the person. Even if properly explained, the performative aspects of the *trial*, the actions of the attorneys and the judge, will be what the jury hears. All these ideas—the feigned pregnancy, the pretend limp, the performative health condition as well as the use of a parking pass or signs telling us not to judge others, as well as the legal routine—fit together to form a network of mistrust, trust, trickery, reality, seen, and unseen illness, injury, impairment, and disability.

Expectations of Illness

In all these examples, an individual has tapped into something important about how the public reacts to and understands illness or, conversely, has failed to recognize these common expectations. The common denominator is that all these individuals know what is expected of them to garner interest or sympathy. The behavioral element is not hardwired but learned in human society. The man with the sign at the bottom of the off-ramp from the highway knows that his cardboard poster might say, "Have a Nice Day", but his clothing and demeanor ask for handouts. Is he faking? Maybe. We do not know. Is he performing? Yes. It is an art form that many have perfected—globally and historically. The local hospital might have patients, young and old, describe their pain today as an emotion and by use of graduated emojis, happy to sad. We are good a demonstrating pain and discomfort; we use it to reach out to our parents for help when we are young and scrape a knee.

The art of being ill is a socially acceptable way of demonstrating pain, and there is the reverse. The fabrication of illness, whether perpetrated on another or by an individual, for social or monetary gain is accomplished because the public believes certain tropes about illness generally, and they weigh proof of illness or disability within a common framework of ideas. If this framework is not intact, the public might also not believe a person who *is* disabled is who he says he is. The unseen disability—gut issues, heart troubles, or other internal problems—leaves the spectator with questions of truth.

This collection of essays explores the art of illness, and the deceptions and truths around health and bodies, from a multiplicity of angles from antiquity to the present. They are divided into three parts on "Conceptualizing Malingering", "Historic Cases of Malingering", and "Regulations and Laws Against Malingering". Furthermore, the authors represent a large swath of the world being from or living in Belgium, Canada, England, France, Germany, Scotland, and the United States bringing a variety of perspectives to this conversation.

Conceptualizing Malingering

The opening section on "Conceptualizing Malingering" brings together four vastly different chapters, each of which defines the idea of the bioethics of malingering for their own field, location, and time period. The first essay is "Malingering in Ancient Greece and Rome" by Lisa LeBlanc. It is startling to learn that the idea of malingering—as a concept of faking illness to get out of work or retire from the army early—was not only understood in ancient Greece and Rome but also legislated. Moreover, playwrights and authors used the concept to their advantage, having characters use the art of faking illness to get out of slavery or uphold their values, by lying to those the audience knew were bad, thereby preserving goodness. The second chapter is Chelsea Silva's "Form, Fraud, and Performance in Middle English Medical Satire". Silva examines the work of a charlatan who owns a parchment filled with lines and figures that seems quite scientific, perhaps even mystical to the medieval patient. A patient, much like today, expected certain things from his physician, and this "formula" made the practitioner appear real. Yet, as we know now, any "formula" or diagram for even the best doctoring could be copied or, more significantly, faked. Silva takes us into this world of medieval medical expertise, magic, and quackery, explaining the organizing principles that shaped the medieval experience of health. In the third paper in this opening section, Irina Metzler brings the medieval and contemporary together. Metzler examines "Pathologising Ecstatic Dance: Reflections on Medieval Dansomnia and the Love Parade in Berlin, 1996". It is striking to see the same terms—"illness", "twitching", "frantic", and "distortions of the body"—in both the records of the fourteenth century and those of the late twentieth. It is not the dancers who are malingering or faking, but rather, it is those reporting on what they witnessed who pathologize the dancers' actions. The reporters, in both time periods, considered the dancers to have some sort of mass mental health disorder. In the Middle Ages, viewers question what might have "[given] rise to this mental plague",[1] and in 1996, reporters saw, "a bunch of sick people. . . . Paths of contagion and methods of treatment are unknown".[2] This might be hyperbole on the part of the twentieth-century reporter, but the point of both writers is clear—to use medical terminology to discredit and malign.

Taking us in a different direction, for the fourth paper in this section on "Conceptualizing Malingering", Herb Leventer asks critical questions about "malingering" for contemporary society. In his chapter,

"Philosophical Paradoxes of Factitious Disorders", Leventer inserts several case studies or study examples throughout to unpack several related disorders for the reader, including factitious disorders, malingering, and Munchausen's disease, among others. He walks through the myriad of ever-changing elements in American Psychiatric Association's *Diagnostic and Statistical Manual of Mental Disorders* since its inception, pointing to cracks in diagnoses and understandings of factitious disorders and malingering. Leventer reminds readers that not all physical and mental issues are, as yet, understood. Contemporary medicine at times over-medicates and over-tests while simultaneously coming often, and oddly, to the conclusion that if the tests show nothing, the patient is fine. The patient is left frustrated at best and labeled as a "malingerer" or with a mental health flag on their record at worst. Leventer concludes with some suggestions on how contemporary medicine might rethink these diagnoses if for no other reason than to be more ethically responsible to patients that genuinely need assistance.

Historic Cases of Malingering

The second section covers several "Historic Cases of Malingering" from the Middle Ages to the beginning of the Modern period. These case studies review the human element in the story of malingering and faking illnesses and the chapters, in the section, focus on a case or two to center their work around the pinpoint of one core theme.

In the first chapter of historic malingering, Emma Trivett delves into the lives of two queens in Scotland who used the idea of pregnancy to stay alive and stay queen in her chapter, " 'Because she pretended to be pregnant and was not': Fake Royal Pregnancies in Medieval Scotland". Once a person rose to the level of the aristocracy, it was a long way to fall if found out. Queen Yolande de Dreux, the second queen of Alexander III, not only faked her pregnancy but also tried to substitute an heir. Queen Margaret Logie, who was married to David II, divorced because she faked her pregnancy. However, these pregnancies were each only recorded in one chronicle and the stories there seem suspect. The chroniclers may have used the idea of the queens lying about the heirs to the throne, much like those witnessing the dancers in Metzler's chapter, above, to discredit and malign them.

The second chapter by Wendy J. Turner, "Treason and Malingering: Faking Frenzy in a Sixteenth-Century English Prison", is a close reading of a case study, some of which were originally state secrets. The case concerns William Hawkyns, a London teacher who ran afoul of the Star Chamber Council under Edward VI. Hawkyns feigns madness for a year while locked in the Tower of London, finally confessing that he and a conspirator had planned treasonous acts against the crown. While the details are vague, faking a mental disorder for such a long time takes its toll and either Hawkyns is injured in the interrogation process or becomes mentally ill under the stress of what he is attempting and ends up in Bedlam Hospital.

Case studies are valuable ways of teasing apart what individuals know, how people behave, or what the attitudes of society are. Carolyn A. Day's chapter examines the life and supposed illness of Princess Sophia, daughter of George III of England. Scandals abound among her family and friends, and Day suggests that this might be Sophia's way of getting attention. With a detailed analysis of the archival evidence, Day carefully recreates what and when Sophia might have been doing to trick the country and her family and friends into believing she was ill.

Regulations and Laws Against Malingering

The final section covers "Regulations and Laws Against Malingering", and, while this part of the book focuses on this topic, certainly other concepts in law concerning malingering have already been discussed by the authors mentioned earlier in the volume. In the first chapter on regulations, Courtney A. Krolikoski considers false beggars, particularly those faking leprosy, in her chapter, "*Faking It*: Thirteenth-Century Bolognese Responses to Feigning Leprosy". Krolikoski notes that the people of Bologna wanted to be charitable citizens, but they also wanted to make sure their funds were going to the truly needy and not impostors. They passed statutes against false beggars entering the city and, at the same time, protected those suffering from what was then called "leprosy". The second chapter on regulations is "*Expertis medicis videatur*: Legal Medical Expertise in the Apostolic Chancery's Assessment of Personal Injury Damages During the Avignon Period (1309–1378)" by Ninon Dubourg. Dubourg takes a close look at the pontifical institution, one of the first entities to assess personal injury. This research investigates how forensic medicine worked in the institution's adjudication process and how that became the model for the Apostolic Chancery at the end of the Middle Ages. She finds that these records demonstrate that physicians were trusted medical experts and advisors on cases, verifying the reports on personal injuries and the damages to be paid. This section concludes with a fabulous chapter by Luke I. Haqq, "Compensatory Damages and the Construction of Injury in Prenatal Torts, 1960–1975". This chapter sifts through the changing use and abuse in law of suits concerning "wrongful conception" and "wrongful life" and how these prenatal and natal torts have led to a culture of parents of children with serious prenatal diseases—sometimes preventable—giving birth and turning around to sue for multimillion-dollar awards based in part on the care of the child, but in large part on their own (the parents') alleged pain and suffering, even when they are happy to have the child in their lives. Haqq argues that this is because the U.S. legal system has a serious flaw and suggests ways to reevaluate the U.S. legal path.

Understanding Health, Ill Health, and Malingering

From the point of view of each individual field, all of the chapters in this volume take on the task of defining malingering or faking illness. A common method among many of these chapters is the use of case studies to provide evidence and support to the arguments. The concept of fraud appears in nearly all of the chapters. Fraud as a topic comes up in LeBlanc's work on Greek and Roman military regulations, Silva's research on medieval medical quacks, Dubourg's study of personal injury damages in medieval Avignon, Krolikoski's examination of regulations against faking so-called leprosy in late medieval Bologna, and in Haqq's examination of intent among those suits for "wrongful" conception or birth. Both Trivett and Turner look at the larger issue of fraud: treason. Leventer's quick look at avoidance of contemporary military obligations also looks at fraud; however, that is not the focus of his chapter. His chapter is a philosophical discussion about how and why to define certain elements, and so-called diseases, that surround patients perceived as malingerers. Metzler's work, like Leventer's, is a look at how perception and terminology can harm or distort the truth of what a person is suffering (or not suffering). This too is a type of "faking" but done so for the benefit of the viewer.

Overall, this book is about health deception and invented health conditions. Many people took this "faking" to the level of an art form, while others imposed medical terminology where there was no illness or injury. Performative life is not new, and neither is malingering, as demonstrated by the chapters presented here that span almost 3,000 years of history. The human elements within these pages also tell the stories of real problems in society: of thwarted attempts to have children, find a job, or explain a real condition; of avoiding the death penalty, work, or military duty; of condemning others for differences, disabilities, dancing, or inability to have children. Some of these cases have health policy implications for contemporary societies. Altogether, they paint a picture of humans doing human actions—cheating, lying, and stealing, but also hiding, surviving, and working. They enable us to see the good as well as the bad, the "malingerers" who are sufferers mislabeled as well as those wanting only attention or to cheat the system.

Notes

1 J. F. C. Hecker, *The Epidemics of the Middle Ages*, transl. B. G. Babington, 3rd ed. (London: Trübner, 1859), p. 88.
2 "die Töne bollern mit der Gewalt eines Preßlufthammers ans Ohr," Rainer Schmidt, "Deutschland, liebes Technoland", *Die Zeit*, no. 30 (July 19, 1996).

Reference List

Hecker, J. F. C. *The Epidemics of the Middle Ages*. Translated by B. G. Babington. 3rd ed. London: Trübner, 1859.
Schmidt, Rainer. "Deutschland, liebes Technoland." *Die Zeit*, no. 30 (July 19, 1996).

Part I

Conceptualizing Malingering

1 Malingering in Ancient Greece and Rome

Lisa LeBlanc

The fear that people are faking illnesses to get out of military duty or to gain additional financial benefits from the government often appears in modern times. These fake illnesses may be complaints of actual problems that have gone away, or they may be entirely fictionalized problems. Since people who are ill are often treated differently from the healthy, those who want at least one aspect of the treatment given to the ill have feigned illness in order to gain those benefits. Records of people malingering go all the way back to ancient times, appearing in Greek and Roman texts. Reasons for malingering, the benefits the individual seeks, have not changed that much over time. Individuals are still trying to avoid unpleasant or dangerous jobs or seeking to gain extra help that they would not get if they were whole. While the explanatory texts show a clear concern with detecting and averting malingering, the narrative texts from the ancient world tended to be more sympathetic to those who feign illness, often presenting the situation as the only or best solution available.

Defining Malingering

The concept of malingering is defined not just by the actions, but also by the motivations for those actions. Malingering does not appear in the *Diagnostic and Statistical Manual of Mental Disorders*, 5th edition (DSM-5) as a mental health diagnosis, but it is listed as a V code (an occurrence when a client meets with a provider for a reason other than disease or injury but that does influence care) under "Nonadherence to Medical Treatment".[1] The DSM-5 describes malingering as "the intentional production of false or grossly exaggerated physical or psychological symptoms, motivated by external incentives such as avoiding military duty, avoiding work, obtaining financial compensation, evading criminal prosecution, or obtaining drugs".[2] The DSM-5 does acknowledge that malingering can sometimes serve as an adaptive behavior, giving the example of a prisoner of war malingering to adapt to the situation.[3]

DOI: 10.4324/9781003452324-3

The DSM-5 also distinguishes between malingering and actual disorders. For instance, malingering requires the presence of external motivations. While factitious disorder is a disorder in which the patient feigns physical or psychological symptoms, it is not done for external reasons. Both conversion disorder and somatic symptom-related disorder lack the external motivations, but they also differ from malingering in that the symptoms are not intentionally created.[4]

Because one of the motivations for malingering is avoiding military duty, the U.S. Uniform Code of Military Justice has its own specific definition of malingering. Article 115 refers to it as "feigning illness, physical disablement, mental lapse, or derangement carried out in a hostile fire zone or in time of war".[5] Thus for the military definition of malingering, the feigning must be motivated by avoiding the danger of war. The term "malingering" was derived from the French *malinger* and was first used in the nineteenth century and was restricted to military use.[6] Halligan, Bass, and Oakley argue that the term "malingering" is often not used in modern psychology because of the negative connotations, and they define malingering, or illness deception, as "the intentional production of false or exaggerated symptoms motivated by external incentives".[7] For all the definitions, the intentionality of the act and the presence of exterior motivations are necessary.

Halligan, Bass, and Oakley point out that the external incentive may go beyond financial benefit, such as that gained in lawsuits or from disability. It can also include improving the quality of life (relying on others to take care of them), avoiding stressful work (such as in the military), avoiding a job that one does not like, avoiding a trial or jailtime, and obtaining drugs by feigning illnesses that need them.[8] In addition to varied motives for malingering, the degree to which malingering is occurring also varies in severity. A four-part typology, created by Lipman, includes "(1) *invention*: where a patient without actual symptoms claims he has, (2) *perseveration*: genuine symptoms previously experienced are alleged to be present, (3) *exaggeration*: symptoms or their associated effects (disabilities) are magnified or embellished, (4) *transference*: where genuine symptoms currently present are falsely attributed to previous or unrelated injuries".[9] Clinical reports indicate that an important characteristic of malingering is that the patient shows restraint. Those who do not exaggerate their symptoms have a better chance of not being discovered. The patient must either exhibit behaviors that are atypical or avoid typical behaviors consistently, but not to excess.[10]

Malingering is a fairly consistent condition, with various sources using the term to explain the motives behind a person intentionally feigning physical or psychological symptoms. Although the term develops much later, the characteristics of malingering are clearly seen in ancient works, both works meant to teach and explain and narrative works meant to entertain.

Explanatory Texts

In the ancient world, there are not many texts that explain malingering. The primary explanatory text in the ancient world comes from Greece, while there are a few in Rome that touch on malingering. In both cases, the main concern is with slaves malingering in order to avoid unpleasant work. While a few of the texts make reference to what to do with malingering slaves from the perspective of agricultural advice, the work that most thoroughly covers malingering is by Galen.

Living in the second and third centuries CE, Galen was a Greek physician and writer. His influence in medicine continued through the seventeenth century. During his career as a physician, Galen moved to Rome and practiced there. He dictated hundreds of texts in which he emphasized observation and experimentation.

In his *Omnia Opera*, Galen includes a section called "Simulation of Disease and How to Detect It".[11] In this work, Galen mentions that there are many reasons for feigning illness, but his primary concern is to outline how a physician should identify such a simulation. He emphasizes that many malingerers both create symptoms and pretend that genuine symptoms continue beyond when they are actually gone. As with modern arguments, he presents signs that someone is feigning, such as refusing treatment. He also proceeds to give two examples of malingering from his own experience, although both of these are examples of feigning physical illness, not mental illness.

The first is a man who pretends to have colic to avoid a citizen's meeting that he felt would be dangerous for him. In this case, Galen was able to identify malingering because the man refused treatment and the colic went away shortly after the meeting despite the individual not changing his diet. In the other case, a young slave complained of a swollen knee in order to avoid having to travel with his master. Galen identified malingering in this case because of the character of the slave (prone to lie) and the fact that that slave had a girlfriend he would not have wanted to leave. Galen confirmed his suspicion that the swelling was induced by drugs by applying a medicine that would reduce swelling but not pain, and the slave claimed the medicine had worked on the pain. Based on his personal experiences, Galen recommended a doctor prescribe bitter medicines and even surgery since someone feigning illness would not be willing to go through these measures whereas someone genuinely in pain would.[12]

There are other sources that acknowledge malingering among slaves, as Galen did. Peter Hunt refers to several Roman agricultural sources that concern themselves with malingering slaves:

On the one hand, several works on agriculture mention the need to take care of slaves who are ill. Slave owners did not want sick slaves to die unnecessarily or to recover slowly because they had been forced, by whipping for instance, to continue to work while ill. On the other hand, to allow one slave to avoid hard work by falsely claiming illness might put slaveholders or farm managers on the slippery slope to supporting many 'sick' and unproductive slaves. Cato's notorious advice that such slaves not be fed full rations or simply be sold would have ensured that malingering was an unattractive option, but who would buy sick slaves and for how much (Cato, On Agriculture 2.4, 2.7)? So a duty assigned to the wife of the estate manager, the vilica—a slave like her husband—was to take care of sick slaves, but also to be sure that they really were sick.

(Columella, On Agriculture 12.3.7; cf. Xenophon, Oeconomicus 7.37)[13]

While feigning a physical illness was easier to get away with, madness would also have been feigned.

The Roman writers made reference to malingerers and ideas of how and why to recognize the feigning of illness, particularly with slaves, because of the impact on farm labor. Cato the Elder lived in the third- to second-century BCE. He was a statesman and orator, and his speeches tended to rail against luxury in Rome. While he wrote on history, medicine, justice, and the military, the only work of Cato's to survive is his work on farming. In *De Agricultura*, Cato mentions, "When the slaves were sick, such large rations should not have been issued".[14] While this may be an attempt to not spend money on sickly slaves,[15] Peter Hunt argues that withholding food from sick slaves is a way to discouraging malingering.[16] As mentioned earlier, this idea is supported by Columella, who writes about the problems of malingering slaves, directing that the estate manager's wife's duty was not only to care for sick slaves but also to make sure that they were genuinely sick.[17]

Of course, it is not just slaves who would feign illness for a particular benefit. The Roman military also had concerns about soldiers faking illness in order to get out of their military service. After serving a particular number of years, usually 20, soldiers were given an honorable discharge with benefits of land and money. However, a soldier who experienced illness or injury could also be granted an honorable discharge. This discharge was only granted after a careful examination to prevent malingering though.[18]

The *Military Laws from Rufus*, authorship uncertain but possibly Rufus of the second to the first-century BCE, outlines how someone who wounds himself to get out of military duty would be punished with death, unless the person was genuinely mad. Furthermore, the work states that anyone who avoids military service will become a slave and anyone who injures his son so his son cannot serve in the military will be exiled. More specific to malingering, however, is the passage that states "*Quicumque metu hostium languorem corporis simulauerit, capite punitory* (Whoever, from fear of the enemy, feigns bodily ailment, shall be punished with death)".[19] In addition, the *Corpus Juris Civilis*, a compilation of the Roman jurists from the second and third centuries CE and collected by Justinian in 534, also discusses military matters despite being civil law. While not as specific to malingering as the *Military Laws from Rufus*, these laws also mention punishments for evading military service, which is slavery, punishment of those who prevent their sons from service either by hiding him or by injuring him as exile and loss of property, and punishment of those who self-injure to get out of military service as death.[20]

In all of the texts that set out to explain malingering, the primary argument is how to identify and prevent it and what punishments are applied. There is little concern about why the individual will malinger, just how to stop it. This is different from the narrative texts where the sympathy is usually with the malingerer. Furthermore, the explanatory texts tend to focus on malingering as tied to illness, implying physical symptoms, whereas the narrative texts emphasize the feigning of mental illnesses.

Narrative Texts

In works of literature, the motivations of characters do allow for such exploration. These works explain that there are valid reasons for individuals hoping to avoid something negative by feigning illness. In these cases, it is often the hero or main character of the narrative who practices the deception, so the reaction to malingering on the part of the author is very sympathetic.

While V. Kuperman studies malingering in contemporary works of literature, some of the conclusions he reaches also apply to ancient texts. The study shows that "In fiction, as in the clinic, malingerers often prefer mental disorders to somatic diseases".[21] This is most likely due to the ease in mimicking mental health issues as well as how difficult psychological malingering is to disprove. The study also shows that fictional malingerers usually create active symptoms as opposed to negative symptoms like mutism and paralysis, which is also true of clinical cases.[22]

Xenophon of Ephesus lived in the second to third centuries BCE in Greece. His only surviving work, "An Ephesian Tale", is one of five ancient Greek romances. In the five books of "An Ephesian Tale", readers meet the ultimate star-crossed lovers. Habrocomes and Anthia are shipwrecked, captured, separated, sold as slaves, tortured, and left for dead several times. At one point in the romance, Anthia is sold to a brothel but is determined to maintain her vow of chastity (which is more a vow of fidelity by today's standards) to Habrocomes. When she is put on display at the brothel, she falls to the ground and mimics the "sacred disease". She tells the brothel keeper,

> Once, when I was still a child, I strayed away from my family during a celebration of a festival vigil, and came upon the grave of a man who had recently died. There it seemed to me that someone leapt out of the grave and tried to lay hold of me. I shrieked and tried to flee. The man was frightful to look upon, and his voice was more horrible still. Finally, when day broke, he let me go, but he struck me on the chest and said that he had cast this disease into me. Beginning with that day I have been afflicted with that calamity which takes divers forms and divers occasions.[23]

The sacred disease in question was epilepsy, which in ancient Greece was believed to be an attack on the brain caused by the gods and was accompanied by psychological disorders. Hippocrates, who denied the role of the gods, presented the disease as one of the brain. It was seen as akin to madness, even possibly the madness that afflicted Hercules. In the story of Habrocomes and Anthia, however, the epilepsy is feigned in order to avoid Anthia's role in the brothel and maintain her fidelity to her husband, Habrocomes. In this, she succeeds. Instead of being required to work at the brothel, she is nursed at the keeper's house until she is strong enough to be sold on as a slave.

We see in this text many of the ideas around malingering. Anthia is a prisoner and is clearly using malingering as an adaptive strategy. Before Hippocrates, the sacred disease was thought to be sent by the gods, although in this case it appears that the sacred disease can be passed on to others by those cursed. While Hippocrates argued that epilepsy had a natural cause, not a divine one, the idea of it as a religious disease did not die out right away. It is not clear which origin Xenophon is drawing on, since Anthia claims she got it by being struck on the chest by a revenant. But to the brothel keeper, this is a realistic claim. Her malingering succeeds, and she is able to be reunited with her beloved without ever being unfaithful to him. Xenophon's sympathy is obviously with Anthia since she overcomes many obstacles, being nearly raped, being thrown into a pit with vicious dogs, and being enslaved and sold, among other obstacles. But the narrative emphasizes Habrocomes and Anthia constantly overcoming their obstacles to remain faithful; therefore, her malingering is a positive thing.

Perhaps one of the most important ancient examples of malingering is that of Odysseus. The story was originally recorded in the *Cypria*, which now survives only in excerpts and summaries, but those pieces provide us with a clear story of a great hero who still simulated madness in order to avoid military service. It was Odysseus who suggested to Tyndareus that he extract an oath from the suitors of Helen of Troy that they will defend the suitor chosen against challenges. Because of this oath, when Helen is taken to Troy by Paris, Odysseus is called upon to join the war. Since Odysseus had received a prophecy that it would take him a very long time to be able to return home and that he would return home having lost all of his crew and goods, he was reluctant to go. There are a few different details in the excerpts and summaries, but they all agree that Odysseus feigned madness in order to avoid the war. Proclus's summary of Cypria tells us, "Odysseus pretends to be insane because he does not / want to go to the war. But they find him out; on advice of Palamedes, / they kidnap his son Telemachus as a threat, thus forcing him to go".[24] This form of madness as well as the means of revealing the deception varies depending on the source of the excerpt. In *The Myths of Hyginus*, Odysseus puts on a cap and starts to plow his field with a horse and ox. Palamedes believes he is faking and puts Telemachus in the path of the plow, saying "Give up your pretense and come and join the allies".[25] At this point, Odysseus stops feigning madness and joins the men leaving for war. In another version of the story, Odysseus raves like a madman. Palamedes once again does not believe him and seizes Telemachus from Penelope and threatens to kill him with a sword. At that point, Odysseus admits that he was feigning madness and agrees to join the others in the war.[26] Later in this version, Odysseus frames Palamedes for treason by planting gold in his tent and having a prisoner forge a letter from Priam to Palamedes. When Agamemnon finds the letter, Palamedes is stoned for treason.[27] Hyginus gives the same information, although he also includes that in the fake letter, Priam offers Palamedes the same amount of gold for betraying the Greeks as Odysseus is buried in the tent.[28] Thus, the failure of Odysseus's attempt to feign madness to get out of going to the Trojan War leads to the death of the man who discovers the deception.

It is interesting that one of the greatest Greek heroes, Odysseus, went to such lengths to avoid war. Some scholars think he may even have foreseen the many suitors attempting to take his kingdom and his wife. Of all the Greek heroes, it seems appropriate that Odysseus, who is regularly known as a trickster, is the one to attempt to feign madness. It is likely that it is Odysseus' trickster nature that allows him to take such actions without losing his status as a hero. In his case, however, he fails in his attempt. Palamedes is able to see through malingering and force him to reveal his deception, which gains him Odysseus' enmity. And, of course, the *Odyssey* shows that Odysseus' concerns and reasons for malingering were valid—his journey home takes 20 years and when he does return home, it is without any of his men or ships.

Another account of malingering occurs in Plutarch's life, particularly the "Life of Marcellus". Plutarch lived in the first century CE and is best known for the biographies of his *Parallel Lives*. The subject of this life,

Marcus Claudius Marcellus, lived several centuries before Plutarch and served as a consul and military leader. At one point in Plutarch's biography, the Romans wanted to annex the city of Engyium in Sicily. Nicias of Sicily was in favor of the annexation and argued for it in the assemblies. Those who opposed this plan proposed to arrest him and turn him over to the Carthaginians, who also wanted to control the city. In order to avoid this, Nicias went to an assembly and started to argue in favor of the Romans. In the middle of his speech, he:

> suddenly threw himself upon the ground, and after a little while, amid the silence and consternation which naturally prevailed, lifted his head, turned it about, and spoke in a low and trembling voice, little by little raising and sharpening its tones. And when he saw the whole audience struck dumb with horror, he tore off his mantle, rent his tunic, and leaping up half naked, ran towards the exit from the theatre, crying out that he was pursued by the Mothers [the goddesses who appear in the town]. No man venturing to lay hands upon him or even to come in his way, out of superstitious fear, but all avoiding him, he ran out of the gate of the city, freely using all the cries and gestures that would become a man possessed and crazed.[29]

That this was planned ahead of time is shown by the fact that his wife escaped the city under the guise of searching for him.

Unlike the previous two narratives, this story is presented as nonfiction, as a biography. But despite the nonfiction status of the text, the sympathy in this case still seems to be with Nicias. In this case, Nicias feigns illness in order to avoid a negative sentence from the assembly. Unlike modern texts, he is not subtle in presenting his symptoms, but for the period, according to Plutarch, this extreme behavior is effective against the superstitious citizens. This story also differs from the others in that it does not directly involve the main character. Nicias is a minor character, used just as an example of Marcellus's fairness. It is to Marcellus that Nicias flees once he is out of the city, and when Marcellus later captures the city and threatens to put the men to death, he spares them for Nicias's sake. Thus, Nicias is tied to the hero and his malingering is used to get Nicias to the hero.

The Greek narrative examples, unlike the explanatory ones, clearly show that malingering is a technique used by good people to avoid negative consequences. Both Anthia and Nicias are threatened by their situation and use malingering as an adaptive behavior to survive the dangerous situations. It could be argued that Odysseus' motivations were also adaptive because of what he knew ahead of time about the consequences of him joining the war. His character, as a trickster, makes malingering appropriate and positive.

There are a few brief references to malingers in ancient Roman comedy, but they are not the emphases of the plays. For example, Plautus uses the idea of feigned madness, but in this case, it is not the "mad" individual who is motivated to practice the deception. In *Casina*, Cleostrata is given a female infant, Casina, as a maid. When the child grows up, Cleostrata's husband and son both fall in love with her. The husband, Stalino, arranges for Casina to marry his bailiff, so he might have access to her. Cleostrata avoids this by substituting someone else, but also in Act 3, Scene 5, another servant of Cleostrata makes up a story to convince Stalino that Casina has gone mad.[30] What is interesting in this play is that Casina herself never appears—the deception of madness is done through others.

In another example, Plautus's *Menaechmi*, a source for Shakespeare's *A Comedy of Errors*, another character feigns madness, this time on stage. Madness runs through the play, caused by the confusion of twin boys with the same name who grew up apart, unaware of one another and who are now in the same town. At one point, several of the characters believe the foreign Menaechmi is the native Menaechmi gone mad, so he decides he will play mad in order to scare them off.[31] At the end of the play, the twins are reunited and the foreign Menaechmi returns to his normal behavior. Like the Greek narratives, Plautus presents malingering as sympathetic. While Casina does not malinger herself, Cleostrata creates the story of her madness to prevent her own husband from being unfaithful to her. Menaechmi feigns madness because he believes he is surrounded by mad people, and he wishes to escape their clutches.

Aristophanes is the exception to the rule. His reference to malingering is extremely brief and actually draws on a legend that had already existed, but he is also the only author who uses malingering for a negative purpose. Aristophanes makes reference to a "cloak thief" in two of his plays, *Acharnians* and *The Birds*. In Aristophanes' *The Birds*, Aristophanes makes reference to Orestes, who will "weave a tunic, so that the righteous cold may not drive him any more to strip other folks".[32] While Orestes son of Agamemnon was legitimately insane due to the Furies in the *Oresteia* by Aeschylus, this Orestes is the son of Timocrates. He would pretend to be mad in order to rob individuals of their cloaks. Aristophanes says, "a certain Orestes, pretending to be mad, used to strip off passer-by; for he was a cloak thief" (Ach 1167).[33] In this case, Orestes is feigning madness in order to steal from others. While this is a very brief reference, Aristophanes essentially makes reference to this character, a liar and thief, as a threat to another character.

It is important to keep in mind that the Roman references are all comedies. Whether they are positive or negative, they are meant to add humor to the play, so they are not really judgment on the behavior. They are a simple plot device to keep the story moving. In *Casina*, it is the switch of brides that deters the husband, not the false madness. In *Menaechmi*, the feigned madness does not last long and tends to blend with the madness of the entire play. In Aristophanes' plays, the thief-malingerer(s) only appears as a threat to other characters.

The text outlining the end of Seneca's life, by the Roman historian Tacitus, while nonfiction, is still presented as a narrative and not an explanatory text, and in keeping with the other narrative texts, it presents Seneca's malingering in a positive light. Seneca, along with Burrus, had worked as a tutor to Nero because of Agrippina's influence, and when Nero first became emperor, Agrippina with the help of Nero's tutors was able to keep Nero under control. Eventually, Nero had Agrippina assassinated, and 3 years later Burrus died, according to contemporary sources at Nero's hand. At this point, Seneca requested permission to retire so that he could devote himself to study, but Nero denied his request. As the political situation worsened, Seneca "had feigned illness and confined himself to his bedroom, subsisting on the most meager diet".[34] The feigned illness only helped for so long, and when Seneca, falsely or not, was implicated in an assassination attempt against Nero 3 years later, he, on orders from the emperor, committed suicide.[35]

While ancient explanatory texts present malingering in a negative light, narrative texts, especially since they explore reasons behind malingering, are far more sympathetic. Roman comedies are not always sympathetic, but their purpose is comedy, not sympathy. The vita of Seneca is much the same, garnering sympathy from readers as a historic individual who used malingering to prolong his life and avoid his overbearing, if not clinically mad, emperor.

A Final Twist

While ancient texts have commented on whether an illness was genuine or feigned, there was a text that offers a third conclusion. The *Pseudepigraphic Writings* of Hippocrates creates a fictional story that presents Hippocrates as the writer of a collection of letters that outline his concern over and investigation into the madness of Democritus.[36] The epistolary collection begins with a letter to Hippocrates from the city of Abdera expressing concern about Democritus' mental state and its impact on the city. Hippocrates writes to several people, preparing to go to Abdera to investigate but also bringing a potion in case the concerns are true.

In the seventh letter of the series, Hippocrates gives his account of his meeting with Democritus. When he first meets him, he finds Democritus writing "A treatise on madness".[37] As they continue to talk, Hippocrates finds Democritus' primary symptom, excessive and unexpected laughter, to be a sign of sanity. Democritus tells him,

I laugh at one thing, humanity, brimming with ignorance, void of right action, childish in all aspirations, agonizing through useless woes for no benefit, traveling to the ends of the earth and her boundless depths with unmeasured desire, melting gold and silver, never stopping this acquisitiveness of theirs, ever in an uproar for more, so that they themselves can be less.[38]

Hippocrates questions whether this is really a subject for laughter, but Democritus responds that if it was not humans' own fault, he would not laugh. Instead, he says, humans are at fault but continue to blame everyone but themselves. After this, Hippocrates returns to the city council and reports that Democritus is not mad but is, in fact, the wisest man alive. His symptom is just a reaction to the futility of the world, and his madness is neither real nor feigned; it is just a man who is misunderstood by the weaker minds around him.

Conclusion

Malingering was clearly an idea that was present in the ancient world. At first, there seems to be a conflict between those writing law—who clearly were against malingering—and those who wrote literature—who at times seem to find malingering helpful in tricky situations. Yet, Greek and Roman authors who wrote about malingering in law or other official documents wrote to prevent fraud among soldiers, slaves, and others. In the explanatory texts, the emphasis is on prevention and punishing when prevention failed, and not in look into why malingering occurred. The explanatory texts were created to deal with the problems that malingering creates; malingering in this light is seen as a negative action, one that is false and in league with liars and cheats.

In ancient literature, the depiction of malingering was used to deceive, yet often in a much more sympathetic light, such as a hero escaping the horrors of captivity or violence through the use of feigned illness or madness. Whether in the prose works of Greece or the plays of Rome, the characters who malinger all have strong motives for their feigning of illnesses, with the exception of Aristophanes whose reference to a malingering character is just in passing and used to shed light on the characters around him. Interestingly, the motives are still ones that appear today—to deflect harm or gain sympathy when captured or trapped (Anthia and Menaechmi), avoid military duty (Odysseus), evade judgment (Nicias), or eschew odious duty (Casina). Since they are all attempting to protect themselves, with the exception of Casina, who was assigned fake madness by her mistress to protect Casina and to deter her husband, the authors' and the audience's sympathies are with the malingerers.

Hippocrates reminds us all, however, that there is a third option to real illness or malingering, which today we would refer to as misdiagnosis. Democritus is fortunate in the fictional Hippocrates' ability to diagnose, especially as in the eighth letter, he points out that the cure Hippocrates brought for his illness would have actually driven him mad.[39] Overall, malingering is acceptable in the texts of the ancient world only in the narratives. In the explanatory texts, malingering is condemned. However, in the narratives, the situations those who malinger are in are extreme, and this is often the only option to save themselves. In the exemplary texts, the writers are looking only at a more general situation. So, the more accepting views in the narratives may be due more to the situation. But this discrepancy in the causes and acceptability shows that writers of the ancient world could adapt malingering to their own purposes.

Notes

1 A V code, also known as "Other Conditions That May Be a Focus of Clinical Attention", are conditions that are not mental health disorders but are conditions that affect the "diagnosis, course, prognosis, or treatment": of a mental health disorder; American Psychological Association, *Diagnostic and Statistical Manual of Mental Disorders*, 5th ed. (Washington, DC: American Psychological Association, 2013) (hereafter, DSM-5), 715.
2 DSM-5, 726.
3 Ibid., 727.
4 Ibid.
5 Peter Halligan, Christopher Bass, and David A. Oakley, "Willful Deception as Illness Behavior", in *Malingering and Illness Deception*, eds. Peter Halligan, Christopher Bass, and David A. Oakley (Oxford: Oxford University Press, 2003), 7.
6 Ian P. Palmer, "Malingering, Shirking, and Self-inflicted Injuries in the Military", in *Malingering and Illness Deception*, eds. Peter Halligan, Christopher Bass, and David A. Oakley (Oxford: Oxford University Press, 2003), 42.
7 Halligan, Bass, and Oakley, "Willful Deception as Illness Behavior", 3.
8 Ibid., 12–13.
9 Ibid., 12. Frederick D. Lipman, "Malingering in Personal Injury," *Insurance Law Journal* (1962): 452.
10 V. Kuperman, "Narratives of Psychiatric Malingering in Works of Fiction", *Journal of Medical Ethics* 32 (2006): 69.
11 This work is translated in Galen, "Galen on Malingering, Centaurs, Diabetes and Other Subjects More or Less Related", translated by Fred B. Lund, *The Proceedings of the Charaka Club*, X (1941): 52–55.
12 Galen, "Galen on Malingering", 52–55.
13 Peter Hunt, *Ancient Greek and Roman Slavery* (Hoboken, NJ: John Wiley & Sons, Inc. 2018), 213.
14 Cato the Elder, *De Agricultura*, transl. W. D. Hooper and H. B. Ash, Loeb Classical Library (Cambridge, MA: Harvard University Press, 1934), https://penelope.uchicago.edu/Thayer/E/Roman/Texts/Cato/De_Agricultura/A*.html: 2.4.
15 C. E. Brand, *Roman Military Law* (Austin, TX: University of Texas Press, 1968), 155–57.
16 Hunt, *Ancient Greek and Roman Slavery*, 213.
17 Ibid.

18 Brad Ballard and Robert W. Enzenauer, "Historical Perspective on Ocular Malingering", *Historia Opthalmologica Internationalis* 2 (2019): 316–17.
19 Brand, *Roman Military Law*, 164–65 (translation is by Brand).
20 Ibid., 179, 185.
21 Kuperman, "Narratives of Psychiatric", 68.
22 Ibid., 71.
23 Xenophon, "The Ephesian Tale", in *Three Greek Romances*, transl. Moses Hadas (New York: Macmillan Publishing Company, 1953), 117–18.
24 Proclus, "Summary of the Cypria", in *The Epic Cycle*, ed. and trans. by Gregory Nagy, https://chs.harvard.edu/primary-source/epic-cycle-sb/, lines 25–27.
25 Hyginus, *The Myths of Hyginus*, trans. and ed. by Mary Grant (Lawrence: University of Kansas, 1960), https://topostext.org/work/206, line 95.
26 Apollodorus, *Library: Epitome*, trans. James George Frazer, Loeb Classical Library (Cambridge, MA: Harvard University Press, 1921), vol. 122, https://www.theoi.com/Text/ApollodorusE.html, 3.7.
27 Ibid., 3.8.
28 Hyginus, *The Myths of Hyginus*, 105.
29 Plutarch, *Parallel Lives: Life of Marcellus*, Loeb Classical Library, trans. by Bernadotte Perrin (Cambridge, MA: Harvard University Press, 2017), vol. V, 20.
30 T. Maccius Plautus, *Casina, or the Stratagem Defeated,* Perseus Digital Library: Tufts University, from *The Comedies of Plautus*, ed. and trans. Henry Thomas Riley (London: G. Bell & Sons, 1912), http://www.perseus.tufts.edu/hopper/text?doc=Perseus%3Atext%3A1999.02.0097%3Aact%3Dintro%3Ascene%3Dsubject.
31 T. Maccius Plautus, *Menaechmi, or the Twin Brothers*, from *The Comedies of Plautus*, ed. Henry Thomas Riley (London: G. Bell & Sons, 1912), Perseus Digital Library: Tufts University, http://www.perseus.tufts.edu/hopper/text?doc=Perseus%3Atext%3A1999.02.0101%3Aact%3D5%3Ascene%3D2; Act 5, Scene 2.
32 Aristophanes, *The Birds*, The Internet Classics Archive (Web Atomics: Daniel C. Stevenson, 1994–2000), http://classics.mit.edu/Aristophanes/birds.html.
33 Vayos Liapis, "Ghosts, Wand'ring Here and There: Orestes the Revenant in Athens", in *Dionysalexandros: Essays on Aeschylus and His Fellow Tragedians in Honour of Alexander F. Garvie*, eds. Douglas Cairns and Vayos Liapis (Swansea: The Classic Press of Wales, 2006), 19.
34 Anna Lydia Motto and John Richard Clark, "Seneca's Last Years", *The Classical Outlook* 50, no. 7 (1973): 78.
35 Ibid.
36 Hippocrates, *Pseudepigraphic Writings*, ed. and trans. Wesley D. Smith (NY: EJ Brill, 1990).
37 Ibid., 77.
38 Ibid., 81.
39 Ibid., 93.

Reference List

Printed Primary

Apollodorus. *Library: Epitome.* Translated and Edited by James George Frazer. Loeb Classical Library. Vol. 122. Cambridge, MA: Harvard University Press, 1921. https://www.theoi.com/Text/ApollodorusE.html.
Aristophanes. *The Birds.* The Internet Classics Archive. Web Atomics: Daniel C. Stevenson, 1994–2000. http://classics.mit.edu/Aristophanes/birds.html.

Cato the Elder. *De Agricultura*. Translated by W. D. Hooper and H. B. Ash. Loeb Classical Library. Cambridge, MA: Harvard University Press, 1934. https://penelope.uchicago.edu/Thayer/E/Roman/Texts/Cato/De_Agricultura/A*.html.

Galen. "Galen on Malingering, Centaurs, Diabetes and Other Subjects More or Less Related." Translated by Fred B. Lund. *The Proceedings of the Charaka Club* X (1941): 52–55.

Hippocrates. *Pseudepigraphic Writings*. Edited and Translated by Wesley D. Smith. New York: EJ Brill, 1990.

Hyginus. *The Myth of Hyginus*. Edited and translated by Mary Grant. Lawrence: University of Kansas Press, 1960. https://topostext.org/work/206.

Plautus, T. Maccius. *Casina, or the Strategem Defeated*. Translated and edited by Henry Thomas Riley. London: G. Bell & Sons, 1912. Perseus Digital Library: Tufts University. http://www.perseus.tufts.edu/hopper/text?doc=Perseus%3Atext%3A1999.02.0097%3Aact%3Dintro%3Ascene%3Dsubject.

———. *Menaechmi, or the Twin Brothers*. Originally in *The Comedies of Plautus*, ed. Henry Thomas Riley. London: G. Bell & Sons, 1912. Perseus Digital Library: Tufts University. http://www.perseus.tufts.edu/hopper/text?doc=Perseus%3Atext%3A1999.02.0101%3Aact%3D5%3Ascene%3D2.

Plutarch. *Parallel Lives: Life of Marcellus*. Loeb Classical Library. Vol. V. Translated by Bernadotte Perrin. Cambridge, MA: Harvard University Press, 1917.

Proclus. "Summary of the Cypria." In *The Epic Cycle*, edited and translated by Gregory Nagy. Revised by Eugenia Lao. Harvard: Center for Hellenic Studies, 2020. https://chs.harvard.edu/primary-source/epic-cycle-sb/.

Xenophon. "The Ephesian Tale." In *Three Greek Romances*, translated by Moses Hadas, 69–126. New York: Macmillan, 1953.

Secondary

American Psychological Association. *Diagnostic and Statistical Manual of Mental Disorders*. 5th ed. Washington, DC: American Psychological Association, 2013.

Ballard, Brad, and Robert W. Enzenauer. "Historical Perspectives on Ocular Malingering." *Historia Opthalmologica Internationalis* 2 (2019): 315–19.

Carroll, Matthew F. "Malingering in the Military." *Psychiatric Annals* 33, no. 11 (2003): 732–36.

Halligan, Peter, Christopher Bass, and David A. Oakley. "Willful Deception as Illness Behavior." In *Malingering and Illness Deception*, edited by Peter Halligan, Christopher Bass and David A. Oakley, 3–28. Oxford: Oxford University Press, 2003.

Hunt, Peter. *Ancient Greek and Roman Slavery*. Hoboken, NH: John Wiley & Sons, Inc., 2018.

Kuperman, V. "Narratives of Psychiatric Malingering in Works of Fiction." *Journal of Medical Ethics* 32 (2006): 67–72. doi:10.1136/jmh.2005.000213.

Liapis, Vayos. "Ghosts, Wand'ring Here and There: Orestes the Revenant in Athens." In *Dionysalexandros: Essays on Aeschylus and His Fellow Tragedians in Honour of Alexander F. Garvie*, edited by Douglas Cairns and Vayos Liapis, 201–32. Swansea: The Classic Press of Wales, 2006.

Palmer, Ian P. "Malingering, Shirking, and Self-inflicted Injuries in the Military." In *Malingering and Illness Deception*, edited by Peter Halligan, Christopher Bass, and David A. Oakley, 42–53. Oxford: Oxford University Press, 2003.

2 Form, Fraud, and Performance in Medieval Medical Satire

Chelsea Silva

In the spring of 1382, Roger Clerk of Wandsworth was sued by the Londoner Roger atte Hacche. The plaintiff declared that Clerk had come to his home and, upon seeing his wife Johanna lying indisposed with a fever, claimed to be knowledgeable and experienced in the art of medicine. In return for an initial payment of 12*d*, Clerk provided the couple with "an old parchment, cut or scratched across, being the leaf of a certain book".[1] Wrapping the parchment in a golden cloth, Clerk asserted that if it were placed around Johanna's neck, it would heal her. The promised healing never occurred and the same parchment was presented to the court as evidence. Asked to clearly identify its virtue, Clerk, who had attended the hearing in person, claimed that the object had a healing prayer against fevers inscribed on it, and recited a garbled version of the prayer himself: "*Anima Christi, sanctifica me; Corpus Christi, salva me; in isanguis Christi, nebria me; cum bonus Christus tu, lava me* [sic]" (Soul of Christ, sanctify me; Body of Christ, sanctify me; Blood of Christ, intoxicate me; [corrupted Latin] since you are the good Christ, wash me).[2] When the parchment was examined, however, the court discovered that the words were nowhere to be found and, moreover, that Clerk himself was illiterate.[3]

This essay is about Clerk's golden fabric and scratched parchment: the form of fraudulent medicine, and its contents. As I will discuss, both legal and literary accounts of medical fraud emphasize its reliance on the shaping *forms* of medicine: on patient expectations about what medicine and its practitioners looked and sounded like. As the structures through which medical care was recognized and enacted, forms are organizing principles that shape experiences of health. Whether textual (such as the remedy), physical or visual (such as the urinal or the uroscopy wheel), or behavioral (such as the bedside examination), medical forms make recognizable the process of treatment. In the case of frauds, however, the actual care that lies within, beyond, or behind those forms is frequently nonsensical or nonexistent, consisting of scratches or intangible ingredients rather than a learned prayer or practical prescription. In their use as vessels for this kind

DOI: 10.4324/9781003452324-4

of content, medical forms signify not only pretensions to medical authority but also the rhetorical expertise of the quack, whose credibility depended not on the efficacy of his cure but on the convincing nature of his performance. The quack's expertise, in other words, was in his ability to perform and to counterfeit: to look, speak, and act in accordance with popular expectations about who a physician was, and what a physician did.

Modern scholarship on the history of quackery has predominantly centered on the social, literary, and professional milieu of the early modern period.[4] This historiographical focus is understandable given the pronounced surge in discourse about medical fraud beginning in the late 1500s. The explosion of quackish stuff—by which I mean both materials produced by quacks and material depicting and denouncing them—was a result of the blossoming print marketplace and the stability and stratification of professional medicine, which increasingly became an arena in which practitioners of diverse ranks jostled for clientele. In the developing commercial medical marketplace of seventeenth- and eighteenth-century England, quackery, particularly in its itinerant forms, became inextricably linked to theatrical production; as M. A. Katritzky has explained, quacks at markets and fairs "sweetened their 'commercial breaks' with free shows involving anything from brief comic or musical routines or a trained animal to a full-length play".[5] As this suggests, the critical tendency to identify quackery as an early modern phenomenon extends to medicine's association with popular dramatic performance, though as scholars including Jody Enders, Claire Sponsler, and Margaret E. Owens have shown, the medieval drama was also deeply concerned with the performative aspects of corporeal signification.[6]

The comparative dearth of scholarship about quackery in medieval Britain is likely also a consequence of its relatively late arrival at medical regulation. England, Scotland, and Ireland therefore present an experience of healthcare distinct from the rest of Europe, where medical practice was regulated much earlier (in Sicily as early as 1140, for example; in Iberia beginning in 1289).[7] England did not enact licensure regulations with any real success until 1512, and Gaelic Scotland and Ireland followed suit much later: Dublin's College of Physicians was not established until 1667, and Edinburgh's not until 1681. In the centuries before licensure, medical regulation happened on a case-by-case basis, almost always as a means of redressing harmful practice rather than preventing it. Especially in the context of comparatively flourishing medical programs in European universities, neither Oxford nor Cambridge prioritized the study of medicine, with the result that very few of their graduates were certified physicians.[8] Even taking into account that many must have obtained some level of university education, if not a degree, Faye Marie Getz has shown that fewer than one percent of all recorded students at medieval Oxford left any record of medical study.[9] The eventual success of the regulation of English medical practice in 1512—following a number of unsuccessful civic appeals in the preceding years—was likely enabled by the founding of the Royal College of Physicians by Thomas Linacre 6 years later, an institution that provided a source of practitioners who were legally qualified not only to practice medicine themselves but also to assess its practice by others. Negotiations of trust between patient and practitioner remained complex even when a patient could rely on a degree or license to indicate a degree of competency. In the years before licensure regulation, until something went wrong and a suit was brought to court, assessing a practitioner's legitimacy was the patient's prerogative.

These earlier (and, admittedly, scarcer) depictions of healthcare fraud illuminate important dimensions of the relationship between healer and patient. This scholarly lacuna is the primary concern of this essay: the role of the medieval quack before the heyday of the printing press and the growth of commercial medicine. The pages that follow emerge from two major questions. First, how did medieval medical practitioners establish their legitimacy and secure the trust of their patients before the introduction of licensing requirements? And second, how do satirical depictions of quack physicians complicate our understanding of those strategies? The first section of this essay discusses the role of performance in the establishment of trust between patient and physician. I move then to the historical and legal context of medical fraud in medieval England, considering civic and judicial responses to charlatan practitioners who made use of those strategies in order to deceive their clients. The essay's final section turns to literary texts that illustrate the role of form in quack medicine, including William Dunbar's *The Feigned Friar* and a number of anonymous mock verse prescriptions. Together, these sources reveal a medieval understanding of textual and material forms as flexible media through which medical authority and identity could be constructed, performed, and assessed.

Performance in the Practitioner–Patient Relationship

Patient confidence in a healer's legitimacy was far from assured, especially before the establishment of professional licensing requirements; as Michael R. McVaugh notes, "the patient had to make sure that the physician knew his business, while the physician had to reassure the patient that he really did deserve to be given the case".[10] One twelfth- or thirteenth-century text attributed to Arnald of Villanova, for example, warns physicians about patients who might attempt to test or trick them by presenting a sample of wine or animal urine in place of human urine for diagnosis. This was of particular concern when uroscopy happened at a distance, often at the physician's own lodging, and not at a patient's bedside. Practitioners are encouraged to take precautions "by which", the text explains, "we can protect ourselves against people who wish to deceive us". It goes on to recommend that the physician exercise his diagnostic skill on the messenger's or patient's face, searching for symptoms not of disease but of deception: "You must look at him sharply and keep your eyes straight on him or on his face; and if he wishes to deceive you he will start laughing or the color of his face will change".[11]

Detecting deception on the part of the patient was just one part of the physician's establishment of competency and authority, an accomplishment that constituted an important element in the negotiation of trust between the two. Securing a patient's confidence and trust involved a *performance* of medical authority in the term's lesser-known Middle English sense: to make, construct, or shape.[12] In textual encounters between practitioner and patient, this is visible in familiar forms such as the imperative recipe text-type (most simply, "take *x* for *y*") and reassuring efficacy phrases such as *probatum est*, "it is proven". In face-to-face encounters, the figure of the physician itself was often the shaping form, the structuring medium through which medical trust was established. In the execution, or performance, of their practice, those who claimed medical expertise shaped themselves into the form of the expert. McVaugh writes that the physician–patient encounter:

> [N]ot only provides a range of information about the patient's condition, it makes it abundantly clear that the physician is a person of impressive learning and skill and ensures that the patient will have confidence in his treatment: as William [of Salecito] goes on to assure us, "this kind of deliberate enquiry establishes the physician as knowledgeable and authoritative to laymen, the friends of the patient, and it confirms the patient and the bystanders in their trust of him, especially if they know little or nothing about medical science anyway; and thus the patient's mind will be set at rest".[13]

When a practitioner failed to adequately secure a patient's obedience and trust, medical relationships soured quickly. In 1433, for instance, the York leech Matthew Rutherford was sued for the extraordinary amount of 40 pounds by the Prior of Guisborough and his canon for mistreatment of the canon's injured leg. In response, the defendant asserted that his recalcitrant patient had not only insisted on continuing an unwholesome diet but had actually thrown away the medicines Rutherford prescribed.[14] An even more striking example is provided by Thomas atte March, who in

1369 sued Walter Leche of Billingsgate for the loss of the middle finger of his right hand, which he had paid Walter 5s to treat (with an additional 1s 8d promised upon its successful cure). The defendant protested that he had tried to apply treatment but that Thomas had first refused to comply and later assaulted his healer with a hatchet "and in the process broke his finger and pulled the bones, nerves, and veins of that finger so much with a pair of pinchers that he caused the damage on himself".[15] Spurred by mistrust between the two parties, such incidents could be harmful to a patient's health and—perhaps of more concern to the practitioner—to his own reputation and livelihood.

To ensure the best outcome possible, practitioners sought to gain their patient's trust through displays of expertise that asserted authority by means of three major elements of performance: speech, appearance and behavior, and material accoutrements. They needed, in other words, to adhere to lay expectations of how "good medicine" sounded, looked, and acted. This was not a matter of universal agreement; as numerous surviving sources attest, practitioners themselves quibbled over what "professionalism" entailed in the sickroom. But the wide variety of surviving advice texts, including established material from classical sources such as Galen, Plato, and Hippocrates, as well as newly authored treatises written with the medieval professional in mind, provides a rich illustration of the shape of practitioners' understanding of medical encounters in the Middle Ages.

The connection between medicine and rhetoric dates from well before the medieval period. Classical Greek texts evince tension between, on the one hand, acknowledgment that some rhetorical maneuvering was necessary in order to have a good relationship with one's patient, and on the other, a wariness of overreliance on performance at the expense of skill. As Stephen Pender has observed, Greek sources denigrate physicians who draw heavily on rhetoric in their practices but also admit to the expectation that they will do so, a reliance furthered by the Platonic insistence on the methodological resonance linking medicine and rhetoric, both of which depended on etiology. Pender explains:

> The rhetor and the physician share a single method, its success determined by the aptitude with which effects (passions aroused in oratory or symptoms of illness) are sutured to causes (the nature of an auditor's soul or the character of illness).[16]

The persistence of this historical connection between medicine and rhetoric is personified in the figure of Mercury, whose appearance in Henryson's *Testament of Cresseid* (c. 1500) embodies the connection between the two; the god is "richt eloquent and full of rethorie, / with polite termis and delicious", clad in a scarlet gown as a "Doctour in physick", bearing in one hand a book and, in the other, boxes filled:

> with fyne electuairis,
> And sugerit syropis for digestioun,
> Spycis belangand to the pothecairis,
> With mony hailsom sweit confectioun.

> [with fine electuaries
> And sugared syrups for digestion,
> Spices belonging to the apothecaries
> With many wholesome sweet confections.][17]

Henryson's Mercury presents an idealized physician: learned, wearing his hood in the style of a "poeit of the auld fassoun" ["poet of the old style"] and his scarlet gown in the manner appropriate to a physician, offering sweet language and sugared medical confections, both of which might serve as a balm to his patients (245). Most importantly, the speaker's closing remark that Mercury is "honest and gude and not ane word culd lie" asserts that the god is incapable of falsehood and deception—an ideal indeed, in the often-risky medieval medical marketplace (252).

In its instantiations in exchanges such as bedside visits and consultations, rhetorical positioning had marked effects on the potentially contentious relationship between patient and practitioner. In part, the practitioner's verbal maneuvering was intended to protect his own reputation, a goal visible in the oft-repeated advice that regardless of the severity of a given case, the physician should, to his patient, promise an easy recovery, and to the patient's friends, describe a dire prognosis. If the patient recovered, his friends would be all the more impressed with the physician's skill. If the patient died, his friends would admit that the physician had predicted the correct outcome from the start. Practitioners are similarly encouraged to capitalize on lay ignorance: "it helps greatly that a term is not understood by the people", writes one medieval author, advising readers that the phrase "obstruction in the liver" is an especially good choice when one is unsure of the real issue.[18] Jargon helped practitioners establish a clear boundary between themselves and those they treated, many of whom would have had some degree of medical knowledge of their own. Particularly for university-educated physicians, the ability to showcase learned knowledge to which lay healers would not have had access provided an important advantage during the later Middle Ages, when competition between classes of practitioners was keen.

Just as a patient's impression of a practitioner could be managed by careful speech, so too could it be manipulated by the practitioner's physical appearance and behavior during consultation and treatment. The

Hippocratic *Praecepta* cautioned physicians to steer clear of overly luxurious dress and perfume, "for excess of strangeness will win you ill-repute, but a little will be considered in good taste, just as pain in one part is a trifle, while in every part it is serious".[19] Physicians were likewise advised to stay away from the wives and daughters of their patients; to accept whatever meal was served by the family, however modest; to show gratitude and appreciation upon taking their leave at the end of the consultation; and to be good-humored and as honest as possible.[20] Much advice of this kind encourages the physician to comport himself in a manner that portrays learnedness and wisdom, even if he is uncertain about the patient's illness, for the benefit of both his own reputation and the morale of the suffering patient. Many texts instruct the physician to project an air of relentless cheer, no matter how dire the prognosis: one treatise suggests that he should enter the room "with a hilarious countenance and a joyful voice saying: 'Hey there, what do you say? What sort of fun are you having?'" This strategy, which Loren MacKinney has called a "somewhat reprehensible . . . [but] clever psychological approach", seems to be intended to benefit the practitioner's purse as much as the patient's spirits; as surviving lawsuits attest, a happy, friendly patient is more likely to pay his bill than an unhappy one.[21]

The conduct of the practitioner had more immediate and vital consequences than good public relations. The importance of patient trust and confidence to medieval medicine had been tacitly acknowledged in 1215, when the twenty-second canon of Lateran IV decreed that a physician sends for a priest, or "physician of the soul", before beginning to treat a patient. This was in part a means of asserting the primacy of spiritual health: Many physical maladies stemmed from spiritual wounds, which being healed might make the physical treatment more efficacious. There was also, however, a practical dimension to this decree. The same canon also notes that by calling for a cleric *prior* to beginning his work, the physician would forestall the potentially fatal dip in morale that might occur should he pause mid-treatment to summon a priest. This emphasis on the link between practitioner comportment and patient survival is made more explicit in the numerous secular guides that advise practitioners about how to act not only during the consultation but also during the more dangerous phases of treatment. The practice of medicine could entail a fair amount of dramatic performance on the part of the practitioner.[22] The fourteenth-century surgeon Guy de Chauliac, for example, recommends distracting a patient during traumatic medical procedures. "If a patient is hemorrhaging", he writes,

[T]ell him to keep his eyes shut, or carry him into a dark room so that he cannot see the blood flowing, cannot even look at red things that might make him think of blood; keep telling him that it isn't flowing any longer, or if it is, that it's good for him that it's still flowing.[23]

Physicians could also rely on material objects to signal their authenticity. Myriad other items beyond the ubiquitous urine flask used patient expectations to encourage trust in a practitioner's ability. Many were practical in nature, including instruments for surgery, cautery, and bloodletting, jars and bandages, and even animals; patients who believed themselves infested with serpents or frogs, for example, were said to be cured when a physician used sleight of hand to convey such an animal into their excrement, showing the patient that the creature had been removed.[24] Other material objects, particularly textual ones, were primarily useful as signals of expertise rather than as direct aids to treatment. Perhaps the most obvious example of these is the folding almanac, a manuscript that was hung from the physician's belt for visibility and ease of use. To consult it, the practitioner would have flipped it upright and unfolded one or more of its leaves into a sheet six or eight panels in size. As Peter Murray Jones has noted, many of the specialized images on those sheets include erroneous information; uroscopies are frequently miscolored, and indication lines like those surrounding the Vein Man often led to incorrect captions. A physician who consulted his almanac performed access to a kind of knowledge that the patient did not possess, presumably fostering trust or, at the least, a healthy respect for the physician's learnedness that might increase the patient's likelihood of following a given treatment.[25]

The explosive proliferation of English medical texts in the later Middle Ages enabled patients to interpret not only their own maladies but also the legitimacy of their attending practitioners in ways that had previously been unthinkable. As Julie Orlemanski has pointed out, the medieval lay populace—particularly those with some wealth—were actively involved in the etiological interpretation of medical signs. By the later Middle Ages, "medicine's explanatory systems were gaining ground", Orlemanski writes, "even if who was able to call on those systems, with what authority, remained a matter for contestation".[26] The pages above have provided a necessarily brief survey of the strategies utilized by medieval medical practitioners to cultivate patient trust in their expertise. The remainder of this essay is concerned with the way that literary and legal texts depict the use of those same strategies by medical frauds. As I will suggest, these texts evince social and civic investment in (and anxiety about) what can be done with versatile signifiers such as Clerk's golden bag or the recipe form. Like legitimate practitioners, the subjects of these lawsuits and poems make use of popular expectations about the form and appearance of medicine. But by filling in those forms with nonsense such as overtly impossible, inadvisable, or outright nonsignifying material, medieval quacks mark medicine as a site of identity production and negotiation for both patient and practitioner.

Legal-Historical Context: Malpractice and Fraud

Though I use the word "quack" (a variant of "quacksalver") here, it should be noted that its use to denote a medical charlatan did not occur until the late sixteenth century.[27] As it does today, the term served more often as a weapon to be directed at others than as a fixed marker of identity. Roy Porter's definition of the word focuses on the fraud's relative separation from the fabric of community medical practice:

> He (or she) was called a quack who transgressed what those in the saddle defined as true, orthodox, regular, 'good' medicine. He who chose to operate as a quack, or had no alternative but to do so . . . had to adopt the behaviour that best enabled him to survive and thrive as an outsider.[28]

As his words suggest, definitional difficulty emerges in large part from the heterogeneous nature of premodern medicine, what Porter calls a "panorama" of "practitioners of many stripes, some more, some less engaged in quackish activities".[29] The medical community of late medieval England was comprised of learned physicians, surgeons, barbers, midwives, oculists, itinerant healers, dentists, apothecaries, and clerics, among others, many of whom were in direct competition for clients.[30] Their training ranged from book-based university education to apprenticeship to personal experience and trial and error. Then, as now, basic levels of medical knowledge were available to most households, meaning that one did not have to identify as a professional in medicine in order to practice it among family and friends. Quack's most straightforward definition—someone who claims expertise in medicine without the appropriate qualifications—is fairly unhelpful when considering the centuries before "appropriate qualifications" had been professionally determined and enforced in England. Many critiques of fraudulence emerged from medieval physicians and surgeons, whose livelihoods suffered from the popular mistrust of medicine engendered by their un- or underqualified counterparts. Though an itinerant barber might consider himself equipped to perform surgery, the same was not necessarily true of other surgeons whose city he visited.

Early civic attempts to govern medical practice focused on just this kind of internal circumspection, calling on committees of respected practitioners to assess the actions of their peers. These inquests were reactive, rather than proactive, and typically occurred only once a practitioner's actions had been called into question by a plaintiff suing for damages following mistreatment. The cases in question often underscore not only differences of opinion about who was qualified for which kinds of practice but also the consequences of practitioner overconfidence on a patient's wellbeing. Such is the 1354 assault case in which fishmonger Thomas de Shene alleged in the king's court that John le Spicer of Cornhill:

> struck him [with a knife] on the shoulder on the right side of the head and there cut his veins and nerves such that the abovesaid veins and nerves were so constricted and withered that his mouth is drawn and enormously twisted and his eye is uprooted, whereby [Thomas] lost most of his vision, hearing, and speech.

John Le Spicer, whose name suggests that he was an apothecary rather than a trained surgeon, maintained that his actions had not been assault but cure: The fishmonger had asked for an ailment to be removed, and he had provided treatment "according to his ability". This was in fact the second time that Thomas had taken John to court over the incident; during the first, a case brought before the mayor's court, an assembly of surgeons examined the "enormous and horrible wound" on the fishmonger's jaw and judged that if John had been "expert" in his knowledge or art at the time he accepted the case, the wound could indeed have been healed.[31] This is far from the only example in which a medical practitioner's actions are depicted as violent, malicious acts by the patients on which they practiced. In 1361, a York tailor accused his barber of imprisoning and mistreating him before extracting a number of his teeth, resulting in 100s of damage.[32] A year before, John atte Ford and his wife Ellen accused William Phillip of maiming Ellen "treacherously and by premeditated assault", having "struck" her palm "such that the same hand's veins and nerves contracted and wholly died" before fleeing the scene. Phillip's version of the story asserted that he was a doctor who had been contracted by the pair to cure Ellen's hand, which he had done to the best of his ability.[33]

Defining medical quackery during a period in which expertise was a flexible and diversely interpreted concept is difficult. What distinguished a fraudulent practitioner from an overambitious one? This is, in essence, a matter of intention; in his use of a golden cloth and fake Latin manuscript as proof of expertise, Clerk deceived Roger and Johanna "falsely and maliciously".[34] His failure to cure was not the result of a practitioner overestimating his own competency, an error that appears to have catalyzed many malpractice suits. Indeed, it would have been difficult for Clerk to *under*estimate his ability, as Riley's *Memorials of London* asserts that he was both illiterate and "altogether ignorant of the art of physic or of surgery".[35] The clearest legal distinction between fraud and malpractice is made visible not in the accusations of bad practice, but in the resultant sentencing. The most common outcome of a guilty verdict in a malpractice suit was financial and focused on the wronged party: Damages were paid to the plaintiff, and the defendant was either fined or imprisoned.[36] As Clerk's case indicates, outright fraud merited a very different response, one that emphasized the broader social danger presented by pretension to medical authority. Accordingly, Clerk was tried not for malpractice or negligence but for "deceit and falsehood" (in Riley's *Memorials*) and for "having pretended to be expert in medicine" (in the *Calendar of Letter-Books*).[37]

In order that no other innocent citizens be misled about his qualifications, Clerk was sentenced to be led:

> through the middle of the City, with trumpets and pipes, he riding on a horse without a saddle, the said parchment and a whetstone, for his lies, being hung about his neck, an urinal also being hung before him, and another urinal on his back.[38]

Clerk's punishment emphasized identity fraud as his major offense. The urinals, sometimes called jordans, would have clearly signaled his pretension to the role of a physician; as Michael R. McVaugh has noted, the urine flask "had the iconic significance of a modern physician's white coat: it represented the expertise, the specialized knowledge possessed by the physician, and the respect that the expertise deserved".[39] The whetstone would have marked him out as a liar more generally.[40] A similar sentence had been carried out the previous year, when a man pretending to be the authority of a physician and an astrologer lied about an oncoming pestilence and was sentenced to be paraded through the city, bedecked with urinals and a whetstone. That account specifies that his punishment occurred in full view of the medical practitioners to whose ranks he had pretended to belong.[41] Together, these accounts suggest that in cases of fraud, it is not (or at least not only) "bad medicine" that is threatening, but the malicious pretension to—the *performance of*—unearned authority.

The public nature of Clerk's punishment, and that of the unnamed astrologer-quack, served many purposes, two of which help us understand the way fraudulent behavior was interpreted within medieval communities. It made their transgressions a matter of city-wide spectacle, marking their actions as an offense against not only the plaintiffs but also the common good.[42] As Katie Normington has noted, in their role as "performative practices which literally 'staged' the city and its rules", these punishments—alongside other public exhibitions such as royal processions and funerary parades—worked to construct both individual and social identities.[43] Their sentences also provided the public with a second opportunity to accurately discern their respective identities from their signifying objects, an interpretive act in which the general populace would have already engaged in theatrical contexts. In her discussion of the "corporeal semiotics" of the quack physician in the fifteenth-century Croxton *Play of the Sacrament*, for example, Sarah M. Owens points out that his threadbare gown and torn hose would have suggested a certain unprofessional carelessness to medieval audiences, while the physiognomic associations of his flat nose and trimmed beard, respectively, indicated lechery and dishonesty:

> When a character like Brundyche is described as 'rough of face' or 'flat-nosed', the author is assuming a level of sophistication in the audience that incorporates at least the basic concepts of humoral and complexion theories. Much as the surgeon is endowed with the authority to know and understand the human body, the audience is equipped to understand various characters and their foibles, through a combination of their actions and their physical appearance.[44]

While the healer reads the patient's ailing body—its color, pulse, urine, motion—the patient also reads the healer's own appearance and behavior. Roger and Johanna had been taken in by the trappings of medical authority Clerk bore, by his claims to experience and knowledge and possession of a Latin prayer and rich golden cloth. His sentencing allowed for a more accurate interpretation, one that revealed the semantic versatility of those material signifiers. This strategy was not restricted to medical practitioners; earlier that year, a London embroiderer and apparent checkers hustler by the name of William Soys was sentenced to the pillory with his doctored playing board displayed beside him; the same day, a Scotsman was also convicted of cheating Londoners with a pair of "false dice", which were hung from his neck during his punishment.[45]

The display of these meaningful objects—the media by which swindlers accomplished their goals—takes on a special resonance in the case of medical fraud. With the addition of the whetstone, Clerk's jordans and parchment were figured not as meaningless objects nor as irrefutable markers of qualification, but as the instruments through which his deception was carried out. Physical *materia medica* was presented as the means by which medical authority was signaled and recognized, and through which it could be revealed as false. In their use of these objects, quacks and the courts that sentenced them capitalized on popular understandings of what medicine looked like and drew on the same strategies of signification that legitimate physicians used to gain the trust of their patients. As I discuss later, this versatility extended beyond material objects to encompass the forms of medicine that structured their usage. Whether the quack is the subject or speaker, these literary accounts emphasize form and performance as the means by which medical authority is constructed—and as the means by which it might be deconstructed by the discerning reader.

Medical Fraud in Satirical Verse

William Dunbar's "The Feigned Friar of Tongland", written in the early sixteenth century, presents a heavily embellished account of the real-life antics of John Damian, abbot of Tongland from 1504 to 1509. There is some opacity around Damian's origins in the historical record. The treasurer's accounts for James IV's reign refer to Damian as "the French leich" and "the French medicinar", while John Leslie's later *Historie of Scotland* provides a more substantial description that identifies him as Italian, not French, and centers his work as a failed alchemist. In addition to his appointment as abbot, Leslie's account goes, Damian had also been provided by the king with the costly materials from which he promised to produce the quintessence. Upon failing, he attempted to regain the king's favor by beating a pair of visiting ambassadors back to France by means of a set of man-made wings. In doing so, the *Historie* explains, Damian attempted to "conterfute" or impersonate King Bladud, a monarch of Roman Britain supposed by Geoffrey of Monmouth to have bedecked himself in feathers in an ill-fated attempt to fly.[46] Damian's 1507 flight was just as short-lived, resulting in a broken leg and presumably some amount of public ridicule.[47]

Dunbar's satirical dream vision presents another, decidedly fictionalized account of the abbot's actions. In it, Damian is a Turk who crosses into Lombardy from his native Tartary, kills a cleric for his clothes to avoid a forced baptism, and proceeds to France, where he assumes the guise of a leech. There his work kills so many of his patients that he is forced to flee to Scotland, where he continues to feign expertise in the practice of medicine with predictable and consistent consequences: "in leichecraft", the poem summarizes, "he was homecyd" (33).[48] The poem concludes with a lengthy and scatological account of Damian's attempted flight, ending with the imposter trapped in a midden, hiding from flocks of enraged birds whose harsh noises awaken the poem's speaker from his sleep.

Dunbar's poem is useful in two distinct ways. First, it presents its subject as a fraudulent physician—among other "feigned" identities, including friar and alchemist—who relies on the material and behavioral trappings of medicine to succeed in his ruse. Second, it takes seriously the confused, jumbled contents of those outer signifiers. In doing so, the poem reveals to readers the precarity of medical authority and the flexibility of its forms. To falsify his identity as a cleric, Damian trades his presumably foreign clothing for the habit of a religious man of Western Europe. When his unholy conduct eventually leads to the revelation of this "dissimulance", (13) he is forced to flee to France and, later, Scotland, and to put his literacy to use in a closely related career path: medicine. In Scotland, he works as an apothecary and barber, letting blood and prescribing purgatives. His rates are exorbitant—a single night's attendance, the speaker notes, would cost a patient both his horse and his hide—and his treatments are violent. But despite a marked lack of actual medical skill, experience, or knowledge, Damian knows the *forms* of healthcare—the shapes and patterns it takes— and possesses the ability to perform them convincingly, drawing on several of the strategies discussed earlier to portray himself as a knowledgeable practitioner.[49]

The material signifier of professional credibility provided in Lombardy by his stolen habit is later, in France and Scotland, obtained using the accoutrements of medical practice: in particular, his iron surgical tools, numerous enough to fill a trunk and rough as unsanded wood, which in his hands transform from instruments of healing to "instrument[s] for slawchtir" (39). Surgical tools are ubiquitous as signifiers of medical practice in medieval illuminations, second only to urinals. The Englishman John of Arderne's *Fistula in ano* is perhaps the best-known text to include detailed illustrations of surgical tools, but it is far from the only one. In a counterpart to the famous image of the Wound Man, whose illustrated body is riddled with knives, arrows, swords, lances, cudgels, sharp branches, axes, and the occasional stinging insect, illustrations of surgical tools offered hope for repair and recovery: a tension between injury and treatment, written on the body and experienced painfully from within it. As the media through which physically traumatic procedures were enacted, surgical tools were an element of medicine with which patients had direct contact both when the tools were utilized on them and when they were required to assist their healer by holding objects themselves, an experience preserved in manuscript illuminations. BL Harley MS 1585, for example, depicts a patient holding a bowl to catch the blood resulting from his nasal surgery; Sloane MS 1975 shows a patient clutching a jar of ointment in readiness for his surgeon to finish utilizing a long needle to treat his cataract.[50] Working as an apothecary, Dunbar's Damian would have possessed weights and measures, sieves, presses, and gallipots; as a barber, he would have owned knives, bandages, and bowls explicitly for bloodletting.[51] As an alchemist—particularly one engaged in the search for the quintessence, an element believed to have myriad uses in medicine—he would have used jars, flasks, crucibles, alembics, and cucurbits.[52] But while these props work for a time, allowing him to maintain the ruse of professionalism, they do not impact his actual ability as a healer or alchemist, only his appearance at competence in those practices.

In Lombardy, Damian's misbehavior (what the speaker calls his "cursit govirnance" [14]) reveals that he is not a truly holy man, regardless of what his stolen habit appears to signify. By the time he reaches Scotland, he appears to have understood that it was not only props but personal conduct that determined the success of his dissimulation: In addition to drawing on material objects, Damian also shapes his behavior to align with popular expectations of legitimate medical practice. He lets blood, gives cures, and prescribes purgatives. His pretension to professionalism is most visible in the steep price he charges for his services. This move frames his labor as remunerative (and therefore professional) rather than altruistic or amateur; as Henri de Mondeville somewhat cynically observes in his *Cirurgia*, "the patient mistrusts whatever is given free of charge. He does not believe that he will be given something of value for nothing".[53] In short, Damian's "fenyt" (17) expertise in medicine adheres to patient expectations about what medical authority looked like. Were it not for his fatality rate, he might be believed to be a successful, if extortionate, physician.

But in Dunbar's poem, Damian's repeated movement through identities—from traveler to religious man, religious man to medical practitioner and alchemist, and failed alchemist to aspiring bird—has consequences. Dunbar presents Damian's flight not as an effort to prove himself to James IV, as Leslie's history has it, but rather as the last in a series of cut-and-run escapes that began with his relocation from Lombardy to France. His position in Scotland is especially visible, and his flight is framed as an attempt to avoid the consequences of his pretension to ecclesiastical, medical, and alchemical competency. Damian's skill at fraudulence is associated with his identity as a "Jow of a grit engyne [ingenuity]", descended from giants (31). His itineracy is consistently and xenophobically framed as an attempt to avoid the punitive consequences of his actions, a formulation that resonates in both medical contexts—practitioners entering cities from rural areas, for example, were often subjected to suspicion and mistrust from city-dwellers—and antisemitic ones, particularly in stories of such as that of the immortal Wandering Jew, sentenced to endless peregrination after heckling Christ before his crucifixion.[54]

The ease with which Damian shifts between identities is mirrored in the uncertainty of his identification by others; indeed, it is precisely the changeable nature of his performance that troubles outside attempts to discern his "true" form. The birds who attack Damian mid-air first attempt to assign him a variety of mythological identities, from Daedalus and the minotaur (both hybrids, in their marriage of animal and human forms) to Mars's blacksmith and Saturn's cook.[55] Others recognize him as a horned owl, a bird like them, but sinister and unwelcome.[56] His inability to convincingly feign these identities, or perhaps his ability to feign them too well, leads to Damian's downfall: The birds batter him so aggressively that he is forced first to defecate over a herd of cattle and then to strip off his feathered wing-jacket and plummet into a mire, where he hides from their assault for 3 days, submerged up to his eyes in filth.

The scatological emphasis in Dunbar's poem has its basis in Damian's actual attempted flight from the battlements of Stirling Castle, which resulted in a broken femur when Damian crash-landed in a midden some distance from the keep. Damian himself allegedly blamed his failure on the inclusion of hen feathers in the wings, arguing that hens are naturally drawn to the midden, not the skies.[57] This tendency towards raw, crude matter is a hallmark of medical satire, a genre that Julie Orlemanski writes "evinces both fascination and furious skepticism toward *phisik*'s vocabulary of materiality".[58] Her discussion of Robert Henryson's satirical "Sum Practysis of Medecyne" focuses on its jumbled use of medical jargon and birdsong, arguing that the poem "conjures two antagonistic limits, or dreams, of language: one, perfect precision and specificity, a complete expression of complete knowledge; the other, pure sound, a language that leaves behind meaning and becomes music".[59]

In its depiction of Damian's fraudulence and its repercussions, Dunbar's poem engages in the second of these conjurations, although the outcome is not musical; instead, jarring and discomposed sound heralds the dissolution of Damian's carefully counterfeited expertise. The poem is largely devoid of the jargon that marks "Sum Practysis". In fact, it is in its most technical moments, when its speaker might use medical terminology to describe the effects of Damian's treatments, that the poem turns instead to more textured and evocative idiomatic expression, offering a figuration of language as malleable and material, capable of being shaped into new and surprising forms. Damian's laxatives cause his patients' hips to shake and shimmy wildly, "hiddy giddy"; his purgations frequently put thieves to death without the expense of a "widdy", or noose (44, 48).[60] This emphasis on sound is inescapable in the second half of the text, which is devoted to the aural and physical tumult of the assailing birds. Damian's time in the midden is defined by sound, language collapsed—or perhaps freed—to noise:

> The air was dirkit with the fowlis
> That come with yawmeris and yowlis,
> With skryking, skrymming, and with scowlis,
> To tak him in the tyde.

These moments provide the sonic equivalent of the rough scratches on the quack Roger Clerk's parchment; by privileging sound over linguistic meaning, the noisy content of the dream reveals the fraudulent nature of Damian's identity. He manipulates the physical and behavioral signals of medical expertise in order to assume the form of a physician, but it is that same capacity for self-fashioning and imposture that ultimately reveals the lack of meaning beneath his performance.

Birdsound in "The Feigned Friar" acts as a bridge between the waking and dreaming worlds, as it does in other dream visions. The speaker in Chaucer's *Book of the Duchess*, for instance, is greeted by the harmonious sounds of birdsong, "so mery a soun, so swete entewnes", as he wakes within a bright dream-chamber.[61] Dunbar's speaker experiences a cruder avian awakening; the birds surrounding Damian's midden are so numerous that they darken the air, and their sounds are "so hiddowis" (125) that they not only jolt the speaker from his sleep prematurely but force him to curse their names for the remainder of his life. Their disruptive clamor persists beyond the narrative bounds of the poem and into the speaker's reality, moving from the immaterial dream-space to the waking world; it reveals the fabricated nature of the story itself, which dissolves into noise that denies the speaker the satisfaction of any resolution. Within the dream vision, birds function as the vehicle for Damian's comeuppance. Outside it, the cacophony of their sound abruptly reveals the poem's truth: that its narrative is an unreal fantasy, and that in his pretension to medical authority Damian is, like the mire in which he lands, full of shit.

Medieval satire recipes evince a similar interest in the kinds of capacious nonsense medical forms can carry, but in these texts, it is the speaker who occupies the role of the quack, offering the reader nonsense in the shape of medicine. The recipe form itself becomes the site of counterfeit, and its contents quickly reveal the ineffectual nature of the speaker's knowledge. As with real-life fraud, the success of the satire recipe depends entirely on its speaker's rhetorical acumen: their ability to convincingly perform expertise. Unlike real cases of fraud, however, successful satire recipes produced laughter; attentive readers participated in the joke, rather than falling victim to it. One nonmedical example is provided by the anonymous Scots poem "Lord Fergus's Gaist", preserved alongside Dunbar's "The Feigned Friar" and Henryson's "Sum Practysis" in the Bannatyne manuscript. The satirical recipe instructs its reader in summoning a spirit, calling for readily obtainable ingredients such as horse teeth, the tails of toads, and bundles of withered sticks, but emphasizing the role of sound rather than signifying language. The conjurer, for example, must sit within a circle and cast holy water "w[ith] pater noster patter patter", a term that transforms a Latin prayer into a collection of well-worn phonemes spoken rapidly and insincerely, or perhaps into the sound of the small footsteps of the poem's titular "littel gaist".[62] The recognizable form of the instructional text gives shape to the crude, sonic materiality of its contents; here, as in Dunbar's poem, the reader is presented not with learned expertise, but with the flexibility of its rhetorical trappings.

In mock medical prescriptions, the material of bodies and language is given a more particular shape in the remedy form. Like Damian's promise to produce the quintessence or to cure a patient's ills despite a lack of medical training, these often promise more than their speaker can reasonably deliver. One satirical recipe opens with an ambitious claim—"Yff a ȝong woman had a c. men take, / I can her ageyne a mayd make" [If a young woman has a hundred men taken / I can her again a made make]—and supplies a lengthy list of necessary but impossible ingredients, including the sound of a bell, the light of a glowworm, and the foot of an eel. This recipe-poem is grounded in many of the traditional elements of the remedy form, even beyond the fundamentals of imperative tone and sequential structure that define most instructional texts. Its speaker is attentive to the concerns of the physician, including the willingness of the patient to follow the prescribed course of treatment (the medicine, he notes, is worthy enough that "she wylle yt take") and emphasizes the importance of compliance with his instructions in preparing the recipe (the speaker instructs readers to "do as I yow telle"). Of the four ingredients for which quantitative measurements are provided, presumably for added verisimilitude, the recipe calls for units of seven and nine, both numerologically significant numbers frequently found in remedies.

Behind this adherence to the expected form of the remedy is the textual equivalent of scratched parchment: a cure entirely dependent on ingredients that either only exist in immaterial form (such as moonlight, the launch of a bird from its perch, or the sound of a bell, horse, or cartwheel) or do not exist at all (such as tallow obtained from a gnat or marrow obtained from a stone). The few parts of the recipe's instructions that do seem possible are inadvisable. A woman seeking to restore her maidenhead should presumably *not* be "leyd in an esy bed", as the poem directs, much less one in a hothouse that would exacerbate an already overheated humoral complexion. The underlying adynative message is that the restoration of one's virginity is as possible as the extraction of blood from a stone—which is to say, not possible at all.[63]

The nonsense matter of mock prescriptions has an internal logic: It demands ingredients or treatments that are either impossible, because they are intangible or do not exist at all, or ill-advised, because they run counter to common understandings of health and the body. In following recipe language to its furthest possible conclusions, to the negation of meaning, the mock prescription engages in a more overt version of the kind of specificity often found in the serious recipes it satirizes. Wellcome MS 405, for example, includes instructions, apparently in earnest, to cure an ailment of the eyes: "Take strawberys noþer to ripe ne to grene & put hem into a lynene cloþ neyþer to ðykke ne to ðynne".[64] Satirical recipes are humorous because they present a harmless, defanged performance of fraudulence: Though their forms announce their medical nature, their contents are manifestly impractical. The pleasure they produce is a result of the shift in power dynamics: These poems break down the boundary between learned expert and amateur, and writer and reader. Like the Londoners who watched Roger Clerk's passage, readers of satire poems are enabled to assess a practitioner's legitimacy for themselves, or at least to participate in the outcome of such an assessment. The layperson, not the so-called professional, becomes the diagnostic authority, even as the texts draw the concept of medical authority itself into doubt.

Literature, of course, only provides a version of medical practice: the experience of healthcare as it might, or might not, have occurred. The reality of every relationship between the medieval healer and the patient was unique and, as the lawsuits discussed earlier demonstrate, individuals could have very different understandings of events even within the locus of a single exchange. By looking at legal, medical, and literary texts together, however, we can begin to draw some conclusions about the way that practitioners performed expertise for their clients, and about the way that patients assessed, accepted, or resisted that authority. These works suggest that even before the establishment of licensure regulation and the development of the commercial marketplace, medical fraud was alive and well in premodern England and Scotland. From convicted criminals to fictionalized frauds like John Damian and the nameless speakers of satire recipes, medieval quacks demonstrably relied on patient expectations about how medicine looked (in its material and textual instantiations) to structure their performance. In endeavoring to appear as much like a legitimate practitioner as possible, the successful quack made such skillful use of medical forms that the inexpert content of those forms was overlooked, at least at first. The eventual discovery of that incoherent, immaterial, and nonsensical substance could transform the quack once again, this time from practitioner into the subject of scorn, laughter, or civic censure.

Notes

1 H. T. Riley, *Memorials of London and London Life in the 13th, 14th, and 15th Century* (London: Longmans, Green, 1868), 464–66.
2 When written correctly, the beginning of the prayer, known as the *Anima Christi* or *Soul of Christ*, reads as follows:

Anima Christi, sanctifica me.
Corpus Christi, salva me.
Sanguis Christi, inebria me.
Aqua lateris Christi, lava me.
Passio Christi, conforta me.
O bone Iesu, exaudi me
Et non me permittas separari a te.

[Soul of Christ, sanctify me.
Body of Christ, save me.
Blood of Christ, intoxicate me.
Water from the side of Christ, wash me.
Passion of Christ, comfort me.
O good Jesus, hearken to me
And do not allow me to be separated from you.]

Clerk's oral version apparently jumbled the fourth and sixth lines, and his testimony asserted that the prayer would act as an antipyretic, when the text as preserved in contemporaneous manuscripts makes no such specific claims. The version above, found in British Library MS Harley 2253, for example, concludes by noting the prayer's usefulness as a means of general remission of sin: "*Qui hanc orationem devote dixerit iiim dies veniale possidebit*" [The person who pronounces this prayer devoutly for three days will gain forgiveness]. *The*

Complete Harley 2253 Manuscript, ed. Susanna Greer Fein (Kalamazoo: Medieval Institute Publications, 2014), vol. 2. Quote found in Riley, *Memorials*, 464–66.

3 Riley, *Memorials*, 464–66. A much-abbreviated account of Clerk's trial and sentencing is found in Letter-Book H of the *Calendar of Letter-Books of the City of London*, ed. Reginald R. Sharpe (London: HMSO, 1907), fol. cxlv. The Letter-Book specifies that the parchment scrap was "an old scroll (*cedulam*) cut or torn across (*eridicatam extransverso*) from a leaf of a book and wrapt in a piece of cloth of gold". This case is also discussed in Sara M. Butler, "Medicine on Trial: Regulating the Health Professions in Later Medieval England", *Florilegium* 28 (2011): 71–94.

4 For example, Roberta Mullini, *Healing Words: The Printed Handbills of Early Modern London Quacks* (Frankfurt: Peter Lang, 2015); M. A. Katritzky, *Women, Medicine, and Theatre 1500–1750: Literary Mountebanks and Performing Quacks* (Aldershot: Ashgate, 2007); David Gentilcore, *Medical Charlatanism in Early Modern Italy* (Oxford: Oxford University Press, 2006); Margaret Pelling, *Medical Conflicts in Early Modern London: Patronage, Physicians, and Irregular Practitioners* (Oxford: Oxford University Press, 2003); Roy Porter, *Quacks: Fakers & Charlatans in English Medicine* (Stroud: Tempus, 2000); Roger King, *The Making of the Dentiste, c. 1650–1760* (New York: Routledge, 1998).

5 Katritzky, *Women, Medicine, and Theatre*, 5.

6 Jody Enders, *The Medieval Theater of Cruelty: Rhetoric, Memory, Violence* (Ithaca: Cornell University Press, 1999); Margaret E. Owens, *Stages of Dismemberment: The Fragmented Body in Late Medieval and Early Modern Drama* (Delaware: University of Delaware Press, 2005); Claire Sponsler, *Drama and Resistance: Bodies, Goods, and Theatricality in Late Medieval England* (Minneapolis: University of Minnesota Press, 1997). As Katritzky has noted, historians of medicine, theatre, and economics have only recently turned their attention to the performative dimension of *fraud* medicine in particular (Katritzky, *Women, Medicine, and Theatre*, p. 8). Katritzky's study provides a valuable examination of the way that itinerant acting troupes could provide early modern women with access to two realms from which they were frequently excluded: professional healthcare and theatrical production. Those studies—like Katritzky's—which do consider early sixteenth-century quacks often rely on accounts from the continent, where the commercialization of medicine and drama alike occurred earlier than in England. A notable outlier is Sarah M. Owens, "Leechcraft/Stagecraft: Performing Bodies in Late Medieval Medicine and Drama" (Ph.D. diss., University of Denver, 2006), which discusses the intersection of quackery and theatrical performance in England.

7 James M. Powell, translator, *The Liber Augustalis or Constitutions of Melfi, Promulgated by the Emperor Frederick II for the Kingdom of Sicily in 1231* (Syracuse, NY: Syracuse University Press, 1971), 131; Edward F. Hartung, "Medical Regulations of Frederick the Second of Hohenstaufen", *Medical Life* 41 (1934): 587–601; Luis García-Ballester, Michael R. McVaugh, and Agustín Rubio-Vela, *Medical Licensing and Learning in Fourteenth-Century Valencia* (Philadelphia: American Philosophical Society, 1989).

8 Padua, which granted four medical degrees in 1407, eight in 1434, and nine in 1450, provides a clear counterexample to the relative scarcity of English medical accreditation. Nancy G. Siraisi has posited that these numbers suggest a medical student body approaching 100 in 1450 (out of a total of 800 enrolled students).

Nine medical degrees were granted that year, out of a total of 93, indicating that medical instruction accounted for about ten percent of the university's activity. Siraisi, *Medieval and Early Renaissance Medicine: An Introduction to Knowledge and Practice* (Chicago: University of Chicago Press, 1990), 64. At Oxford, on the other hand, only 94 individuals taught medicine or were awarded a degree in the subject from 1300 to 1499, though the university granted 500 doctorates in theology in the 1300s alone. Medical numbers were even lower at Cambridge. Carole Rawcliffe, ed., *Sources for the History of Medicine in Late Medieval England* (Kalamazoo: Medieval Institute Publications, 1995), 60.

9   Faye Marie Getz notes that:

> a medical degree was not required for a practitioner to serve as a physician to an elite patron, which must have diminished the numbers of men willing to endure the lengthy process of certification. This did not necessarily mean that a physician without a medical degree had never studied medicine in a university, but only that he had not completed formal requirements for a degree.

Getz, "The Faculty of Medicine Before 1500", in *The History of the University of Oxford, II: Late Medieval Oxford*, eds. J. I. Catto and T. A. R. Evans (Oxford: Oxford University Press, 1992), 373–405; Getz, *Medicine in the English Middle Ages* (Princeton: Princeton University Press, 1998), 69.

10   Michael McVaugh, "Bedside Manners in the Middle Ages", *Bulletin of the History of Medicine* 71, no. 2 (1997): 203.

11   Henry E. Sigerist, "Bedside Manners in the Middle Ages: The Treatise *De Cautelis Medicorum* Attributed to Arnald of Villanova", *Quarterly Bulletin of the Northwestern University Medical School* 20, no. 1 (Spring 1946): 139. McVaugh contests the attribution to Arnald and suggests a date of composition in the twelfth century rather than the late thirteenth, observing that as the medical profession evolved, assessment, diagnosis, and treatment increasingly happened at the bedside, rather than at a distance. McVaugh, "Bedside Manners", 211–12.

12   *MED*, s.v. "performen, v[erb]". One could, for example, perform a tower, a bridge, or an orchard; in Lydgate's *Troy Book*, King Meryon is well-performed, or well-shaped, "by kynde". Lydgate, *Lydgate's Troy Book: A.D. 1412–20*, vol. I, ed. Henry Bergen (EETS e.s. 97, 1906), 2.4954.

13   McVaugh, p. 213, quoting William of Saliceto, *Summa conservationis*, in Cambridge MS Trinity College Cambridge 1202, fol. 1va.

14   C. H. Talbot and E. A. Hammond, *Medical Practitioners in Medieval England: A Biographical Register* (London: Wellcome Historical Medical Library, 1965), 213–14.

15   The National Archive (Public Record Office), ms KB 27/434, as found in Robert C. Palmer, *English Law in the Age of the Black Death, 1348–1381: A Transformation of Governance and Law Studies in Legal History* (Chapel Hill: University of North Carolina Press, 1993), Appendix 7, section k. Both cases are also discussed in Butler, "Medicine on Trial," 85–86.

16   Stephen Pender, "Between Medicine and Rhetoric", *Early Science and Medicine* 10, no. 1 (2005): 44. See also: Pankaj K. Agarwalla, "Training Showmanship: Rhetoric in Greek Medical Education of the Fifth and Fourth Centuries BC", in *Hippocrates and Medical Education*, ed. Manfred Horstmanshoff (Leiden: Brill, 2010), 73–85.

17   Denton Fox, ed., "The Testament of Cresseid", in *The Poems of Robert Henryson* (Oxford: Clarendon Press, 1981), ll. 240–49.

18 This prognostic advice appears in numerous sources, including Alberto de Zan-cariis, though perhaps earliest in the Anonymous Salernitanus, "De adventu medici ad aegrotum libellus", edited by Salvatore Renzi in *Collectio Salerni-tana*, vol. II (Napoli: Filiatre Sebezio, 1853) alongside the note about the term "obstruction". McVaugh, "Bedside Manners", 204; Manuel Morris, "Die Schrift des Albertus de Zancariis aus Bologna" (Diss., University of Leipzig, 1914), 17–18. The treatise was first published in Salvatore de Renzi, *Collectio Salernitana: ossia documenti inediti, e trattati di medicina appartenendi alla scuola medica Salernitana*, vol. II (Naples: Filiatre Sebezio, 1853), 74–80.

19 Precepts, X. In *Hippocrates*, trans. W. H. S. Jones (Cambridge: Harvard University Press, 1868), vol. I, 240.

20 See n. 7 above.

21 The quoted treatise is an extended version of "De adventu" and appears in Bibliotèque Nationale, Paris, BN MS Lat. 7091; L. C. MacKinney, "Medical Ethics and Etiquette in the Early Middle Ages: The Persistence of Hippocratic Ideals", *Bulletin of the History of Medicine* 26, no. 1 (1952): 26. The Latin text is published in de Renzi, *Collectio Salernitana* V (1859): 348–49.

22 Or perhaps on the part of a public performer or reader; one fifteenth-century banns advertising the services of an itinerant physician concludes with the state-ment "I telle ȝow nouȝth alle his heste scyensses it were to longg to spekyn off". On this manuscript (BL Harley MS 2390), see Linda Ehrsam Voigts, "Fif-teenth Century English Banns Advertising the Services of an Itinerant Doctor", in *Between Text and Patient: The Medical Enterprise in Medieval and Early Modern Europe*, eds. Florence Eliza Glaze and Brian K. Nance (Firenze: Sismel, 2011), 245–77, at 267.

23 Guy de Chauliac, *Guigonis de Caulhiaco (Guy de Chauliac), Inventarium sive Chirurgia Magna. Volume 1: Text*, ed. Michael R. McVaugh, Studies in Ancient Medicine 14 [1] (Leiden: Brill, 1997), VI.2.7, 375. Christopher Bon-field notes that the renowned English surgeon John Arderne says something similar, observing that cheering and comforting words from a surgeon bolstered a patient's ability to withstand the trauma of surgery. See "The First Instru-ment of Medicine: Diet and Regimens of Health in Late Medieval England", in '*A Verray Parfit Praktisour': Essays Presented to Carole Rawcliffe*, eds. Linda Clark and Elizabeth Danbury (London: Boydell and Brewer, 2017), 119, n. 140.

24 Robert Burton, *Anatomy of Melancholy* (Oxford: John Lichfield, for Henry Cripps, 1628), for example, recalls the sixteenth-century physician Felix Plat-ter's attempt to cure a colleague, an attempt that failed because of the patient's knowledge of the sleight-of-hand trick: "Platerus would have deceived him, by putting live frog's into his excrements; but he, being a physician himself, would not be deceived" (part. I, sect. 3.1.2).

25 Peter Murray Jones, "Image, Word and Medicine in the Middle Ages", in *Visu-alizing Medieval Medicine and Natural History, 1200–1550*, eds. Jean A. Giv-ens, Karen M. Reeds, and Alain Touwaide (Aldershot: Ashgate, 2006), 1–24, at p. 11. This possibility is also discussed by Julie Orlemanski in "Physiognomy and Otiose Practicality", *Exemplaria* 32, no. 2 (2011): 194–218. Karen Eileen Overbey and Jennifer Borland describe the folding almanac as a "participatory space of knowledge," a material object whose movement enabled an affective connection between physician and patient". Orlemanski, "Diagnostic Perfor-mance and Diagrammatic Manipulation in the Physician's Folding Almanacs", in *The Agency of Things in Medieval and Early Modern Art: Materials, Power and Manipulation*, eds. Grażyna Jurkowlaniec, Ika Matyjaszkiewicz, and Zuzanna Sarnecka (New York: Routledge, 2007), 144–56, at 145.

26 Julie Orlemanski, *Symptomatic Subjects: Bodies, Medicine, and Causation in the Literature of Late Medieval England* (Philadelphia: University of Pennsylvania Press, 2019), 58.

27 Stephen Gosson, *Schoole of Abuse* (London: Thomas Woodcocke, 1579), refers to "A quackesaluers budget, of filthy receites." *OED*, s.v. "quacksalver, n."

28 Porter, *Quacks*, 11.

29 Porter argues that in addition to their isolation from the main body of medical practice, quacks were frequently marked by a tendency towards self-promotion; one-off relationships with patients (as opposed to longer, durative relationships formed over the course of multiple interactions); and a reliance on the sale of mysterious cures. Porter, *Quacks*, 11.

30 In Gaelic Scotland and Ireland, medical practice was slightly less heterogeneous, since some family lines produced medical practitioners as a matter of succession. As the Flemish scientist Johann Baptista van Helmon observed,

> the noblemen of Ireland grant a field to a member of their household who takes care of their health . . . This person will have a book left to him by his ancestors, stuffed full of remedies. So whoever inherits the book inherits the field.

The fourteenth-century resurgence of Gaelic society in Ireland—and the thriving Gaelic highlands of Scotland—meant that medical dynasties, sometimes called medical kindreds, exerted a shaping force in regional medical practice from the later Middle Ages well into the seventeenth century. Quote in Pierce Grace, "Medicine in Gaelic Ireland and Scotland, c. 1350—c. 1750," *Irish Historical Studies* 44, no. 166 (2020): 201–23.

31 TNA KB 27/375, in Palmer, *English Law*, Appendix, 7a.

32 TNA CP 52/35, in Palmer, *English Law*, Appendix, 7d.

33 TNA KB 27/399, in Palmer, *English Law*, Appendix, 7c. Phillip was found guilty and arrested; the court awarded John and Ellen £30 in damages.

34 Riley, *Memorials*, 465.

35 Riley, *Memorials*, 465–66.

36 In 1310, for example, Master John of Curnbull was sued following his failure to heal a patient's leg. He was found guilty and forced to pay a hefty fine of thirty pounds (approximately £18,500 in today's currency). Some decades earlier, two other English physicians were imprisoned after being found guilty in a malpractice suit that determined they had provided fatal doses of medication to two different patients. Joseph Schatzmiller, *Jews, Medicine, and Medieval Society* (Berkeley: University of California Press, 1994), 80, 182 n. 5; the latter case is also discussed in Palmer, *English Law*, Appendix 7. A more moderate example is provided by a 1377 case in which three surgeons assessed the work of a practitioner named Richard Cheyndut and determined that, "owing to his lack of care and knowledge," his patient was in danger of losing his left leg; Cheyndut was "committed to prison"—though the record does not indicate for how long—but the plaintiff was awarded damages in the amount of 50s only (equivalent to a little more than £1,500 today). A. H. Thomas, ed., *Calendar of the Plea and Memoranda Rolls of the City of London: Volume 2, 1364–1381* (London, 1929), Roll A 22: 1376–77, 231–44.

37 Riley, *Memorials*, 464; *Calendar of Letter-Books*, fol. cxlv.

38 Riley, *Memorials*, 466. The account in Letter-Book H agrees with this in all details except one: It records that Clerk was sentenced to the pillory rather than the mobile display of a public parade (see fol. cxlv).

39 McVaugh, "Bedside Manners", 203. This recognizability rendered urinals especially fit for mocking; a satirical letter in the National Library of Wales MS Brogyntyn ii.1 describes a sick man who sends his urine to the leech in a urinal so large it is scarcely able to fit through the door, "save as grace was þe hovs was wyde ynowȝe". The letter is published in Nancy P. Pope, "A Middle English Satirical Letter in Brogyntyn MS. II.1", *American Notes and Queries* 18, no. 3 (2005): 35–39.

40 Whetstones were used to identify liars in legal and punitive contexts as early as 1364. Joel B. Smith, "Lying for the Whetstone: A Saying and its Links with Folk Life and Tradition", *Folk Life: Journal of Ethnological Studies* 42, no. 1 (2003): 54–60.

41 "In conspectu cunctorum physicorum et cirurgiorum". Thomas Walsingham, *Quondam Monachi S. Albani, Historia Anglicana*, series *Chronica monasterii S. Albani*, ed. H. T. Riley (London: Longman, Green, etc., 1864), vol. II, 63.

42 As Madeline Pelner Cosman has noted, Clerk's trial signaled that his offense was against both Roger atte Hacche and his wife Johanna, as well as against the mayor and the wider city community of London. "Roger Clerk violated not only one man's trust", she points out, "but also London's civic code forbidding practice of the unlearned and the unlicensed". Cosman, "Medieval Medical Malpractice: The Dicta and the Dockets", *Bulletin of the New York Academy of Medicine* 49, no. 1 (1973): 22–47, at 31–32.

43 Katie Normington, *Medieval English Drama: Performance and Spectatorship* (Cambridge: Polity Press, 2009), 49.

44 Owens, "Leechcraft/Stagecraft", 59.

45 Riley, *Memorials*, 455–76.

46 John Leslie, *History of Scotland* (org. title: *De origine, moribus, et rebus gestis Scotorum libri decem* (Rome, 1578), 76. Geoffrey of Monmouth's account has Bladud impacting the ground so violently that he is scattered into countless fragments.

47 In his preface to the *Compota theasaurariorum*, James Balfour Paul notes that Damian's failure to take wing evidently did no serious damage to his relationship with James IV, as his name continues to appear in the royal treasury accounts for several years following the attempted flight in 1507 (lxxvi-viii). James Balfour Paul, ed., *Compota theasaurariorum regum scotorum: Accounts of the Lord High Treasurer of Scotland* (Edinburgh: H. M. General Register House, 1900), vol. II.

48 All quotations of Dunbar's poem have been taken from John Conlee's TEAMS edition of the text; line numbers are cited parenthetically. William Dunbar, *William Dunbar's Complete Works: Poems Public and Private* (Kalamazoo: Medieval Institute Publications, 2004).

49 Although literacy was not required to succeed—at least temporarily—as a quack, as the example of the illiterate fraud Roger Clerk attests, it must have helped. Dunbar's speaker notes early on in the poem that Damian "couth wryte and reid" (12). *William Dunbar's Complete Works*.

50 The illuminations are found in BL Harley MS 1585 (fol. 9v) and BL Sloane MS 1975 (f. 93r) respectively, and are reproduced in Peter Murray Jones, *Medicine in Medieval Illuminated Manuscripts* (London: The British Library, 1998), 79, 80.

51 On the material objects utilized by professional apothecaries, see Patrick Wallis, "Consumption, Retailing, and Medicine in Early Modern London", *The Economic History Review New Series* 61, no. 1 (2008): 26–53.

52 The Scottish crown's treasurer's report attests that the real Damian received, among numerous other royal payments, £3 for "glass flacatis [flasks] and stuf"

in January 1504 and 24s. for the purchase of twelve urinals the following July. *Compota thesaurariorum*, 416, 446.

53 The exchange of payment for medical services rendered also afforded the legal protection of the court. Luis García-Ballester, "Medical Ethics in Transition in the Latin Medicine of the Thirteenth and Fourteenth Centuries: New Perspectives on the Physician-Patient Relationship and the Doctor's Fee", in *Doctors and Ethics: The Earlier Historical Setting of Professional Ethics*, eds. Andrew Wear, Johanna Geyer-Kordesch, and Roger French (Amsterdam: Rodopi, 1993), 38–71, at 51.

54 The account of the Wandering Jew is included in a number of medieval chronicles, including Roger of Wendover's thirteenth-century *Flores historiarum*. [Roger, of Wendover, *Flores Historiarum: The Flowers of History, from the Year of Our Lord 1154 and the First Year of Henry the Second, King of the English* (London: Longman & Co., 1886–9).] Tension between itinerant and fixed medical practitioners only heightened over time. In the mid-seventeenth century, Margaret Cavendish, for example, described the removal of one troupe of itinerant quacks from Antwerp, following conflict with local practitioners:

> [T]he magistrate Commanded them out of the Town, for fear of the Plague, which was then in the City, although some said, the Physicians through Envy to the Mountebank, Bribed them out; the truth is, they had Reason, for the Mountebank was then so much in Request, as most of the People made him their Doctor, and Jaen Potage (for so the Fool was named) was their Apothecary.

Margaret Cavendish, *CCXI Sociable Letters* (London: William Wilson, 1664), 407–8, as found in M. A. Katritzky, *Women, Medicine, and Theatre: Literary Mountebanks and Performing Quacks* (London: Routledge, 2007), 14.

55 The mention of Vulcanis evidently refers to Damian's face, which was streaked and blackened like a smith's, thanks to his alchemical labors (51). "Saturn's cook" is a more ambiguous reference, which could reinforce the image of Damian's fire-blackened visage but could also recall Saturnus's association with the Greek Cronus, the Titan who consumed his own children. Theresa Tinkle, "Saturn of the Several Faces: A Survey of the Medieval Mythographic Traditions", *Viator* 18 (1987): 289–308.

56 Owls are often associated with Jews; the night-dwelling bird, as William the Clerk's *Bestiare divin* puts it,

> lives in the darkness and has the air of being a supporter of the devil. It is the figure of evil Jews who do not believe in Jesus Christ, the true sun. Jews lived in the darkness, and the true believers in the light.

("*vit dans les ténèbres et a tout l'air d'être un suppôt du diable. C'est la figure des mauvais Juiss qui n'ont pas volulu croire en Jésus-Christ, le vrai soleil. Les Juiss ont vécu dans les ténèbres, et les vrais croyants dans la lumière*".) See *Le Bestiaire Divin De Guillaume, Clerc De Normandie*, ed. M. C. Hippau (Caen: Chez A. Hardel, 1852), 97–98. Owls are frequently depicted beset by other attacking birds, both in literature such as *The Owl and the Nightengale* and in art, for which see Mariko Miyazaki, "Misericord Owls and Medieval Anti-Semitism", in *The Mark of the Beast: The Medieval Bestiary in Art, Life, and Literature*, ed. Debra Hassig (New York: Garland, 1999), 23–59.

57 Leslie, *Historie*, 76.
58 Orlemanski, *Symptomatic Subjects*, 83.
59 Ibid., 112.
60 *Dictionary of the Older Scottish Tongue*, s. v. "hiddy-giddy, adj." ("from a riming jingle", possibly associated with "heid" and "giddy", meaning topsy-turvey), and s. v. "widdy".
61 Larry Benson, *The Riverside Chaucer*, 3rd ed. (Oxford: Oxford University Press, 2008), 309.
62 The poem survives in the Bannatyne MS (Edinburgh, NLS Advocates MS 1.1.6), fols. 114r-5r, and is published in *Early Popular Poetry of Scotland and the Northern Border*, ed. David Laing (London: Reeves and Turner, 1895), vol. 1, 284–88.
63 This poem is found in a copy of Caxton, *Mirrour of the World* (1481), written by a later reader in 1520. It is published in *Reliquiae antiquae: Scraps from Ancient Manuscripts*, eds. Thomas Wright and James Orchard Halliwell (London: J. R. Smith, 1845), 250–51. Another satirical recipe, intended for the nearly blind, instructs the reader to put the impaired man in a sealed, smoky house and wait until his eyes begin tearing before filling them with "brymston and sope". If after this treatment the patient's sight is not so improved that he can see "as well at mydnyȝt as at none", the speaker proclaims that he shall lose his right arm. The poem is recorded in Oxford, Bodleian Library MS Eng. poet. e.1, fol. 21v.
64 London, Wellcome MS 405, fol. 20r. Despite the text's overspecific demands, it is possible to make this particular remedy, and the others in its manuscript are practical in nature, suggesting that its writer intended it to be used.

Reference List

Archival Sources

British Library, London

BL MS Harley 2253, *Anima Christi* or *Soul of Christ*.
BL Harley MS 1585, Pseudo-Hippocrates, *Epistula ad Antiochum regem*
BL Harley MS 2390, 15th-century manuscript on ink and alchemical medicine.
BL Sloane MS 1975, Medical and herbal miscellany.

The National Archive, Kew, London

TNA KB 27/375, King's Bench, Court Record.
TNA KB 27/399, King's Bench, Court Record.
TNA KB 27/434, King's Bench, Court Record.
TNA CP 52/35, Court of Common Pleas Record.

Other Archives and Libraries

Bibliothèque nationale de France, Paris, BN MS Lat. 7091, "De adventu."
Bodleian Library, Oxford. Bod. Lib. MS Eng. poet. e.1.
The National Library of Scotland, Edinburgh, Advocates MS 1.1.6, Bannatyne Manuscript.

The National Library of Wales, NLM MS Brogyntyn ii.1, A Middle English Miscellany.
The Wellcome Trust Library of Medicine, Archives: Wellcome MS 405.
Trinity College Cambridge MS 1202, fol. 1va, William of Saliceto, *Summa conservationis*.

Printed Primary

Alberto de Zancariis (1280–1348). Morris, Manuel. "Die Schrift des Albertus de Zancariis aus Bologna." Diss., University of Leipzig, 1914.
Anonymous Salernitanus, "De adventu medici ad aegrotum libellus." In *Collectio Salernitana: ossia documenti inediti, e trattati di medicina appartenendi alla scuola medica Salernitana, Volume II*, edited by Salvatore Renzi, 74–80. Napoli: Filiatre Sebezio, 1853.
Balfour Paul, James, ed. *Compota Theasaurariorum Regum Scotorum: Accounts of the Lord High Treasurer of Scotland*. Vol. II. Edinburgh: H. M. General Register House, 1900.
Benson, Larry. *The Riverside Chaucer*. 3rd ed. Oxford: Oxford University Press, 2008.
Burton, Robert. *Anatomy of Melancholy*. Oxford: Iohn Lichfield, for Henry Cripps, 1628.
Calendar of Letter-Books of the City of London. Edited by Reginald R. Sharpe. London: HMSO, 1907.
Cavendish, Margaret. *CCXI Sociable Letters Written by the Thrice Noble, Illustrious, and Excellent Princess, the Lady Marchioness of Newcastle*. London: William Wilson, 1664.
———. "CCXI Sociable Letters." In *Women, Medicine, and Theatre: Literary Mountebanks and Performing Quacks*, edited by M. A. Katritzky. London: Routledge, 2007.
Caxton, William. *Mirrour of the World*. Edited by Oliver H. Prior. Paris: Alain Lotrain, 1520.
———. *Mirrour of the World*. Westminster and London: William Caxton, 1481.
Chauliac, Guy de. *Guigonis de Caulhiaco (Guy de Chauliac), Inventarium Sive Chirurgia Magna. Volume 1: Text*. Edited by Michael R. McVaugh. Studies in ancient Medicine, 14 [1]. Leiden: Brill, 1997.
The Complete Harley 2253 Manuscript. Edited by Susanna Greer Fein. Translated by Susanna Greer Fein, David Rabin, and Jan Ziolkowski. Vol. 2. Kalamazoo: Medieval Institute Publications, 2014.
Conlee, John, ed. *William Dunbar's Complete Works: Poems Public and Private*. Kalamazoo: Medieval Institute Publications, 2004.
Early Popular Poetry of Scotland and the Northern Border. Vol. 1. Edited by David Laing. London: Reeves and Turner, 1895.
Fox, Denton, ed. "The Testament of Cresseid." In *The Poems of Robert Henryson*. Oxford: Clarendon Press, 1981.
Gosson, Stephen. *School of Abuse*. London: Thomas Woodcocke, 1579.
Hippocrates. Vol. I. Translated by W. H. S. Jones. Cambridge: Harvard University Press, 1868.
Le Bestiaire Divin De Guillaume, Clerc De Normandie. Edited by M. C. Hippau. Caen: Chez A. Hardel, 1852.

Leslie, John. *Historie of Scotland*. Org. title: *De origine, moribus, et rebus gestis Scotorum libri decem*. Rome, 1578.

Lydgate. *Lydgate's Troy Book: A.D. 1412–20*. Vol. I. Edited by Henry Bergen. Early English Text Society, e.s. 97, 1906.

Powell, James M., trans. *The Liber Augustalis or Constitutions of Melfi, Promulgated by the Emperor Frederick II for the Kingdom of Sicily in 1231*. Syracuse, NY: Syracuse University Press, 1971.

Reliquiae Antiquae: Scraps From Ancient Manuscripts. Edited by Thomas Wright and James Orchard Halliwell. London: J. R. Smith, 1845.

Renzi, Salvatore de. *Collectio Salernitana: ossia documenti inediti, e trattati di medicina appartenendi alla scuola medica Salernitana, Volume II*. Naples: Filiatre Sebezio, 1853.

———. *Collectio Salernitana*. Vol. V. Naples: Filiatre Sebezio, 1859.

Riley, H. T., ed. *Memorials of London and London Life in the 13th, 14th, and 15th Century*. London: Longmans, Green, 1868.

Roger, of Wendover. *Flores Historiarum: The Flowers of History, From the Year of Our Lord 1154 and the First Year of Henry the Second, King of the English*. London: Longman & Co., 1886–9.

Thomas, A. H., ed. *Calendar of the Plea and Memoranda Rolls of the City of London: Volume 2, 1364–1381*, 231–44. London, 1929, Roll A 22: 1376–77.

Walsingham, Thomas. *Quondam Monachi S. Albani, Historia Anglicana*. Series: *Chronica monasterii S. Albani. Volume II*. Edited by H. T. Riley. London: Longman, Green, etc., 1864.

Secondary Sources

Agarwalla, Pankaj K. "Training Showmanship: Rhetoric in Greek Medical Education of the Fifth and Fourth Centuries BC." In *Hippocrates and Medical Education*, edited by Manfred Horstmanshoff. Leiden: Brill, 2010.

Bonfield, Christopher. "The First Instrument of Medicine: Diet and Regimens of Health in Late Medieval England." In *'A Verray Parfit Praktisour': Essays Presented to Carole Rawcliffe*, edited by Linda Clark and Elizabeth Danbury. London: Boydell and Brewer, 2017.

Butler, Sara M. "Medicine on Trial: Regulating the Health Professions in Later Medieval England." *Florilegium* 28 (2011): 71–94.

Cosman, Madeline Pelner. "Medieval Medical Malpractice: The Dicta and the Dockets." *Bulletin of the New York Academy of Medicine* 49, no. 1 (1973): 22–47.

Enders, Jody. *The Medieval Theater of Cruelty: Rhetoric, Memory, Violence*. Ithaca: Cornell University Press, 1999.

García-Ballester, Luis. "Medical Ethics in Transition in the Latin Medicine of the Thirteenth and Fourteenth Centuries: New Perspectives on the Physician-Patient Relationship and the Doctor's Fee." In *Doctors and Ethics: The Earlier Historical Setting of Professional Ethics*, edited by Andrew Wear, Johanna Geyer-Kordesch, and Roger French. Amsterdam: Rodopi, 1993.

García-Ballester, Luis, Michael R. McVaugh, and Agustín Rubio-Vela. *Medical Licensing and Learning in Fourteenth-Century Valencia*. Philadelphia: American Philosophical Society, 1989.

Gentilcore, David. *Medical Charlatanism in Early Modern Italy*. Oxford: Oxford University Press, 2006.

Getz, Faye Marie. "The Faculty of Medicine Before 1500." In *The History of the University of Oxford, II: Late Medieval Oxford*, edited by J. I. Catto and T. A. R. Evans, 373–405. Oxford: Oxford University Press, 1992.

———. *Medicine in the English Middle Ages*. Princeton: Princeton University Press, 1998.

Givens, Jean A., Karen M. Reeds, and Alain Touwaide, eds. *Visualizing Medieval Medicine and Natural History, 1200–1550*. Aldershot: Ashgate, 2006.

Grace, Pierce. "Medicine in Gaelic Ireland and Scotland, c. 1350—c. 1750." *Irish Historical Studies* 44, no. 166 (2020): 201–23.

Hartung, Edward F. "Medical Regulations of Frederick the Second of Hohenstaufen." *Medical Life* 41 (1934): 587–601.

Jones, Peter Murray. "Image, Word and Medicine in the Middle Ages." In *Visualizing Medieval Medicine and Natural History, 1200–1550*, edited by Jean A. Givens, Karen M. Reeds, and Alain Touwaide, 1–24. Aldershot: Ashgate, 2006.

———. *Medicine in Medieval Illuminated Manuscripts*. London: The British Library, 1998.

Katritzky, M. A. *Women, Medicine and Theatre 1500–1750: Literary Mountebanks and Performing Quacks*. Aldershot: Ashgate, 2007.

King, Roger. *The Making of the Dentiste, c. 1650–1760*. New York: Routledge, 1998.

MacKinney, L. C. "Medical Ethics and Etiquette in the Early Middle Ages: The Persistence of Hippocratic Ideals." *Bulletin of the History of Medicine* 26, no. 1 (1952).

McVaugh, Michael. "Bedside Manners in the Middle Ages." *Bulletin of the History of Medicine* 71, no. 2 (1997): 201–23.

Miyazaki, Mariko. "Misericord Owls and Medieval Anti-Semitism." In *The Mark of the Beast: The Medieval Bestiary in Art, Life, and Literature*, edited by Debra Hassig. New York: Garland, 1999.

Morris, Manuel. "Die Schrift des Albertus de Zancariis aus Bologna." Diss., University of Leipzig, 1914.

Mullini, Roberta. *Healing Words: The Printed Handbills of Early Modern London Quacks*. Frankfurt: Peter Lang, 2015

Normington, Katie. *Medieval English Drama: Performance and Spectatorship*. Cambridge: Polity Press, 2009.

Owens, Margaret E. *Stages of Dismemberment: The Fragmented Body in Late Medieval and Early Modern Drama*. Delaware: University of Delaware Press, 2005.

Owens, Sarah M. "Leechcraft/Stagecraft: Performing Bodies in Late Medieval Medicine and Drama." Ph.D. diss., University of Denver, 2006.

Orlemanski, Julie. "Physiognomy and Otiose Practicality." *Exemplaria* 32, no. 2 (2011): 194–218.

———. *Symptomatic Subjects: Bodies, Medicine, and Causation in the Literature of Late Medieval England*. Philadelphia: University of Pennsylvania Press, 2019.

Overbey, Karen Eileen, and Jennifer Borland. "Diagnostic Performance and Diagrammatic Manipulation in the Physician's Folding Almanacs." In *The Agency of Things in Medieval and Early Modern Art: Materials, Power and Manipulation*, edited by Grażyna Jurkowlaniec, Ika Matyjaszkiewicz, and Zuzanna Sarnecka, 144–56. New York: Routledge, 2007.

Palmer, Robert C. *English Law in the Age of the Black Death, 1348–1381: A Transformation of Governance and Law Studies in Legal History.* Chapel Hill: University of North Carolina Press, 1993.

Pelling, Margaret. *Medical Conflicts in Early Modern London: Patronage, Physicians, and Irregular Practitioners.* Oxford: Oxford University Press, 2003.

Pender, Stephen. "Between Medicine and Rhetoric." *Early Science and Medicine* 10, no. 1 (2005): 37–64.

Pope, Nancy P. "A Middle English Satirical Letter in Brogyntyn MS. II.1." *American Notes and Queries* 18, no. 3 (2005): 35–39.

Porter, Roy. *Quacks: Fakers & Charlatans in English Medicine.* Stroud: Tempus, 2000.

Rawcliffe, Carole, ed. *Sources for the History of Medicine in Late Medieval England.* Kalamazoo: Medieval Institute Publications, 1995.

Schatzmiller, Joseph. *Jews, Medicine, and Medieval Society.* Berkeley: University of California Press, 1994.

Sigerist, Henry E. "Bedside Manners in the Middle Ages: The Treatise *De Cautelis Medicorum* Attributed to Arnald of Villanova." *Quarterly Bulletin of the Northwestern University Medical School* 20 (Spring 1946): 136–43.

Siraisi, Nancy G. *Medieval and Early Renaissance Medicine: An Introduction to Knowledge and Practice.* Chicago: University of Chicago Press, 1990.

Smith, Joel B. "Lying for the Whetstone: A Saying and Its Links with Folk Life and Tradition." *Folk Life: Journal of Ethnological Studies* 42, no. 1 (2003): 54–60.

Sponsler, Claire. *Drama And Resistance: Bodies, Goods, and Theatricality in Late Medieval England.* Minneapolis: University of Minnesota Press, 1997.

Talbot, C. H., and E. A. Hammond. *Medical Practitioners in Medieval England: A Biographical Register.* London: Wellcome Historical Medical Library, 1965.

Tinkle, Theresa. "Saturn of the Several Faces: A Survey of the Medieval Mythographic Traditions." *Viator* 18 (1987): 289–308.

Voigts, Linda Ehrsam. "Fifteenth Century English Banns Advertising the Services of an Itinerant Doctor." In *Between Text and Patient: The Medical Enterprise in Medieval and Early Modern Europe*, edited by Florence Eliza Glaze and Brian K. Nance. Firenze: Sismel, 2011.

Wallis, Patrick. "Consumption, Retailing, and Medicine in Early Modern London." *The Economic History Review New Series* 61, no. 1 (2008): 26–53.

3 Pathologising Ecstatic Dance

Reflections on Medieval Dansomnia and the Love Parade in Berlin, 1996

Irina Metzler

In the Middle Ages, John Chrysostom wrote (paraphrased), 'For where there is a dance, there also is the Devil',[1] and in the twentieth century, Emma Goldman wrote, 'It's not my revolution if I can't dance'.[2] At the opening of the twenty-first century, Lyn Gardner, writing a piece called 'The devil in the dance' for *The Guardian*, wrote the following:

> Once upon a time, in the lurid Middle Ages of the modern journalist imagination, in the not-so-distant past, hundreds of thousands of people took part in frenzied outdoor orgies and wild displays of dancing that lasted for weeks. People would dance themselves into a state of elation, tearing off their clothes, laughing, weeping and having sex with strangers. Some participants died of heat stroke and exhaustion, others just had a jolly good time, found release, and then returned to their old lives. A bit like weekend clubbers.

Thus, the medieval outbreaks of so-called dancing manias were positioned as cases of individual and mass hysteria, but also compared to the modern club night. The subjects of this collection of essays, malingering and invented illness, tend to be applied as labels to persons who are *not in* fact ill, but who for one reason or another are feigning sickness. Here, I wish to turn to the opposite situation, to people who are not ill, and do not consider themselves ill, yet are labelled ill. Therefore, the focus of this essay is on the medicalisation of dance, on how certain types of dance, depending on the social context, were seen by commentators as being akin to illness, rather than purportedly legitimate dance (such as ballet, folk dance, ballroom dancing), and how the pathologisation of the activity labels it as deviant.[3] Two specific instances have been selected for the purposes of the present research: the specific Dansomnia of 1374 and the Love Parade in Berlin 1996. Though separated by time as well as geography— the Dansomnia was located in what is now Belgium and France— there are similarities between the two events. These similarities are to be

DOI: 10.4324/9781003452324-5

found in the descriptions by nonparticipants, that is the commentators, historians and journalists, rather than in the events as such. One aim of this chapter was to outline the problem of Dansomnia as an object of study, by pointing out that the milieu and time-specific perspective of the observer dictates the response toward the phenomenon. Some similarities can be found between the events, of course, such as in the mass character of the dances or in the ecstatic element common to both. But it is the reaction of the viewer–commentator that is strikingly similar, and the gaze of 600 years ago medicalised as much as the gaze of 1996.

Dansomnia has over the past two centuries been interpreted variously according to theories pertaining to the history of religion and medicine, thus polarised between cult and illness, a tension which Gregor Rohmann sought to resolve by applying the emic approaches pioneered by anthropologists, and by researching the subject with the aid of the fields of medicine, dance and ritual, and religion and mythology.[4] After the medieval sources first noted the phenomenon, the 'second invention' of Dansomnia during the nineteenth century was instrumental to how a specifically German historiography shaped the history of the concept. The so-called dance manias of the late Middle Ages have fascinated historians since the nineteenth century, when the physician J. C. Hecker became the first modern scholar to propose, not surprisingly considering his profession, that the dancers were driven by some 'inward morbid condition which was transferred from the sensorium to the nerves of motion'.[5] The search for a retrospective *medical* diagnosis has continued ever since, to the detriment of alternative causations. For instance, an article in a dedicated public health journal of 1997 firmly located the dances within a disease model and described the 'Dancing Plague' as 'a public health conundrum'.[6] The baffled journalists of 1996 struggled with positioning the novel event of the Love Parade, settling ultimately on somewhere between an epidemic of mass hysteria and public order offence.

Medieval Dansomnia

In the summer of 1374, the appearance of certain dancers was noticed in the Low Countries and northern France by the lay and ecclesiastical chroniclers; apparently, these dancers were originating from the cities of the Rhine region and spreading into France and Flanders. Some of the dances were called the dances of St John or of St Vitus because of their 'Bacchantic' leaps and jumps[7], which characterised them, and 'which gave to those affected, whilst performing their wild dance, and screaming and foaming with fury, all the appearance of persons possessed'.[8] At Aix-la-Chapelle in 1374, men and women 'continued dancing, regardless of the bystanders, for hours together in wild delirium, until at length they fell to the ground in a state of exhaustion'.[9] Whilst dancing they are oblivious to their surroundings, they shriek, scream and 'rave'—note the use of rave in its older meaning of manic behaviour—and they have visions that 'according as the religious notions of the age were strangely and variously reflected in their imaginations'.[10] And again, the people dancing these dances came to Flanders like those possessed, as the chronicler Gilles de Roya puts it.[11] People danced and leaped, as the Liège Chronicle of 1402 stated, and they were possessed by demons; when the spirit descended into their limbs they were unable to cease dancing and leaping, when it reached their pelvis they were cruelly tortured, and because of this they had small sticks with which they beat themselves about the navel; this calmed their sorrow a little bit, and they threw away their sticks; they had a terrible appearance.[12] The dancing was supposedly preceded by an epileptic fit, with people foaming at the mouth and then suddenly jumping up and starting to dance 'amidst strange contortions'.[13]

The diagnosis of epilepsy as a trigger for the dancing mania was made in the nineteenth century by the medical historian Hecker, who in turn appeared to have received the idea from a fourteenth-century chronicle,[14] demonstrating that the medieval commentators were already medicalising the phenomenon as a way of explaining what they could not otherwise understand. Madeleine Braekman attempted a more modern diagnosis of the dancing mania, also noting the similarity of body movement between the people afflicted with Dansomnia and epilepsy.[15] Whether such diagnostic efforts are valid or useful is not relevant for the purposes of the present argument, suffice it to note that the phenomenon of a public, mass display of dancing was and still is seen as *necessitating* a medically informed explanation. Medieval people themselves appeared to see their dancing as a condition requiring cure, in this case through the agency of the Virgin and selected saints, such as St Lambert, or St Bartholomew who specialised in the treatment of nervous disorders, cramps, convulsions or possessions.[16] Braekman did not regard the diagnosis of (demonic) possession proffered by some medieval contemporaries as part of a truly medical explanation: 'Dans une société dominée par la religion et où la médecine a peu de place, l'Eglise explique les maladies nerveuses comme des cas de possessions diaboliques dont elle seule peut guérir'.[17] ('In a society dominated by religion and where medicine has little place, the Church explains nervous diseases as cases of diabolical possessions that only it can cure'.) However, I do not believe this modern separation of religion and medicine is accurately reflecting medieval views on this matter. There was no strict dividing line between what we would term medicine and religion; one only has to think of the imagery of Christ the Healer to realise that the Church quite clearly saw its role as a healing, and by extension a medical, institution. It is very much a feature of modern, industrialised society to think of strict delineations between so-called scientific disciplines on the one hand

and religion on the other. For the medieval world, where religion was all-encompassing, such a distinction would have been meaningless.

Dancing took place in towns and villages, where sometimes the dancers took over religious houses.[18] Dancing was a mass phenomenon, the allegedly possessed dancers 'assembling in multitudes', and they also frequently 'poured forth imprecations' against the clergy and 'menaced their destruction'.[19] It was this element of anti-clericalism that was probably the deciding factor in achieving the pronouncement of heresy over the dancers by the ecclesiastical authorities. Furthermore, the dancers 'intimidate' other people to not make any footwear other than square-toed shoes, because they had a 'morbid dislike' of the then fashionable pointy-toed shoes. This should be seen not as a sign of the backwardness or untrendiness of the dancers, but as a conscious statement against conspicuous consumption, since the pointy shoes, requiring so much more (unnecessary) material, would generally have been worn by the fashion-conscious wealthy. This element of social protest and anti-consumerism, to put it in modern parlance, is borne out by the observation that the clergy are keen to exorcise the dancers lest the 'disease' spread from the poor, 'for hitherto scarcely any but the poor had been attacked',[20] to affect those from the higher classes as well.

The predominantly lower class participants in dancing were even joined by housewives (one must think of this as eliciting the response in the fourteenth-century equivalent of a shock-horror style gutter press headline today); beggars took advantage of the means opened to them of new ways of getting money from people; children left their parents, and servants their masters, to take part in the dancing. Worst of all, unmarried women 'were seen raving about in consecrated and unconsecrated places, and the consequences were soon perceived'.[21] The appearance of masses of people dancing *per se* was deemed bad enough, but the *sorts* of people dancing were even more worrying to the ecclesiastical and secular authorities, as the above aspects of the perceived breakdown of the established social order show. Thus, the sociologist Robert Bartholomew concluded that the Dansomnias, including tarantism, were not illnesses but forms of expressing social discontentment.[22] Hecker, gazing from a nineteenth-century perspective, reiterated medieval concerns about Dansomnia, since he picked up the idea that the spreaders of the disease are 'idle vagabonds' who mimic the symptoms for their own advantage 'seeking maintenance and adventures' without being 'really affected' by it;[23] he combined a social with a medical explanation for the phenomenon by reasoning that 'in maladies of this kind the susceptible are infected as easily by the appearance as by the reality'.[24] Dancing, music and large, public festivities have always carried a subversive element with them:

The idea of uncontrolled, wild dancing as something dangerous stays with us: the club must be licensed for entertainment; the rave strictly policed. The idea of people enjoying themselves, whirling like banshees out of control is deeply unsettling to authority.[25]

Medicalising the actions of the participants in such actions is one way of regaining control. The application of the disease label is one of the most powerful weapons in the arsenal of those who rule. In the past, medieval heresy was often described by the church authorities as being like cancer on the body of the faithful; most recently in our time, the unvaccinated were accused of spreading disease, sometimes nefariously by asympotomatic means.

Bacchanalia

Dancing as a mass spectacle, as perceived mania, was not entirely new to the fourteenth century. The popular (in the sense of by the people) dancing manias have been seen in conjunction with the clerical dances that were sometimes performed in church by the clergy throughout the Middle Ages, and which the authorities tried in vain to suppress and stifle.[26] The Dance of St John, as the dancing mania was sometimes called, linked dancing with the veneration of John the Baptist by 'all sorts of strange and rude customs',[27] which were already noticed, and forbidden by, St Augustine in the late fourth century: people should not commit excess and sing profane songs at the festival of St John.[28] His contemporary Peter Chrysologus (380—450) did not hesitate to speak of the pest of dancers (*saltatricum pestis*),[29] and canon 53 of a church council held between 343 and 381 reminded Christians assisting at weddings not to leap and dance;[30] also the specific character of dances, circumstances, when and where, were singled out for particular attention.[31] At the end of the fourth century, the archbishop of Constantinople, John Chrysostom (the 'golden mouthed'), pronounced categorically: 'For where there is a dance, there also is the Devil'.[32] And by 1209, canon 17 of the synod held at Avignon reiterated the injunction against dancing in churches on the vigils of saints' feasts;[33] lastly, canon law expressly forbade priests and other clerics to dance.[34] Hecker commented with regard to the activities around the feast of St John: Bacchanalian dances, which have originated in similar causes among all the rude [sic] nations of the earth, and the wild extravagancies of a heated imagination, were the constant accompaniments of this half-heathen, half-Christian festival.[35] He went on to conjecture, that since the appearance of the Dansomnia in 1374 was in July, around the time of St John's feast day, and the dancers uttered John's name, 'the wild revels of St. John's day . . . gave rise to this mental plague, which thenceforth has visited so many thousands with incurable aberration of mind, and disgusting distortions of body'.[36] Coincidentally, the 1996 Love Parade in Berlin was also held in the month of July. The Love Parade as a modern St John's bacchanalic feast, perhaps? The notion of the 'long hot summer' certainly goes back a long way.

An instance of another dancing event related to a saint's feast, again held in summertime, on the first day of August, was reported by Gerald of Wales, writing shortly after 1188, at the church of St Eluned in southern Wales. There people, mainly 'young men and maidens', dance in the churchyard singing traditional songs until they suddenly 'leap in the air as if seized by frenzy'.[37] The dancers further transgress by miming 'with their hands and feet' the movements of the work they normally do, 'in full view of the crowds', something which is contrary to the commandment on Sabbath days,[38] that is the commandment not to work. Gerald of Wales already commented that by participating in these festivities the dancers were absolved and pardoned and their sinful state was mended by the experience. Following suit, Gregor Rohmann interpreted this as a mimetic example of the search for the reintegration of the sinner into a state of grace.[39] An alternative explanation can be found in Nancy Caciola's essay on wraiths, revenants and rituals in medieval culture, who has also cited this episode and instead suggested that such dances may have had an apotropaic function, to ensure the dead stayed within their own realm and did not trouble the living, furthermore conjecturing that the living may have danced with the dead on these special occasions in rituals that preceded the better-known *danse macabre*.[40]

Other dancing mania-like phenomena predating the 1374 events can be found at Erfurt in 1237, when more than a hundred children danced and jumped their way to Arnstadt; at Utrecht in June 1278 with people dancing on a bridge across the river until it collapsed; and most significantly at Kolbigk near Bernburg in 1027.[41] At Kolbigk, some peasants disrupted the Christmas Eve service by dancing and brawling in the churchyard, whereupon the officiating priest, Ruprecht, cursed them that they would dance and scream unceasingly for a whole year. Here is a case where dancing is most definitely perceived as transgressive and has to be duly punished. Maybe this story had some influence over how 300 years later dancing was equally positioned as a transgressive activity, and the participants were punished in the sense that they were afflicted by an illness. Since the contemporary medieval accounts of mass, communal public dancing were written not by the dancers themselves, but by nonparticipants, who additionally were worried about apparent breakdowns of social order, it is not surprising that what is never raised as an issue is that perhaps people danced, especially in the warm days of summer on the feast of St John, for the simple, if banal, reason that dancing is *fun*.

This quality of fun has already been highlighted by Barbara Ehrenreich, whose book on ecstatic rituals and festivities involving feasting, masking and dancing holds the telling subtitle of being 'a history of collective joy'. Her self-professed mission statement was 'to speak seriously of the largely ignored and perhaps incommunicable thrill of the group deliberately united in joy and exaltation'.[42] For Ehrenreich, the pleasure gained from participation in an ecstatic ritual was something that was part of the human condition for millennia, but that had declined over the last few centuries (i.e. since the advent of industrialisation, the Enlightenment, secularisation and other so-called progressive developments). In that, ecstatic rituals followed the same trajectories as the decline of community, which Ehrenreich felt necessitated the same scholarly interest. 'The loss of *ecstatic* pleasure, of the kind once routinely generated by rituals involving dancing, music, and so on, deserves the same attention accorded to *community*, and to be equally mourned'.[43] The final death knell for communal, ecstatic dancing, speaking from the post-pandemic position of 2022, is of course the biophobic, antimaterialist legacy of the virtual, that is digital interaction bequeathed to most of Western society by lockdowns and antisocial distancing. The disdain for all things physical that seems to summarise the zeitgeist of 2022 has, in a rather ironic way, given that the zeitgeist also abhors racial, gender or other privilege, returned to a view held by Europeans over the last four or five centuries, namely that encounters with the exotic, deviant and primitive Other always demonstrate the superiority of the European over the 'savage', since the European is rational, controlled and superior, whilst in their physicality the primitive is childish, irrational and impulsive. From the first encounters of Europeans with the inhabitants of the places they conquered or explored, the activities of the indigenous people came to the European imagination 'to focus on the image of painted and bizarrely costumed bodies, drumming and dancing with wild abandon by the light of a fire'.[44] To 'let oneself go', to dance with 'wild abandon', is to relinquish one's rationality and thereby superiority.

> As horrified witnesses of ecstatic ritual, Europeans may have learned very little about the peoples they visited (and often destroyed in the process). . . . But they did learn, or imaginatively construct, something centrally important about themselves: that the essence of the Western mind, and particularly the Western male, upper-class mind, was its ability to resist the contagious rhythm of the drums, to wall itself up in a fortress of ego and rationality against the seductive wildness of the world.[45]

The class element of medieval Dansomnia events has already been mentioned earlier, but now, following the rise of first anthropology in the late nineteenth century and then the medical sciences, notably psychiatry and psychology in the early twentieth century, the road could be paved for a pathological interpretation of ecstatic dance: dance as a contagious disease.

Music

The power of music as a force in Dansomnia is recognised already by fourteenth-century contemporaries. The dancers were accompanied by minstrels playing upon noisy instruments which incite and encourage people to dance. As Hecker commented:

> [I]t may readily be supposed that, by the performance of lively melodies, and the stimulating effects which the shrill tones of fifes and trumpets would produce, a paroxysm, that was perhaps but slight in itself, might, in many cases, be increased to the most outrageous fury.[46]

As will be seen later, this nineteenth-century interpretation of 'intoxicating' music is not too far removed from the British government's attitude in the 1990s to repetitive music, in both cases ascribing to music a power to influence people's behaviour and especially to incite people to a behaviour that is deemed transgressive. Hecker believed that 'soft harmony' was used to:

> calm the excitement of those affected, and it is mentioned as a character of the tunes played with this view to the St. Vitus's dancers, that they contained transitions from a quick to a slow measure, and passed gradually from a high to low key'.[47]

Additionally, with regard to a phenomenon called tarantism (the name is derived from tarantula, the spider whose bite is meant to have caused it), which appeared in fifteenth-century Italy, music, and especially music progressing from slow to fast measure, was also regarded as influencing the people afflicted by tarantism. A contemporary, the Neapolitan lawyer Alexander ab Alexandro (1461–1523), described the effects of music as making otherwise unsophisticated country people dance gracefully, and how in the summer (note that season again) cities and villages were filled with the sounds of fifes, clarinets and Turkish drums, and how especially the sound of a drum would incite people to ever more violent movements so that their dancing 'was converted into a succession of frantic leaps'[48] until the music stopped, whereupon people would fall to the ground exhausted. One could argue that since it was not just the music *per se* that provided the impetus to dance, but the music of a certain kind and made by specific instruments, that therefore the transgressive aspect of St John's dance, or St Vitus's, or even tarantism, was not deemed to be in the music or dancing as such but in their particular expression. It is doubtful that public, even mass-attended, performances of church music, for example Gregorian chants, would have elicited the same concern and disapproving comments from either contemporaries or later observers as the various dancing manias did.

One way for the observers, commentators and authorities trying to explain the dancing—to make it less threateningly transgressive by labelling it—is to medicalise it, since a medical explanation fits in well with the philosophies of late medieval ecclesiastical and secular authorities. And with the nineteenth-century gaze, as the following statement by Hecker testifies:

> That patients should be violently affected by music, and their paroxysms brought on and increased by it, is natural with such nervous disorders; where deeper impressions are made through the ear, which is the most intellectual of all the organs, than through any of the other senses.[49]

Hecker asserted that at that time, i.e. the late fifteenth and early sixteenth centuries, there was a generally held belief that music and dancing would further distribute the poison causing the disease of tarantism throughout the body and drive it out through the skin, but it had to be expelled completely; otherwise, it became a chronic disorder.[50] People from all walks of life, not just from the medically informed class of contemporary commentators, can therefore use the rationale that dancing, if not actually curing them outright, at least alleviates their disease.

Love Parade

Fast-forward to 1996. In July of that year, some 600,000 (or 750,000, depending on which newspaper reports one cites) people partied freely at the Love Parade, dancing through the streets of an only recently re-unified Berlin. Back in 1989, the last year of a cold war, walled Berlin, DJ Dr Motte[51] (alias Matthias Roeingh) and 150 of his friends staged the first event, and in the intervening years, it grew to become the largest free dance festival for rave, techno or whatever else the cognoscenti wish to term the music. Thanks to a loophole in German law the festival could be staged as a demonstration, thereby not requiring any payments for the use of municipal streets, nor payments for the policing of the event or waste disposal, the latter issue being of particular concern to the German media, which focused on the huge mountains of discarded drinks cans left by the party-goers as the main reason of public concern, rather than any public order issues as would be expected of the media in the United Kingdom had a similar event has been staged in, say, London. Even 5 years later, in 2001, the media labelled the Love Parade a controversial event primarily on the grounds of alleged environmental damage, not as a public order issue.[52] Already in 1996 the lack of any real political motivations had been lamented in some of the more liberal German press. As Rainer Schmidt of *Die Zeit* put it: 'For fun, demonstrated to the scale of a generation for fun's sake, still brings out in a cold sweat every old revolutionary of '68. . . .

When someone dances so much do they still want to vote?'.[53] The importance of being *homo ludens* is still regarded as vastly inferior to the importance of being earnest when it comes to so-called political activity.

The first Love Parade was labelled a harmless event by the media, since it could be seen as a childish display where semi-naked youths hopping about followed a noisy van.[54] By 1996, the event and its participants were being almost ridiculed and the earlier theme of infantilisation was expanded. The ravers were described as 'wriggling'[55] on floats with high-powered sound systems. In another magazine, the participants were described as a 'twitching and wriggling dance-mass'.[56] 'Twitching and wriggling' appeared to be the most common phrase used by journalists to describe techno/rave dance, as yet a third German magazine[57] made use of the same label. 'Thousands twitch in a collective de-cramping', the media stated breathlessly in 1997 at the repeat performance, noting that this modern state of intoxication has been described by cultural historians as a 'culturally ineradicable desire for trance'.[58]

The music is seen as assaulting the dancers, the 'sounds are hitting the ear with the force of a pneumatic drill'[59], and the body of the dancer can only cope through crisis management by switching off the brain and twitching in self-defence, hands and feet moved by reflexes, the body wobbling.[60] Fellow dancers were seen by this particular journalist as participants in 'Technotopia' who, instead of chatting each other up, dance each other up [*tanzen sich an*] whilst displaying enraptured-ecstatic faces [*entrückt-verzückte Blicke*]. All these observations led the journalist to conclude that techno is a medical condition, a disease both real in the reactions it provokes somatically, and a metaphorical illness in the contagion of participation:

> We see hundreds of thousands of semi-naked people who, whilst laughing, force their body to perform movements reminiscent of epilepsy ("dancing"). Do we have here a bunch of sick people who meet each other in the capital for a demonstration of joyous lunacy? The answer is brief and emphatic: yes. For techno is a virus. Namely one of an especially nasty variety. Paths of contagion and methods of treatment are unknown. It nests itself in the body, unnoticed, and proliferates until the entire nervous system is infected.

> [*Wir sehen hunderttausende Halbnackte, die lachend ihre Körper zu epileptisch anmutenden Bewegungen nötigen ("tanzen"). Haben wir es also mit einem Haufen Kranker zu tun, die sich in der Hauptstadt zu einer Demonstration glücklichen Irsinns treffen? Die Antwort lautet kurz und schmerzlos: ja. Denn das Techno ist ein Virus. Und zwar der ganz fiesen Art. Übertragungswege und Heilungsverfahren sind unbekannt. Es nistet sich unmerklich ein und wuchert, bis das ganze Nervensystem infiziert ist.*][61]

Writing now, 26 years after the Love Parade and 2 years after the world shut down due to another virus, the so-called COVID pandemic, the viral symbolism is particularly telling. That journalist in 1996 could think of no worse disease metaphor than a virus to label and describe the abhorrent physical effects of ecstatic dance.

The tone of this article was reiterated by another journalist, who stated that for the raver techno is a drug that only functions at 100 decibels and has a minimum of 130 beats per minute and as little vocals as possible:

> [I]t has to drive into the whole body, not just the ears. Techno is machine music, and the raver is the human machine; a twitching nervous system that converts music for so long until it triggers the emission of pleasurable feelings in the brain, a feeling nobody but the raver believes in.[62]

Somehow the German media back in 1996 failed to pick up on the enhanced experience linked to the drug ecstasy, something a year later was analysed in the British press.[63] Yet more: 'The entire organism of the raver is now in a state of alarm, alerted by the music which does not let him rest until he is in trance and his brain announces bliss'.[64]

As an aside, not just professional journalists homed in on what was perceived as the addictive nature of techno. *Focus* magazine quoted an A-level student from Bavaria who wanted to see a law passed banning all kinds of techno/rave music, as such music was a grave danger to young people who 'are unscrupulously drawn into the vicious circle of techno-music and enslaved by it'.[65]

Returning to the previously analysed theme of medicalisation, it emerges that images of erotic and religious ecstasy are not lacking either, as the author of one article referred to the DJ's use of music as driving the ravers to the brink of rapture until due to pleasurable pain the dancers can only issue high-pitched screams.[66] The object of attending the Love Parade for hundreds of thousands of people, according to *Der Spiegel*, was to dance themselves into a trance.[67] The characteristics of a mass demonstration were also alluded to, the ravers' arms shooting up in a wave of collective howls of ecstasy[68]—the mention of masses of arms raised and the sound of thousands of voices cannot fail, for a certain type of (German) reader at least, to evoke images of other mass demonstrations in Germany's past, the infamous Nürnberg rallies, though here, as in all the articles examined, specifically the perceived *non-political* nature of the event was emphasised. But, rest assured, any direct allusions to Nazi mass-rallies were rapidly dismissed in this journalist's concentration on the hedonistic and ecstatic aspects of the Love Parade, albeit once again medicalising the movement of dance: the collective twitches and the mass trances.[69] Furthermore, body cult and especially so-called primitive or tribal body decoration in the form of body piercing were expounded on and analysed, as if to emphasise the anthropological primitivism of the dancers. *Der Spiegel* also followed the linking of rave with primitivism made by some theorists: 'Techno is like voodoo, as the techno-critics say, and the music is as simple as in the past when shaggy-haired people danced ecstatically to the music of drums'.[70]

In the United Kingdom, too, the medicalisation of the dance movement had found its way into the media. A video by the band Prodigy to accompany their number one hit *Firestarter* received 'a record number of complaints' after being shown on Top of the Pops. Apparently the sight of band member Keith Flint 'shivering and shaking (some would say *dancing* [journalist's emphasis])' was frightening small children.[71] In addition to the fevered medical description of Flint's dance, the then-current vogue for rushing to the protection of children from perceived moral harm, and the consequent infantilisation of adult society, had also found its place in this particular analysis of rhythmic movement. But then the United Kingdom is, after all, the country which introduced a law in 1994 with the Criminal Justice Bill which specifically singled out listening to 'repetitive beats' as socially (and politically) subversive.[72]

Whether organisers or party-goers ever intentionally tried to be subversive pre-1994 through their dance is another issue, but it is interesting to note that amongst the huge conglomerate-type businesses that constitute the vast majority of legally sanctioned rave events post-1994 some aspects of social and political subversion survive, notably in the form of collectives like Exodus, based around Luton, who expanded in a cultural rather than in a business sense to link dance events with socio-political direct action: 'Not just concerned with putting on parties, they are committed to channeling [sic] profits and energy into rebuilding derelict properties for the homeless'.[73] The relevance of this was expressed by Exodus themselves in that they named their events not just plain old raves but 'community dances'—thereby linking dance, millenarian-utopian ideas, community and individual empowerment, the same as the anti-consumerist, anti-clerical dancers in the fourteenth century, perhaps?

To add a note to the complexity of the medicalisation of these dance movements, consider that medicalisation is a hallmark of those in positions of power trying to assert themselves over the powerless, especially in modern times. As Ivan Illich stated, in 'some industrial societies social labelling has been medicalized to the point her all deviance ha to have a medical label'.[74]

Primitivism Positioned

One final note on both medieval Dansomnia and modern techno/rave concludes this essay. The aspect of primitivism that observers and commentators ascribed to techno and rave culture is found equally in the elements of deviance attributed to medieval Dansomnia by the nineteenth- and twentieth-century historians. The dances performed by the medieval people were not seen as legitimate expressions of dance because the accompanying music, the rhythms and the body movements themselves did not conform to what these historians, and the contemporary medieval authorities before them, know and acknowledge as dance. By turning to what some modern scholars have written with regard to anthropology one may find explanations for the meaning of dance that position dance within a dialectic of the socio-culturally acceptable and the deviant in a more meaningful way. For example, Judith Lynne Hanna has tried to discuss dance after a fashion that recognises the cultural specificity of movement, music and event, and therefore allows dance to be positioned as a socially informed activity. She observes: 'Ethnocentrism has reigned, and false dichotomies have been drawn between 'primitive' and nonprimitive' dance. . . . Focus on the promotion of social harmony has neglected dance's disharmonious consequences'.[75]

In both medieval Dansomnia and 1990s techno parades dance can be viewed as 'disharmonious', in the sense that it has been turned into a deviant, transgressive activity, because it is not the right kind of dance, and subsequently has been medicalised, due to the gaze of authority's need for explaining and thereby disciplining the transgression. Hanna allows dance to function both within and without the delineations of socially accepted norms: 'Dance may mirror or refract social and political structures and techno-environmental factors. However, it may also be a generative force, a processual agent, reflecting 'anti-structure' even going beyond what Peckham refers to as the human's 'rage for chaos', the need to experiment with novelty within the safety of an artistic, 'pretend' situation'.[76] On the theme of trance and ecstatic dance, Hanna has some interesting points to make. As she proposes:

> Altered states of consciousness may be induced by socialized responses to the contextual situation, by auto-suggestion, and by physical behaviour such as energetic dancing, which may alter brain wave frequencies, adrenalin, and blood-sugar content, and induce giddiness through high speed or sensory rhythmic stimulation in more than one sensory mode. Kinesthetic stress, overexertion, and fatigue, also increase susceptibility to rhythm.[77]

Hanna's choice of the word 'giddiness' is especially interesting, since giddy, which now means mad or foolish, was originally in its Old English meaning related to possession by a god (*guðam*), and therefore similar to enthusiasm, in its original Greek meaning (entheos [ἔνθεος] = filled by a god).[78]

The verdict by Hanna is still an explanation phrased in the language of medico-biological theories, but neither does it exclude socio-cultural elements, nor is the description of the body's biological functionings used as a way of pathologising and thereby disciplining dance. Applied purely speculatively, this theory can offer some insight on medieval Dansomnia, allowing for both Hecker's medical analysis[79] as well as providing a place for the possession, attributed to Dansomnia by medieval authors. The parallels of techno/rave with dance as described in anthropological terms are made by proponents of techno themselves, not just by the disciplining voice of outside commentators. So the Swiss author Patrick Walder on techno: 'The DJ is the shaman, the dealer the medicine man. Raves are the dance rituals of industrialised society. Ecstasy is the magic potion for it'.[80] Modern techno/rave dance, seen as an expression of primitivism by the extraneous gaze, is doubly subversive in this context, in that not only it is deviant *a priori* by being primitive, but that, by appropriating this label for itself, techno culture turns the intended derogation into a positive asset for itself.

My interpretative approach here hinged around the ludic qualities of dance, a concept of dance, especially of public and communal dance, as 'ecstatic dissent'[81] which opened up the possibility, pure and simple, that dancing might be fun. The various commentaries and interpretative layers do nothing better than to disguise this banal but eminently plausible explanation: amongst a multitude of reasons, people also danced for the joy of it.

Notes

1 John Chrysostom, Homily 48 on Matthew. This paraphrase is often quoted. The original is much longer, this one is the quote from the online of New Advent: "For though the daughter of Herodas be not present, yet the devil, who then danced in her person, in theirs also holds his choirs now, and departs with the souls of those guests taken captive." See no. 4, https://www.newadvent.org/fathers/200148.htm.

2 This, too, is an often-"quoted" paraphrase of Emma Goldman. She writes of a "boy" who cannot understand why she is dancing when he thinks that behaviour is not befitting of a revolutionary. She writes,

I insisted that our Cause could not expect me to become a nun and that the movement should not be turned into a cloister. If it meant that, I did not want it. 'I want freedom, the right to self-expression, everyboy's right to beautiful, radiant things'. Anarchism meant that to me, and I would live it in spite of the whole world—prisons, persecution, everything. Yes, even in spite of the condemnation of my own comrades I would live my beautiful ideal.
Living My Life (New York: Alfred A. Knopf, 1931), 56.

3 On the history of medieval dancing generally see Julia Zimmermann, *Teufelsreigen—Engelstänze. Kontinuität und Wandel in mittelalterlichen*

Tanzdarstellungen (Mikrokosmos 76) (Frankfurt: Peter Lang Verlag, 2007); Jeremy Barlow, *A Dance Through Time: Images of Western Social Dancing from the Middle Ages to Modern Times* (Oxford: Bodleian Library, 2012); Gerald Siegmund, "Auf Biegen und Brechen. De-Formierter Tanz und manieristische Körperbilder," in *ReMembering the Body: Body and Movement in the 20th*, eds. Aleida Assman, Jan Assman, Gabriele Brandstetter, et al. (Berlin: Hatje Cantz Publishers, 2000), 136–70; Jan Bremmer and Herman Roodenburg, with intro. by Keith Thomas, *A Cultural History of Gesture from Antiquity to the Present Day* (Cambridge: Polity Press, 1991).

4 Gregor Rohmann, *Tanzwut. Kosmos, Kirche und Mensch in der Bedeutungsgeschichte eines mittelalterlichen Krankheitskonzepts* (Göttingen: Vandenhoeck & Ruprecht, 2013); also idem, "The Invention of Dancing Mania: Frankish Christianity, Platonic Cosmology, and Bodily Expressions in Sacred Space," *The Medieval Journal* 12, no. 1 (2009): 13–45.

5 J. F. C. Hecker, *The Epidemics of the Middle Ages*, transl. B. G. Babington, 3rd ed. (London: Trübner, 1859), 12. Tarantism, the phenomenon straddling the very late medieval and early modern period, is another subject for the medical gaze; see J. F. Russell, "Tarantism," *Medical History* 23 (1979): 404–25. Other examples of the medicalising view are to be found mainly in the German literature (given that most of the dancing manias are documented for the German region, this interest by German scholars is perhaps not surprising), such as Egon Schmitz-Cliever, "Zur Frage der epidemischen Tanzkrankheit des Mittelalters," *Sudhoffs Archiv für Geschichte der Medizin und der Naturwissenschaften* 37 (1953): 149–61, who calls the dances a mass hysteria and psychic epidemic (p. 153); Egon Schmitz-Cliever and Herta Schmitz-Cliever, "Zur Darstellung des Heiltanzes in der Malerei um 1500," *Medizinhistorisches Journal* 10 (1975): 307–16; R. H. R. Park and M. P. Park, "Saint Vitus' Dance: Vital Misconceptions by Sydenham and Bruegel," *Journal of the Royal Society of Medicine* 83 (1990): 512–15, who promote rheumatic fever mixed with a hefty dose of 'religious superstition' as the origin for the late medieval dances; and most recently the magisterial *Habilitationsarbeit* by Rohmann, *Tanzwut*, 2013.

6 L. J. Donaldson, J. Cavanaugh, and J. Rankin, "The Dancing Plague: A Public Health Conundrum," *Public Health* 111, no. 4 (1997): 201–4.

7 Hecker, *Epidemics of the Middle Ages*, 80.

8 Ibid.

9 Ibid.

10 Ibid., 81.

11 Gilles de Roya, "*Annales Belgici*: 'de dansers wandelden in Vlaenderen als verhoede lieden', cited by M. Braekman, 'La dansomanie de 1374: heresie ou maladie?'," *Revue du Nord*, 63, no. 249 (1981): 341.

12 Liege Chronicle:

> Dansabant ac saltabant ibi. Obsessi erant a demonibus et quando spiritus descendebat in crura eorum, non poterant contineri a dansatione et saltu; quando autem ascendebat in parvum ventrem, tunc torquebantur dure, et ideo habebant tuellas et parvos baculos, unde stringebant se circa umbilicum fortiter, et trudebant vel faciebant se trudi pugnis in ventre parvo, et sic cessabat dolor eorum aliquantulum projiciebantque a longue baculos suos et habebant terribilem aspectum.

> (cited by Braekman, "La dansomanie," 342)

13 Hecker, *Epidemics of the Middle Ages*, 81.

14 Ibid, note 4. Hecker bases his diagnosis on a contemporary account by the Sponheim Chronicle of 1374.

15 Braekman, "La dansomanie," 343.

16 'Les danseurs recherchent une thérapeutique dans l'appel aux saints et à la Vierge', ibid.

17 Braekman, "La dansomanie," 345–46.

18 Hecker, *Epidemics of the Middle Ages*, 82.

19 Ibid.

20 Hecker, *Epidemics of the Middle Ages*, 83.

21 Ibid., 84. Note the nineteenth-century euphemistic allusion to pre-marital sex and the birth of illegitimate children.

22 Robert E. Bartholomew, *Exotic Deviance: Medicalizing Cultural Idioms— From Strangeness to Illness* (Boulder: University Press of Colorado, 2000), who in his chapter 'Medieval Dancing Manias as History-Specific Variant of "Mass Psychogenic Illness": A Critique and Reappraisal', pp. 127–52, based on anthropological evidence takes issue with the medicalised views of Hecker and Backman.

23 Ibid.

24 Ibid.

25 Lyn Gardner, "The Devil in the Dance," *The Guardian*, January 27, 2001.

26 See inter alia Jeannine Horowitz, "Les danses cléricales dans les églises au Moyen Age," *Le Moyen Age* 45 (1989): 279–92; also Rohmann, *Tanzwut*.

27 Hecker, *Epidemics of the Middle Ages*, 87.

28 'Nec permittamus solemnitatem sanctam cantica luxuriosa proferendo polluere', quoted by Hecker, *Epidemics of the Middle Ages*, 87, n. 2.

29 Peter Chrysologus, sermon CXXVII, *Patrologiae Latinae*, ed. Migne, 52: 552, cited by Braekman, "La dansomanie," 350.

30 Cited by Braekman, "La dansomanie," 350.

31 Ibid.

32 Cited by E. Louis Backman, *Religious Dances in the Christian Church and in Popular Medicine*, transl. E. Classen (London: Allen & Unwin, 1952), 25; also Barbara Ehrenreich, *Dancing in the Streets: A History of Collective Joy* (London: Granta Books, 2007), 74.

33 Cited by Braekman, "La dansomanie," 350.

34 *Decretals*, 1. III, vol. I, can. 12, in: Braekman, "La dansomanie," 350 and note 69.

35 Hecker, *Epidemics of the Middle Ages*, 88.

36 Ibid. Hecker continued his line of reasoning by drawing on social and economic factors, the extreme impoverishment of some people along the lower Rhine due to flood, famine and oppression (pp. 89–90), culminating in his explanation for the somatic location of the dancing mania's worst symptoms (p. 90): Due to hunger and bad food, the bowels of starving people were the areas attacked by pain, which could lead them to the behaviour (beating their stomachs) described above as part of the Dansomnia. On midsummer as a special time, involving both the Christian feast of St John and pagan solstice celebrations, associated with disorder and rebellion outside of the control of the church, see Sandra Billington, *Midsummer: A Cultural Sub-Text from Chrétien de Troyes to Jean Michel* (Medieval Texts and Cultures of Northern Europe 3) (Turnhout: Brepols, 2001).

37 Gerald of Wales, *The Journey Through Wales*, transl. Lewis Thorpe (New York: Harmondsworth, 1978), 92.
38 Ibid.
39 Rohmann, *Tanzwut*, 241–42.
40 Nancy Caciola, "Wraiths and Revenants in Medieval Culture," *Past & Present* 35 (1996): 3–45.
41 Hecker, *Epidemics of the Middle Ages*, 90; see also Edward Schroder, "Die Tänzer von Kolbigk," offprint from *Zeitschrift für Kirchengeschichte*, 17, 1896.
42 Ehrenreich, *Dancing in the Streets*, 16.
43 Ibid., 19.
44 Ibid., 1. Ehrenreich's entire first chapter (pp. 1–20) presents the historiographic overview of how explorers and later anthropologists, sociologists and psychologists have described the dancing they encountered—the red thread running through this is that for Western observers there was always something inherently uncomfortable, if not to say uncanny in a Freudian sense, in the physicality of ecstatic dance rituals.
45 Ehrenreich, *Dancing in the Streets*, 9.
46 Hecker, *Epidemics of the Middle Ages*, 98. For a modern perspective on the negative power of music see James Kennaway, *Bad Vibrations: The History of the Idea of Music as a Cause of Disease* (Aldershot: Ashgate, 2012), which treats the period from c.1700 onwards, since the suggestion that music was a cause of the mental and physical illness was a rare idea before the late eighteenth century. A more positive appraisal of music in general is given by Robert Jordain, *Music, the Brain and Ecstasy* (New York: William Morrow, 1997).
47 Hecker, *Epidemics of the Middle Ages*, 98 and p. 99 note 1. Hecker attributes the description of the calming effects of music to a text from 1650.
48 Alexander ab Alexandro, *Genialium dierum*, libri VI, Lugdun. Bat. 1673, 8vo., lib. II, ch. 17, p. 398, cited by Hecker, *Epidemics of the Middle Ages*, 108 and note 1.
49 Hecker, *Epidemics of the Middle Ages*, 96.
50 Ibid., 108–9, and pp. 112–15 for the effects of different types of music on tarantism in the sixteenth and seventeenth centuries.
51 The DJ received his moniker, according to one anecdote (cited in M. Fischer, M. von Uslar, C. Kracht, A. Roshani, T. Hüetlin, and A. Jardine, "Der pure Sex. Nur besser.," *Der Spiegel* 29 (1996): 98), because after a long night's raving, in the early hours when Dr Motte took over the controls his records cured the exhausted ravers, so they gave him the honorific "Doctor"—the DJ as shaman, the music as medicine. Voices from within the rave culture subsume the medical language of the commentators, or is it perhaps the other way round?
52 John Hooper, "Controversy Rains on Berlin's Love Parade," *The Guardian*, April 9, 2001.
53 'Denn Spaß, bloß um des Spaßes willen in Generationenstärke demonstriert, treibt noch jedem Altachtundsechziger den Angstschweiß auf die lichte Stirn und apokalyptische Gedanken in das Springerhausdemo-verklärte Hirn. Wer so viel tanzt, will der noch wählen?', Rainer Schmidt, "Deutschland, liebes Technoland," *Die Zeit*, no. 30 (July 19, 1996).
54 Uli Hauser and Frauke Hunfeld, "Die Raff-Parade," *Stern*, no. 30 (July 18, 1996): 140–42. The authors refer to the first Love Parade at which 'noch 150 Jugendliche halbnackt hinter einem lärmenden Kleinlaster hopsten . . .'.
55 'Tieflader und Sattelschlepper des Zuges, vollgestellt mit 15 00 Watt-Boxen und zappelnden Ravern . . .', ibid., 141.

56 C. Gottwald, D. Horstkötter, U. Plewnia, R. Vernier, and A. Wolfsgruber, "Big Fun, Big Business," *Focus* 28 (1996): 58: 'die zuckende und zappelnde Tanzmasse'.

57 Cordt Schnibben, "Die Party-Partei," *Der Spiegel* 29 (1996): 92: 'zappelten und zuckten'.

58 'Tausende zucken in einer kollektiven Entkrampfung. Ein moderner Rauschzustand, den Kulturwissenschaftler gerne als "kulturhistorisch unausrottbares Trancebedürfnis" beschrieben haben.' Martin Scholz, ' "Schlafen können wir unser ganzes Leben". Zwischen Kommerz, Volksfest und Techno-Ekstase: Sieben Raver aus Frankfurt im Trubel der Love-Parade', *S/R/D*, 14 July 1997.

59 'die Töne bollern mit der Gewalt eines Preßlufthammers ans Ohr', Schmidt, "Deutschland, liebes Technoland."

60 'Dem Körper bleibt nur noch Krisenmanagement. Hirn ausschalten und Notwehrzucken. Die Reflexe bewegen Hände und Füße . . . wackele ich weiter . . .', ibid.

61 Ibid.

62 Schnibben, "Die Party-Partei," 93:

[E]s muß in den ganzen Körper fahren, nicht nur in die Ohren. Techno ist Maschinenmusik, und der Raver ist die Menschmaschine; ein zuckendes Nervensystem, das Musik so lange umsetzt, bis es im Hirn ein Glücksgefühl ausschüttet, an das keiner glaubt außer dem Raver.

63 Richard Benson, 'And the rave parties on', *The Guardian*, August 7, 1997.

64 Unknown author, *Der Spiegel*, 30, 1996, p. 93: 'Der gesamte Organismus des Ravers ist jetzt im Alarmzustand, alarmiert von einer Musik, die ihn nicht ruhen läßt, bis er in Trance ist und sein Gehirn Glück meldet'.

65 Quoted in C. Gottwald et al., 'Big Fun, Big Business', *Focus*, 28, 1996, p. 56: young people are 'skrupellos in den Teufelskreis von Techno-Musik hineingezogen und hörig gemacht'.

66 'Er fährt die Musik mit sphärischen Klängen immer wieder an den Rand der Erlösung, bis die Raver aus lustvollem Schmerz nur noch schrille Schreie ausstoßen', Schmidt, "Deutschland, liebes Technoland."

67 Schnibben, "Die Party-Partei," 92: 'um sich drei Tage lang in Trance zu tanzen'.

68 '. . . und tausende Arme schnellen in einer Woge kollektiven Glücksgejohles nach oben', Schmidt, "Deutschland, liebes Technoland."

69 'Zuckt hier nicht das Kollektiv? Rauscht hier nicht die Masse?', ibid.

70 Schnibben, "Die Party-Partei," 93: 'Techno sei wie Voodoo, sagt der Techno-Kritiker, und die Musik sei so einfach wie früher, als Zottelige ekstatisch zu Trommelmusik tanzten'.

71 Andrew Smith, "Please Don't Call Us Techno," *The Sunday Times*, November 3, 1996.

72 The reaction of the authorities to dance is actually not new, in this case. Already back in the fourteenth century, the laws of the town of Maastricht forbade dancing 'in the streets and in the churches, in houses and everywhere else' (cited by Braekman, "La dansomanie," 342).

73 Alex Bellos, "Let Our People Go-Go . . .," *The Guardian*, April 15, 1997.

74 Ivan Illich, *Limits to Medicine. Medical Nemesis: The Expropriation of Health* (Harmondsworth: Penguin, 1977), 55.

75 Judith Lynne Hanna, "To Dance Is Human. Some Psychobiological Bases of an Expressive Form," in *The Anthropology of the Body* (= A. S. A. Monograph 15), ed. John Blacking (London, New York and San Francisco: Academic Press, 1977), 211.

76 Hanna, "To Dance Is Human," 216–17. The term anti-structure is derived from V. W. Turner, *Dramas, Fields and Metaphors: Symbolic Action in Human Society* (Ithaca: Cornell University Press, 1974); M. Peckham, *Man's Rage for Chaos: Biology, Behaviour and the Arts* (Philadelphia: Chilton, 1965).
77 Hanna, "To Dance Is Human," 218. For the modern view on ecstatic dance music and trance-inducing states see Matthew Collin, *Altered State: The Story of Ecstasy Culture and Acid House* (London: Serpent's Tail, 2009).
78 s.v. 'giddy', C. T. Onions, ed., *The Oxford Dictionary of English Etymology* (Oxford: Clarendon Press, 1966). See also Thomas Bossius, Andreas Häger, and Keith Kahn-Harris, eds., *Religion and Popular Music in Europe: New Expressions of Sacred and Secular Identity* (London: I. B. Tauris, 2011) on how music and religion may be intertwined, in that music has been used to celebrate the gods, express belief and enable such believers to experience the divine.
79 See note 26 above.
80 Patrick Walder cited in: C. Gottwald et al., "Big Fun, Big Business," *Focus* 28 (1996): 62. 'Der DJ ist der Schamane, der Dealer der Medizinmann. Raves sind die Tanzrituale der Industriegesellschaft. Ecstasy ist der Zaubertrank dazu.'
81 Ehrenreich, *Dancing in the Streets*, 20.

Reference List

Alexandro, Alexander ab. *Genialium dierum*, libri VI, Lugdun. Bat. 1673.
Anonymous. *Der Spiegel*, 30 (1996): 93.
Barlow, Jeremy. *A Dance Through Time: Images of Western Social Dancing From the Middle Ages to Modern Times*. Oxford: Bodleian Library, 2012.
Bartholomew, Robert E. *Exotic Deviance: Medicalizing Cultural Idioms—From Strangeness to Illness*. Boulder: University Press of Colorado, 2000.
Bellos, Alex. "Let our people go-go . . ." *The Guardian*, April 15, 1997.
Benson, Richard. "And the Rave Parties on." *The Guardian*, August 7, 1997.
Billington, Sandra. *Midsummer: A Cultural Sub-Text From Chrétien de Troyes to Jean Michel*. Medieval Texts and Cultures of Northern Europe 3. Turnhout: Brepols, 2001.
Blacking, John, ed. *The Anthropology of the Body*. London: Academic Press, 1977.
Bossius, Thomas, Andreas Häger, and Keith Kahn-Harris, eds. *Religion and Popular Music in Europe: New Expressions of Sacred and Secular Identity*. London: I.B. Tauris, 2011.
Bremmer, Jan, and Herman Roodenburg, with intro. by Keith Thomas. *A Cultural History of Gesture From Antiquity to the Present Day*. Cambridge: Polity Press, 1991.
Caciola, Nancy. "Wraiths and Revenants in Medieval Culture." *Past & Present* 35 (1996): 3–45.
Chrysostom, John. Homily 48 on Matthew. New Advent, "Fathers of the Church." https://www.newadvent.org/fathers/200148.htm.
Chrysologus, Peter. Sermon CXXVII, *Patrologia Latinae*, ed. Migne, 52. Paris: Garnier, 1850.
Collin, Matthew. *Altered State: The Story of Ecstasy Culture and Acid House*. London: Serpent's Tail, 2009.
Donaldson, L. J., J. Cavanaugh, and J. Rankin. "The Dancing Plague: A Public Health Conundrum." *Public Health* 111, no. 4 (1997): 201–4.

Ehrenreich, Barbara. *Dancing in the Streets: A History of Collective Joy.* London: Granta Books, 2007.

Fischer, M., M. von Uslar, C. Kracht, A. Roshani, T. Hüetlin, and A. Jardine. "Der pure Sex. Nur besser." *Der Spiegel* 29 (1996): 98.

Gardner, Lyn. "The Devil in the Dance." *The Guardian*, January 27, 2001.

Gerald of Wales. *The Journey Through Wales.* Translated by Lewis Thorpe. New York: Harmondsworth, 1978.

Goldman, Emma. *Living My Life.* New York: Alfred A. Knopf, 1931.

Gottwald, C., D. Horstkötter, U. Plewnia, R. Vernier, and A. Wolfsgruber. "Big Fun, Big Business." *Focus* 28 (1996): 56–62.

Hauser, Uli, and Frauke Hunfeld. "Die Raff-Parade." *Stern*, no. 30 (July 18, 1996): 140–42.

Hecker, J. F. C. *The Epidemics of the Middle Ages.* Translated by B. G. Babington. 3rd ed. London: Trübner, 1859.

Hooper, John. "Controversy Rains on Berlin's Love Parade." *The Guardian*, April 9, 2001.

Horowitz, Jeannine. "Les danses cléricales dans les églises au Moyen Age." *Le Moyen Age* 45 (1989): 279–92.

Illich, Ivan. *Limits to Medicine. Medical Nemesis: The Expropriation of Health.* Harmondsworth: Penguin, 1977.

Jordain, Robert. *Music, the Brain and Ecstasy.* New York: William Morrow, 1997.

Kennaway, James. *Bad Vibrations: The History of the Idea of Music as a Cause of Disease.* Aldershot: Ashgate, 2012.

Kommerz, Zwischen. "Volksfest und Techno-Ekstase: Sieben Raver aus Frankfurt im Trubel der Love-Parade." *S/R/D*, July 14, 1997.

Louis Backman, E. *Religious Dances in the Christian Church and in Popular Medicine.* Translated by E. Classen. London: Allen & Unwin, 1952.

Onions, C. T. *The Oxford Dictionary of English Etymology.* Oxford: Oxford University Press, 1966.

Park, R. H. R., and M. P. Park. "Saint Vitus' Dance: vital misconceptions by Sydenham and Bruegel." *Journal of the Royal Society of Medicine* 83 (1990): 512–15.

Peckham, M. *Man's Rage for Chaos: Biology, Behaviour and the Arts.* Philadelphia: Chilton, 1965.

Rohmann, Gregor. *Tanzwut. Kosmos, Kirche und Mensch in der Bedeutungsgeschichte eines mittelalterlichen Krankheitskonzepts.* Gottingen: Vandenhoeck & Ruprecht, 2013.

———. "The Invention of Dancing Mania: Frankish Christianity, Platonic Cosmology, and Bodily Expressions in Sacred Space." *The Medieval Journal* 12, no. 1 (2009): 13–45.

———. *Tanzwut. Kosmos, Kirche und Mensch in der Bedeutungsgeschichte eines mittelalterlichen Krankheitskonzepts.* Göttingen: Vandenhoeck & Ruprecht, 2013.

Roya, Gilles de. "*Annales Belgici:* 'de dansers wandelden in Vlaenderen als verhoede lieden,'" cited by M. Braekman, "La dansomanie de 1374: heresie ou maladie?'" *Revue du Nord* 63, no. 249 (1981): 341.

Russell, J. F. "Tarantism." *Medical History* 23 (1979): 404–25.

Schmitz-Cliever, Egon. "Zur Frage der epidemischen Tanzkrankheit des Mittelalters." *Sudhoffs Archiv für Geschichte der Medizin und der Naturwissenschaften* 37 (1953): 149–61.

Schmitz-Cliever, Egon, and Herta Schmitz-Cliever. "Zur Darstellung des Heiltanzes in der Malerei um 1500." *Medizinhistorisches Journal* 10 (1975): 307–16.

Schmidt, Rainer. "Deutschland, liebes Technoland." *Die Zeit*, no. 30 (July 19, 1996).

Schnibben, Cordt. "Die Party-Partei." *Der Spiegel* 29 (1996): 92–93.

Schroder, Edward. "Die Tänzer von Kolbigk," offprint from *Zeitschrift für Kirchengeschichte*, 17, 1896.

Siegmund, Gerald. "Auf Biegen und Brechen. De-Formierter Tanz und manieristische Körperbilder." In *ReMembering the Body: Body and Movement in the 20th*, edited by Aleida Assman, Jan Assman, Gabriele Brandstetter, et al., 136–70. Berlin: Hatje Cantz Publishers, 2000.

Smith, Andrew. "Please don't call us techno." *The Sunday Times*, November 3, 1996.

Turner, V. W. *Dramas, Fields and Metaphors: Symbolic Action in Human Society.* Ithaca: Cornell University Press, 1974.

Zimmermann, Julia. *Teufelsreigen—Engelstänze. Kontinuität und Wandel in mittelalterlichen Tanzdarstellungen* (Mikrokosmos 76). Frankfurt: Peter Lang Verlag, 2007.

4 Philosophical Paradoxes of Factitious Disorders

Herb Leventer

In the seventeenth century, Thomas Sydenham writes:

> [I]t is necessary, in describing any disease, to enumerate the peculiar and constant phenomena apart from the accidental and adventitious ones. . . . Outlying forms of the disease, and cases of exceeding rarity, I take no notice of. They do not properly belong to the histories of disease. No botanist takes the bites of a caterpillar as a characteristic of a leaf of sage.[1]

But Franz Kafka shows how such a monocausal view of disease can facilitate the dismissal as "fake" of unusual symptoms with no apparent cause:

> Gregor Samsa . . . found himself transformed in his bed into a gigantic insect. . . . Well, supposing he were to say he was sick? But that would look suspicious . . . since during his five years' employment he had not been ill once. The chief himself would be sure to come with the sick-insurance doctor, would reproach . . . his laziness and would cut all excuses short by referring to the insurance doctor, who of course regarded all mankind as perfectly healthy malingerers. And would he be so far wrong on this occasion? Gregor really felt quite well. . . . He remembered that often enough in bed he had felt small aches and pains, probably caused by awkward postures, which had proved purely imaginary when he got up, and he looked forward eagerly to seeing this morning's delusions gradually fall away.[2]

Shakespeare, too, writes of trust and subtleties and truth—all things to be considered in this article as it takes up the issue of factitious disorders.

> When my love swears that she is made of truth
> I do believe her though I know she lies,
> That she might think me some untutored youth,

DOI: 10.4324/9781003452324-6

Unlearned in the world's false subtleties.
Thus vainly thinking that she thinks me young,
Although she knows my days are past the best,
Simply I credit her false-speaking tongue:
On both sides thus is simple truth suppressed.
But wherefore says she not she is unjust?
And wherefore say not I that I am old?
O love's best habit is in seeming trust,
And age in love loves not to have years told.
Therefore I lie with her and she with me,
And in our faults by lies we flattered be.
—Shakespeare, Sonnet 138[3]

Edward Snow says the sonnet "displaces the language of 'true versus false' with a more subtle and humane ethical vocabulary".[4] My aim in this chapter is to do the same for factitious disorders.

We All Have Factitious Disorders[5]

Since 1951 when Richard Asher gave the name "Munchausen's disease"[6] to those rare patients who faked illness to justify their frequent use of medical services, the number of articles on it in the medical literature has steadily increased. It is not clear whether the number of actual patients has also increased[7] or whether it is only the willingness of physicians to apply that label to increasing numbers of their patients, especially after the label "factitious disorder" for milder cases of such deception was officially recognized by the DSM-III,[8] the 1980 edition of the American Psychiatric Association's *Diagnostic and Statistical Manual of Mental Disorders*.

My thesis is that "factitious disorder" [FD] is a useless if not empty diagnostic category, and should no longer be used. Like most diseases, it is a socially constructed category, not a natural kind. It is normal that each society will identify certain phenomena as "diseases," and that those identifications should change. From the time of Galen to the eighteenth century, there were only two major mental illnesses: melancholy [caused by an excess of black bile] and mania [caused by an excess of green bile]. By the mid-twentieth century, there were a few dozen; in 1952 that rose to 60 in the first edition of DSM.[9] In 1968, there were 182 in DSM-II, in 1980 there were 265 in DSM-III, in 1994 there were 297 in DSM-IV, but in 2013 there were only 157 in the DSM-5.[10] No one thinks that human psychology has fluctuated so widely in such a short time.

Similar fluctuations have appeared in physical diseases. There are only a few dozen infectious diseases that *are* natural types and do not have to be socially constructed—a good example is measles, where a single cause, a viral infection, produces a single set of symptoms, small red spots and fever, with a uniform prognosis and treatment (or, in this case, prevention by vaccination). For the other 13,000 diseases listed in ICD-9, there is great variation in the degree of social construction, and even more so when ICD-10 increased that number to 68,000.[11] The main justifications[12] for creating a new diagnostic category are: to help the clinician distinguish his patient's symptoms from other categories, identify the cause, or predict the prognosis, or suggest a treatment (or, if that is not known, at least a palliative or preventive). If the proposed new category accomplishes none of these four goals, the clinician is left with just some "medically unexplained symptoms" [MUS].

My main reason for opposing the identification as "factitious" of the subset of MUS that are intentionally created is the impossibility of making that distinction in all but a tiny number of egregious cases. "Intentionality" and "deception" are complex mental states, not simple "yes" or "no" states. They are tricky to define philosophically. Physicians have no special expertise in recognizing them. Even detectives, lawyers, and judges, who *are* trained to identify them, have a difficult time accomplishing it. They all lament that there is no reliable lie detector test, no "truth serum". There *is* a special profession of forensic psychologists, who have developed various "symptom validity tests",[13] but the accuracy of their diagnoses is still controversial. The attempt to identify the few hundred actual deceptive fakers would require harming millions of innocent patients,[14] who will be shamed into avoiding treatment, and will lose trust in the profession's promise to care for the ill (and so, e.g., will be less likely to follow public-health measures in the next pandemic). The situation is reminiscent of the search for "voter fraud". In the United States, there are an infinitesimal number of cases; but to catch them, authorities would disenfranchise the millions of innocents who simply failed to include their middle initial in the voter rolls, or who do not have the proper photo ID. More important, and less visible, authorities would also reduce general trust in the honesty of elections.

MUSs are common in clinical practice. At least a fifth of all patients leave their doctor's office with no diagnosis, prognosis, explanation, or treatment of the symptoms that brought them in for a consultation.[15] This is not as big of a problem as it sounds. Most symptoms resolve and disappear on their own in a week or two.[16] And, usually, a doctor can exclude most of the known and dangerous possibilities: It is *not* a brain tumor, or heart attack, or cancer. In and of itself, that reassurance is enough for most patients. But not all. Many patients insist on an answer, and keep returning, or shopping around for another doctor or an alternate emergency room in hopes of getting a real diagnosis. Given the fact that every year, there are hundreds of millions of visits to the doctor in the United States, if only one in a hundred of the 20% of undiagnosed patients keep seeking an answer, that is a large number—hundreds of thousands of patients each year. It is these patients that the frustrated physician is tempted to tell: "it's all in your head". The frustrated physician wants them to admit that they are exaggerating symptoms. Often, it is these patients that physicians will label as having "factitious disorders".

The difference, then, between MUS and FD is *not* anything about the symptom-complaint-illness itself, but rather a breakdown in the relationship between the patient—now seen as illegitimately demanding—and the doctor—now seeing himself as justifiably frustrated by the patient's refusal to accept the evidence produced by many tests that there *is no* disease to be identified.

MUS, though, cannot be more frequent now than before sophisticated contemporary testing. It is more likely that the *medical profession has changed its idea of what a* successful *diagnosis* (or really, a successful explanation) looks like. Contemporary medical practitioners are no longer satisfied with vague explanations like "a sore throat" as a diagnosis, asking better questions, like "[W]hat kind of sore throat?" and "[W]hat caused the sore throat?" They no longer consider a diagnosis that is merely a description of the symptom—like back pain, tiredness, or stomach ache—to be adequate. The disease should be named for the causal agent—ruptured disc, underactive thyroid, acid reflux—that, for most of the history of illnesses, had not been necessary for the patient, or often the physician, to know. But the contemporary physician is confident that he will usually be able to identify a cause. This increase in confidence occurred in the United States and Europe gradually between the late nineteenth and late twentieth centuries. It is described as the "birth of the clinic" by Michel Foucault and as the "laboratory revolution" by Bruno Latour.[17] In academic medicine, it is the approach that the 1916 Flexner report mandated to reorganize all American medical-school curricula along the scientific-rational model of the early twentieth-century German hospitals. It replaced the traditional physical examination based on an extensive interview of the patient alongside a battery of scientific measurements of the chemical components of the blood and urine, the use of new tools such as the stethoscope and speculum, and new technologies such as the microscope and x-ray. All of these helped the physician gain access to previously inaccessible and even invisible parts[18] of human anatomy and physiology. The data from the tests were much more informative than the verbal report from a patient of their symptoms. The patient could not be expected to know anything about his internal anatomy—certainly not about his internal chemical balance—and his "feeling" was less reliable than the results of scientific instruments. This led to clinicians devaluing patients' testimony[19] and overvaluing test results. When tests revealed no cause for a symptom, it was an easy step to assume that the patient's symptomological claim was unreliable at best, deceptive at worst. All the more so since the general prejudice of contemporary society has been to devalue oral testimony as "hearsay" and overvalue eyewitness testimony especially when it takes the form of a permanent record: a written document or a photograph.[20]

All of this is unfair to the patient, who still has symptoms, perhaps pain, and surely was in the best position to describe what she was feeling. Her insistence that there must be a hidden cause that could be revealed if only the doctor looked deeply enough. After all, patients paid attention to changes in medical practice, and there were always more tests and they had the answers, right? The contemporary medical establishment has insisted that patients seek out pathologies *before* they become apparent, including screening bodies with yearly physical exams, regular colonoscopies, and PSA tests for unlikely pathologies. Physicians would test her blood for signs of future disease. Seek out and "cure" the "silent killers" of elevated blood pressure or high cholesterol *before* they became visible.

Since physicians praise patients who participate in all the recommended screenings, who go for a yearly physicals even though they are healthy, why condemn them for insisting on being treated for real symptoms, just because a doctor has not succeeded in finding a physical cause? The blatant *inconsistencies* of standard medicine's treatment of MUS should be noted: The single most common MUS in the world—headache—has almost never been labeled "factitious", or, for that matter, as an MUS. Much the same, the most common symptom that brings people to a dermatologist: atopic dermatitis. But the almost as common irritable bowel syndrome, not to mention fibromyalgia, chronic fatigue syndrome, PTSD, and many other vague complaints have until recently been dismissed as basically factitious. In general, "the terminology used to describe medically unexplained symptoms is highly inconsistent and varies between countries, between specialties and disciplines, over time and between individuals".[21] It is no wonder that the estimates of the prevalence of MUS vary widely. Published estimates range from 3 to 50 percent of the various patient populations with MUS.[22] I have used "about 20%" as a convenient shorthand, but there is no accurate count. The point here is that it is not a "few". In the United States with over three hundred million people, there are clearly millions of individuals who fall into that category, however defined.

The MUS patient challenges the physician's professional identity; because, in ignorance of the cause, the doctor is unable to find or guess a cure, and so he is stymied. All he can do is order more tests in an attempt to discover a cause. There will always be another test, however expensive or erroneous, which makes it difficult to call it quits. After all, the profession obligates him to care even if he cannot cure. Only some chronic conditions are well enough known and socially accepted for continued palliative procedures ("caring") to be acceptable. But when the symptom is pain—an invisible and unmeasurable symptom—a second professional obligation of the physician kicks in: he is a gatekeeper, part of whose job is:

> to guard the system against unauthorized intruders who may mask their state of dis-ease such that it is made to appear as [real] disease. . . . [But] only bona fide (properly diagnosed), card carrying (insured) patients are welcomed into the medical system. Others, those suffering but not officially "diseased" or adequately insured, are treated like second-class citizens, if not immigrants suspected of being illegal aliens.[23]

And, therefore, are not deserving of compassion. The felt obligation to save healthcare dollars for the "really" sick is one of the drivers behind the attempt to transfer many of those blamelessly suffering MUS into the category of the deceitful, intentional (and thus blameworthy) fakers, and it makes sense from the gatekeeper-side of the doctor's job. This explains why so many of the articles on FD include, usually as an unfootnoted assertation, the supposed fact that these patients create an excessive financial burden on hospitals. Even the sympathetic anthropologist Nichter cannot refrain from commenting that one such patient, who had 14 ER visits in 2 years, "cost the state health care system a quarter of a million dollars for physical ailments which are physically suspect".

Before continuing to disentangle the inter-related phenomena of MUS, FD, malingering, somatization, and hypochondria, I should address a few questions that clinicians reading this might have. First, I am not a physician. I have never seen an actual case of factitious disorder or had a clinical encounter with a patient with MUS. My training is in the history and philosophy of science, and I teach ethics and medical humanities at a medical school. My knowledge is all from books. I quote reports from many actual clinicians, but also from philosophers, psychologists, anthropologists, historians, and poets (like my epigraph from Shakespeare). What these humanists do is suggest other ways of analyzing the problems raised by disease and medicine. They see different structures of analysis and complexities in the seemingly obvious assumptions about what different ways of acting, feeling and being are all about. In short, a medical humanist like me reminds the clinician that medicine is an *art* as well as a *science*. Second, since most diseases are not mono-causal, but are complexes of many factors interacting in composite environments, they produce atypical outcomes in nonstandard patients. The flexible and imaginative approach of the artist, then, can often be useful as a supplement to the scientist's ideal world. The ideal world might not be the one all patients inhabit. Their lived reality is often quite a different one from that of the scientist, and humanists can often see both worlds, which might be useful in aiding physicians to better understand their patients with supposed MUS.

Rasmussen asks the interesting question: Why was the diagnostic category MUS invented in the first place? He answers: because practicing doctors considered all of the various examples to share a single anomaly. Unlike all other medical diseases, MUS were all cases of *symptoms* appearing *without* the simultaneous appearance of any physical *signs* that might have caused it. But this is a common misconception and is not true of most diseases. Headaches, not to mention most mental disorders, also do not present with any measurable physical signs. And most diseases that are mainly biological also have an important psychological and social component, which is necessary for the disease to appear. Not everyone whose antibodies prove that the COVID virus has colonized his body has any actual symptoms of a disease, and physicians really do not know why. MUS is an artifact of the survival of the traditional *bio*medical view of disease and a rejection of the bio*psychosocial* paradigm. Even worse, it represents a now-outdated view of what a "biomedical" cause is.

The two largest groups with MUS are those with autoimmune reactions (about 23 million) and those with "rare" mostly genetic disorders (about 30 million).[24] What both have in common is that they are systemic rather than localized and so hard to detect. Their action is dependent on coexisting environmental factors, from stress, to multiple genes, to chemical and bacterial metabolites. In short, they have multifactorial causes, and, therefore, are good examples of the insight that psychological and social factors often have equally necessary causes along with the traditional purely biological, anatomical, and genetic causes of disease. Such complex causal mechanisms are well known and are not usually considered "medically unexplained", as indicated by the following two examples, which are clearly "medically unexplained" in the sense that the cause in each case is unknown—and there is no cure or treatment beyond palliation—and yet the complaints have been accepted as "real".

Atopic dermatitis, the first example, is the most common of these. These are skin irritations causing rash and, more annoyingly, itch. There is no cure, but most go away on their own, with only palliative care like lotion to soothe and reduce scratching. Physicians do not know exactly what causes them, but it is thought to be a combination of an anomalous immune reaction caused by an inherited flaw in a gene controlling the activation of immunoglobulin E in combination with an environmental irritant.

Rheumatoid arthritis, the second example, is a chronic joint pain disease of uncertain origin, probably a combination of genetics (though only 1 in 20 people with that genetic marker actually have the symptoms), autoimmune reaction (though 20 % of patients with the symptoms do not have the RA factor antibody in their blood), and unknown environmental triggers. The other symptoms are all vague: fatigue, malaise, low-grade fever, weight loss; and, confusingly, many viral infections produce the same symptoms.

The Rheumatoid Arthritis Society specifies that you must have any four of the seven main symptoms or signs (and not necessarily the one actual lab test—for RA factor antibodies) to "have" the disease.

The patients with MUS who are most frequently labeled as FD is in the millions: perhaps ten million with post-traumatic stress syndrome (PTSD), another ten with irritable bowel syndrome (IBS), one million with chronic fatigue syndrome (CFS or ME) in any given year, and millions with sick-house syndrome. These are all considered "suspicious" because there is so much individual variability in response to the same putative triggers or causes. The fact that half of a family is not sickened by whatever chemicals or molds there might be in a house is not proof that the half who *are* experiencing nausea and tiredness are faking their symptoms. This is similar to the phenomenon of differential response to the same medicine or the same trauma. Two people may have the exact same x-ray photo of their slipped disk or torn meniscus, with one in severe pain, and the other oblivious. That is why prophylactic diagnostic full-body MRIs are not recommended. Every person's body has small anomalies that look problematic but are just normal variations. Physicians or technicians are more likely to find a harmless variation than to detect a real problem. Yet, there are three "clinics" in shopping malls near me, run by a company called AffordableScan, offering MRI scans for a thousand dollars each. Similarly, there are companies offering genetic analysis of hundreds of genes, to produce a "polygenic risk score", despite the rejection of such screenings by professional medical societies. Medicine has become democratized enough for these types of companies to flourish.

One might even ask why Americans are not as concerned with the opposite phenomenon of "medically insignificant signs in the absence of symptoms", which should be called MISAS (pronounced "misses")[25]; although, it is usually referred to as "incidentalomas".[26] A recent example comes from some research that concludes: "there is no evidence that routine skin examinations have any effect on melanoma mortality". This was a five-year study at the University of Pittsburgh Medical Center, where primary care doctors at the Center were encouraged to do full body screens of their 600,000 patients. This resulted in doubling the number of early melanomas discovered, but produced no decline in mortality. "Surveillance intensity was a driver of increased detection of *histologically worrisome but biologically benign disease*". The histologic diagnosis that the cells biopsied were malignant melanoma "may be correct, but the prediction of malignant *behavior* incorrect because of the limitations of histological tools to predict an inherently unpredictable future".[27]

There is a lot of surprising uncertainty and refreshing modesty to unpack in the above summary. (1) Why should a "biologically benign" lesion be called a "disease"? (2) What are the "limitations of histological tools"?

They must be significant if half of the cells that meet the criteria of being malignant turn out not to "act" in a malignant way. (3) What causes the prognosis to be "inherently unpredictable in half the cases"? It seems that there must be some confounder, some necessary additional cause to facilitate the malignant action of those cells.

None of this is surprising in the story of disease in general. We already know that many microbes do *not* produce the symptoms of disease in many of the people infected: TB (30%),[28] dengue (80%), and COVID (60%) are the most widespread infections for which we have recent figures. Microbiologists have long abandoned Koch's postulates, which even Koch himself realized were not statistically true. Figures like these are the best arguments against the purely biological view of disease; social factors (like poverty) and psychological factors (like stress) have an enormous influence on whether a "lesion" (anatomic, chemical, genetic, microorganism) actually causes disease. The connection of "sign" to "symptom" is neither one-directional nor simple.

There is a general desire in our society "to make visible the invisible" through the normalization of universal screening. There are negative as well as positive consequences to what at first sight seems like the admirable goal of seeking the truth. The good side has been given the name "precision" or "personalized" medicine. The bad side is the encouragement of hypochondria and illness behavior characterized as "factitious".

Precision medicine jumped to prominence in 2015 when the NIH funded a program to enroll a million people in a giant database and to collect as much medical data as possible on them. The goal was to obtain detailed diagnoses, especially genetic, in order to determine more precisely the response of individuals to medications and to discover why some individuals responded worse than others to the same cancer chemotherapies. Clearly, there were variations in responses to treatments. The effects of any treatment are definitionally statistical—what works for a certain percentage of the group being tested? Young and old, pregnant and not, male and female, black and white, rich and poor, obese and underweight, smoker and nonsmoker—responded differently. The profession first paid attention to this type of population study in pediatrics. Since drugs are rarely tested on children, the proper dosage for them had to be guessed; this used to be "half the adult dose"; but obviously, that was too crude. Mass observational studies were the answer.

As for hypochondria and FD, the connection of these conditions to the normalization of universal screening is less obvious, especially given that everyone is encouraged by the "myth of transparency". Recent work in neuropsychology, though, made the connection between hypochondria/FD and universal screening. Gyorgy Buzsaki's experiments demonstrate that perception is an active rather than passive neurological process. This insight was applied specifically to FD by Mark Edwards.[29] His argument is: A person's perception of his own symptoms is just a specific case of all of a person's perception of the world. The seventeenth-century view, developed by Descartes and Locke, was that our brain is like a blank tablet, a *tabula rasa*, on which the outside world "writes". Our body has different nerves that receive these impressions and then send them to the brain, which coordinates them and interprets them as members of a category you have already come across. It used to be thought that our nerves were passive, like the strings of a piano, silent until struck, and, when struck, produced a sound that they had been structured to make. But new neuropsychology has discovered that the brain's perception is much more active. Though most nerves are passive recipients, a small number of the most important ones are like radar, constantly transmitting probes to the sensory nerves, and quickly fitting their feedback into larger interpretive categories that have already been stored by experience in the brain. A problem occurs when there is a discrepancy between an incoming signal, which detects a vague discomfort which might be a pain, and the continuous "radar" probe feedback from the same area that does not detect any of the usual causes for that pain. The interpretive part of the brain quickly decides that the pain report is probably caused by what usually has caused it in the past. The next step is controversial: After deciding that the vague original distress signals are really signs of a specific and previously known disease, it automatically and subconsciously *enhances* that interpretation by *adding* specific features of that previous signal to what the body actually feels. It is as if the cortex confabulates proof to back up the interpretation it has already decided upon.

Gyorgy Buzsaki gives a good neurophysiological defense of this explanation. But this is really a "localization" of a phenomenon that psychologists identified 50 years ago, starting with Nisbett and Wilson's simple experiment. Subjects were asked to choose one of four identical items and then explain their choice. They all confabulated a reason. Jonathan Haidt has recently done similar work. Lisa Bortolotti concludes that the pervasiveness of such confabulations, made with no intention to deceive, should change our moral stance toward both irrational and delusional beliefs, which she sees as similar. Tahir Rahman is more explicit and applies this to the confabulations and exaggerations made by patients to support their self-diagnoses with factitious disorders. He cites Carl Wernicke's 1892 creation of the idea of the "extreme overvalued idea", to distinguish conditions like anorexia or jealousy from real mental illnesses, which are not just false, but also unshareable and associated with a disintegration of personality. In Rahman's summary "an extreme overvalued belief is one that is shared by others in a person's cultural, religious or subcultural group . . . relished, amplified and defended . . . [and thus should be] differentiated from an obsession or a delusion".[30]

This is like the well-known "confirmation bias", where you "see" what you expect to see. Or to put it in terms of the common medical algorithm: when you hear hoofbeats, you should think "horses" not "zebras". Rare diseases are rare, and so should be the last thing you suspect in diagnosis. The most efficient procedure is to use a decision tree that starts with the most common diseases; only after excluding all of those, do you consider the rare ones, or conclude that it is either a real symptom that remains "unexplained" or meaningless "noise" that should be ignored.

Since I do not think that FD is significantly different from the much larger group of MUS, I will not discuss the changing definitions of FD in the DSM and ICD or the various textbooks of psychiatry. Similarly, though, FDs are usually discussed along with malingering. Malingering is a crime, it is faking a disease for some direct, material, and obvious benefit: originally used in a military context to avoid the dangers of battle. Only in the late nineteenth century, when social insurance was introduced, did it extend to gaining monetary reward like early retirement pension or disability pay to make up for your inability to work. The temptation to lie about disability was obvious. The physician was the most obvious person to distinguish a real from a fake claimant. The fact that most physicians at the time were politically conservative made it easy for them to support the establishment's view that the norm should be a willingness to work and serve in the military; their suspicions of those who sought to avoid either of those obligations seemed obvious.[31]

Yet before government sickness benefits made faking illness rational, in Hector Gavin's *On Feigned and factitious diseases, chiefly of soldiers and seaman, on the means used to simulate or produce them, and on the best modes of discovering impostors*, a 400-page Rabelaisian encyclopedic listing of hundreds of ways of feigning illness and published in London in 1838, six of his 11 reasons for feigning are cases where there is no tangible benefit. These are what would soon be called hysterics and now are called factitious disorders. These include those "influenced by the principle of imitation", wanting to "excite interest", "hysterical fanatics", and the classic FDs. As he writes, "persons not at all in poverty . . . who assume the semblance of disease from some *inexplicable causes*: these are chiefly females".[32] That puzzlement about illness behavior being "inexplicable" reappears in all but the military context.

It explains a lot of the frustration that doctors feel when confronted with MUS. It also makes it convenient to lump MUS patients in with another group, the fifth of Gavin's 11 types of malingerers, whose behavior is so atypical for "civilized" people in nineteenth-century England: the "undeserving poor". In Gavin's words, these poor "prefer idleness to industry [and thereby] deprive the deserving of the benefits intended for them, by defrauding . . . workhouses, hospitals, asylums, dispensaries".

I am encouraged in my view that FD is rare by a paper on malingering that Richard Asher published seven years after he introduced FD into modern medicine with his invention of Munchausen's syndrome. Regretting the widespread use of the Munchausen label, he described the diagnosis of malingering in its "pure" form as "a very rare condition" that is often a cover for the doctor's ignorance of an unusual condition. Asher gives an example of a misdiagnosis he himself had made: One Sunday, he decided to give his wife a rest by waking and dressing his two-year-old daughter after her nap, then taking her for a walk. But, as they began, his daughter started walking with a ridiculous scissor gait, fell a few times, started crying, and said her legs hurt. Asher, a psychiatrist, recognized this as an "aggressive demonstration against the father figure" to which he decided it would be wrong to submit. They had a wretched afternoon. When they got home, his wife undressed the daughter for her evening bath, and cried out: "Richard! You've put both her legs thru the same hole in her knickers!" He continues: "I can still remember, after those tortured limbs had been freed from the crippling garments, how that gay naked figure raced to the bathroom without a trace of malingering"; it taught him to be cautious in diagnosing malingering as well as hysteria, because "there are too many cases of apparent malingering turning out to be . . . organic disease". Surprisingly, he refers back to his old Munchausen's essay, mentioning that the same rarity and caution is true of Munchausen's: "never in the history of medicine have so many[doctors] been so much annoyed by so few [patients]". And he all but throws up his hands in despair by admitting "Nobody can yet answer the two fundamental questions: a) Why do they do it? B) How can we stop them doing it?"[33]

I shall now try to answer Asher's questions by going outside the purely biomedical context and show how some recent work in philosophy—on perception, lying and deception, testimony, and ethics—might shed light on some paradoxes of feigned illness. I offer four psychodynamic narratives that fit different types of factitious diseases. This will not reduce their incidence. It should, though, facilitate a more humane treatment of patients labeled as FD by the medical profession.

Two Recent Cases That Have Been Labeled "Factitious"

In the first illustration, Maria, who faked epilepsy, had numerous epileptic seizures from age 5 to 14, when they were finally controlled by medication; as a result, she was mildly learning disabled. She missed school while in and out of the hospital, made no friends, and rarely left her house where, as an only child, she was lovingly cared for by her devoted parents. In her late 30s, her mother died of a stroke, and at age 42, her father also died. She continued to live alone in the family home. Her parents had set up a fund to provide for her and had arranged brief daily visits from a caregiver. Her social worker arranged a volunteer job as a greeter at a supermarket, where her pleasant demeanor made her popular. But, at age 45, her seizures returned and recurred every few months, even though the dosage of her anti-seizure medication was increased. Since her blood tests revealed a normal amount of seizure medication in her system, she was admitted to the hospital for a 24-hr video observation. That evening, she looked in the hall to make sure no one was coming, threw some magazines on the floor, carefully lay down, and yelled "help!" When no one came, she repeated the performance and, as a nurse rushed in, she started to shake in imitation of an epileptic seizure. When the nurse calmly talked to her, the shaking stopped, she got up and continued conversing with the nurse. Next morning, when the neurologist tried to discuss it, she immediately fell to the floor and began to shake again, and even later, refused to acknowledge any faking.

In the second example from 2016, some CIA operatives in the U.S. Embassy in Havana experienced strange symptoms: a feeling of pressure in their heads, often accompanied by high-pitched sounds. In the next few years, hundreds of other embassy employees in dozens of countries experienced similar symptoms. Brain MRIs revealed no anomalies. Since the CIA concluded that there was no evidence of foreign power acting, nor of the existence of any weapon to beam microwaves at individuals, the most likely cause was mass hysteria, or some unknown medical reaction to some unknown factor in the environment.

These two cases represent two extremes on the spectrum of illnesses labeled factitious. Maria is close to the really extreme and rare Munchausen's syndrome (perhaps a thousand in the United States), where repeated simulations of actual harm are performed. The Havana syndrome is closer to PTSD and chronic fatigue syndrome (which are widespread—millions of cases). These two illustrations, though, share a single probable cause. They are the result of a subconscious attempt to make sense of an MUS by fitting symptoms into a known medical context. This is similar to Freud's explanation of hysteria, where the anxieties troubling the patient were not so much unknown as unacceptable—sexual urges and fantasies. The way chosen by the patient to avoid the pain they caused was to subconsciously *convert* them into less socially unacceptable acts, which produces the bizarre symptoms of hysteria. The factitious patient, though, has a different goal. It is not shame she wishes to avoid, but it is a desire to avoid the pain of not knowing what is causing her vague anxieties, by fitting those anxieties into the narrative of something medical that she had previously experienced (for Maria) or some phenomenon that was a socially approved source of fear, like a Cold War attack by the Russians (for the CIA agents in Havana).

Paradoxes of Perception

Underlying this explanation are some paradoxes in the process of perception, and the naïve view that there is only one "real" reality to be perceived. For example, many people carry in their wallet a picture of their significant other. The photo of my wife in my wallet is a blurry, out-of-focus, Impressionist-style candid photo of my wife smiling; I chose it instead of a formal sharply focused one because it represents what she is to me, how I perceive her—bubbly, happy and outgoing, the joy of my life. Paul Churchland, the neuro-philosopher, whose work consists in measuring blood flow and glucose metabolism in different parts of the brain during different tasks, and by people with different mental pathologies (with the goal of localizing them in parts of the brain), carries a PET scan of his wife's head, showing a perfectly normal pattern of blood flow. What is most significant to him about his wife is her totally normal brain. Neither of us has a "standard" view of our wives. Clearly, there is no "correct" or objective picture of one's wife. Or rather, the standard in our society is that the boring, formulaic sharply focused studio portrait of a formally dressed and posed person, is the "correct" image. This example demonstrates the trend in recent philosophical discussions of "truth" of not asking the question "Is it true?" but instead asking "Is it helpful in understanding the thing?"

In a medical context, perception is the precursor of diagnosis for the purpose of cure. Supposedly, a person can decide what type of thing something is only after perceiving it and that process seems to be straightforward. Early Modern people thought of the eye as a camera, the lens transmitting to the brain an exact reflection of what is really there. But there are some problems with this view. We tend to perceive what we already think is there. The classic case is seventeenth-century preformationism: the theory that there was a miniature adult in the seed of every living thing. This theory predisposed people looking through the newly invented microscope to "see" a little man, a "homunculus", inside every sperm. The Dutch microscopist Hartsoeker even included in his 1694 book, a drawing of that man curled up in the head a single sperm. It is unlikely that he was pretending; he almost certainly did "see" (if only in his imagination) what he drew. Similarly, until the 1950s, it was thought that humans had 24 pairs of chromosomes; every textbook with a photo of the nucleus dutifully noted the 24, and readers who studied the photos thought they saw 24. But by 1960, everyone saw only 23.

People usually "see" only what their brain tells them they should see. As in one standard medical text by Robert Thomas, MD, from 1825, after noting that hysteria afflicted mostly "women of a delicate habit", it proceeds to affirm that "on dissection, its morbid appearances are confined principally to the uterus and ovaria". The similar disease of hypochondria, it asserts, afflicts mostly men, is caused by a loss of energy in the brain and often leads to abdominal problems. Not surprising, then, that "on dissection, the abdominal viscera are enlarged . . . and turgescence is observed in the brain". Clearly, Dr Thomas's expectations guided his eyes.[34] It is a well-known phenomenon—Hamlet used it to ridicule Polonius ["see yonder cloud that's almost in shape of a camel?"].

Kuhn was impressed by the persistence of such prejudices and identified this structural bias, this hold that "normal" science had on most scientists, as the main impediment to scientific progress. Only when the dissonance of the new evidence that contradicted the traditional became extreme did some scientists make revolutionary postulates, to open their eyes, to really see and explain their new observations. He thought that there was little hope to convince the skeptics. Science could advance only when the old believers died off; they were not amenable to more demonstrations or explanations.

Magritte's canvas of an artist painting an eagle, while looking at his model—an egg—illustrates this paradox of seeing what you know is there, rather than what is physically registering on your retina. Maria is like Magritte, vividly seeing the eagle; her doctors and nurses can see only the egg.

Philosophers of art have done much interesting work to elaborate on the complexities of perception as well as the mistake of thinking there is a one-to-one relationship between the object in reality and the representation of it in one's brain. One paradox is the seeming contradiction of saying about a portrait both (1) "that is a face" and (2) "that is not a real face, just a painting of a face". Magritte painted the iconic visual of this in his painting of a pipe, entitled "This is not a pipe". Ernst Gombrich "solved the problem with his example of the hobby horse".[35] For the child, it is a functional replica of a horse, a toy that he treats as if it were a horse in order to play with it. It does not have to be accurate: He would be happy picking up a mop by the handle and yelling "giddy-up". At one level, he knows the toy is not a horse and does not even look like one, but the child can simultaneously act as if it were a horse, without seeing this as a contradiction. Something similar is going on with optical illusions. A silhouette of a white vase against a black background turns into a silhouette of two black faces against a white background. We can see both, but never simultaneously.

We can think of Maria as having this double perspective. For example, according to her therapist, she had lots of anxieties about her lonely life without her parents. She interpreted those anxieties as signs of her previous epilepsy. Instead of going to her doctor and saying she feared her epilepsy had returned, she performed a return of the symptoms, since that made sense of her feelings. Of course, at one level she knew she was producing the symptoms, but at a stronger level, it was a performance of symptoms that she was sure, based on her past experience, would have happened anyway. That is why she could so innocently refuse to accept the video evidence that she had carefully staged her seizure.

Varieties of Truth

Doctors and even family members of people like Maria often react in a huff of righteous indignation when they "prove" that the patient has been lying. But lying is so pervasive a form of social interaction, that this is unfair. We should always ask what role her deception is playing in her life. (Incidentally, as every good mother quickly learns, you should never ask, "Why did you hit Johnny over the head with your shovel?" That is a good way of ending rather than opening up a conversation.) Many people have woken up and thought, "I could use a 'mental health' break", and called in sick; a practice they started in grade school when, the morning of an examination, they told their parent that they had a tummy ache, then placed the thermometer near the light bulb when she wasn't looking, to ensure the necessary high temperature. Or learned that the correct answer when your wife asks "Does this dress make me look fat?" is never "Yes". Or shamelessly told our child about the tooth fairy or Santa Claus. It is normal to act as if truth-telling is optional, or rather, that "truth" is a continuum, rather than an all-or-nothing concept.

Why should we expect patients to be any different? Psychiatrists assume that their patients will be unreliable narrators. Freud supposedly once quipped: "The patient says that the witch in his dream is *not* his mother, therefore she *is* his mother". Psychotherapy is seen as the long process of unpeeling the layers of protective deceptions to reveal the underlying truth of what really happened. So why don't we treat the lies of the factitious patient the same?

One doctor at Brigham and Women's Hospital in Boston found that "unreliable and inconsistent" recall is common among his patients (they remembered less than half of their previous visits, and for a fourth of the visits that they did recall, there was no record in their chart that it had actually occurred). Unsurprisingly, their recall was worse for "information that is perceived as personally threatening or socially undesirable, for example, the number of sexual partners, recreational drug use, or an abortion". And it was worst of all if they had "anxiety or depression, pain or bodily distress".[36]

In fact, there is an interesting literature in current philosophy that tries to redefine "truth" in a way more consonant with the way we actually use it, creating almost a "phenomenology of truth". Typical is Sebastian Gardner, who talks about "motivated self-deception" as a "reasonable form of irrationality". He sees self-deception as only a weak form of lying. It involves holding two beliefs, one of which you know is a false belief, but is useful in helping you avoid some painful realization. In our case, this would be Maria's false belief that she has epilepsy, which she knows how to deal with, rather than loneliness and anxiety, which she is incapable of handling. So we should not think of her as being delusional, or immorally lying; rather we should realize that she is really just making a mistake in logic: "they mistakenly take themselves to have solved their real problem in solving their psychological problem, or, to put it another way, they fail to make a proper distinction between psychological and real problems".[37]

Catherine Elgin presents a more general redefinition of truth. She starts from the paradox that science "unabashedly relies on models, idealizations and thought experiments that are known *not* to be true". Galileo's laws describe motion in a vacuum, or on a frictionless plane, none of which actually exist in nature, both of which had to be approximated. Statistics can be seen as basically rounding off the messy skew of observed measurements. But the inaccuracy of these models is not an inadequacy, "quite the opposite: their divergence from truth or representational accuracy *fosters* their epistemic functioning". They should be thought of as "felicitous falsehoods" or metaphors in that "they exemplify features they share with their targets and therefore afford epistemic access to aspects of their targets that are otherwise overshadowed". They advance understanding because they are "true enough". Of course, "we should not *believe* felicitous falsehoods . . . rather, we should *accept* them and use them as a basis for inference or action". We should not take "truth" to be an absolute, an all or nothing; it is more useful to view it as having a threshold, like similar concepts of "reliability" and "justification".[38]

One of Elgin's examples of a useful falsehood is particularly relevant to factitious disorders: The problem is to exactly predict the flow of air over an airplane wing. However,

> it is possible to derive a second-order partial differential equation that exactly describes this . . . the equation, being non-linear does not admit of an analytic solution. We can formulate the equation, but no one knows how to solve it.

Aeronautical engineers "prefer a first-order partial differential equation that [only] approximates the truth, but admits of an analytic solution" because it is a close enough approximation to allow the design of airplanes. "Since the approximation is more useful than the truth . . . it is preferable, . . . A felicitous falsehood thus . . . may make contributions that the unvarnished truth cannot match": it advances understanding of the domain you are really interested in (airplane design). Similarly, if we are interested in helping Maria, the "truth" of her seizure may be less important than learning what part her misunderstandings play in her own life. And to generalize, in all MUS and chronic conditions, teasing out just how the dozens of interacting physical changes are producing the symptom may be like working on an equation that is theoretically impossible to solve, and so trying to solve it may be an inefficient use of the doctor's time.

Psychodynamic Theories of Factitious Disorders

Bad Faith—Sartre

Maria's factitious epilepsy could be seen as an example of her acting in the "bad faith" described by Sartre in *Being and Nothingness*.[39] Recall that Sartre's concern was with people's authenticity, with the paradox that most men live their lives negating, betraying their own inner selves. They do this voluntarily, using their freedom to give up their freedom. Continual denial of their true selves seems to be the norm for all mankind. Sartre examines the psychodynamics of this bad faith toward oneself. Though such actions have "in appearance the structure of falsehood . . . what changes everything in bad faith is that it is from myself that I am hiding the truth". He rejects Freud's idea that self-deception is unconscious, caused by a split brain, where the ego is separate from and overrides the id. This explanation is unsatisfactory, he says, because it merely reifies rather than explains the split by giving names to the two warring parts of one's self. Sartre gives several examples where self-deception seems more conscious than unconscious.

His strongest case is the woman whose marital disappointment has made her frigid. Sartre quotes some cases from Stekel's book *The Frigid Woman*, where the husband reveals to the psychiatrist that "his wife had given objective signs of pleasure, but the woman, when questioned, fiercely denies them", but admits to thinking of her household budget during sex and even during orgasm, to distract herself from the pleasure she experiences, in order to prove to herself that she really is frigid: She does arithmetic while climaxing in order to deny that she feels pleasure. For Sartre, this is on the borderline between conscious and unconscious action. He invents the term "translucency of consciousness" to describe it, and compares it to playacting. (Elsewhere, he uses "putting yourself to sleep" as an example of similar action on the borderline between intentional and unconscious.) In any event, acting in a way that you know is the opposite of what you actually feel is clearly "bad faith" whether you admit it to yourself or not.

His most famous example is the waiter in a café:

[H]is movement is a little too precise, a little too rapid . . . he bends forward a little too eagerly . . . is too solicitous to the customer. He carries the tray like a tightrope walker. All his behavior seems to us a game. But what is he playing? He is playing at being a waiter. The child plays with his body to explore it; the waiter plays with his condition in order to realize it. This obligation is imposed on all tradesmen. The public demands ceremony . . . there is the dance of the grocer, tailor, auctioneer . . . by which they endeavor to persuade their clientele that they are nothing but a grocer, tailor.

The waiter not only knows that his essence is much more than just his job as a waiter, but he also knows that his customers do not want to see the rest of the real him, so he suppresses the extraneous parts of his true self in the easiest way possible: by "mechanically making the typical gestures of an imaginary café waiter". Presumably, what Sartre wishes is for each waiter to do his waiter-ing in his own way, with his own peculiar gestures, rather than to force his actions into some cliched format. Authenticity would and, for Sartre, should produce hundreds of ways of doing any job.

Sartre considers the normal way society functions—expecting people to adopt pre-made modes of doing things—to be a problem. He doesn't seem to realize that it is inconvenient, inefficient, and disruptive for each member of society to invent his own way of acting in each role. It is as if Sartre thought it would be inauthentic of a "musician" to play music that Beethoven already composed; you should "be your own self" and play only what you compose or can improvise. But for most of us, there is nothing wrong if the ratio of composers to performers (or playwrights to actors . . .) is tiny. Each can be fully authentic, as can Maria, in giving her own performance of the standard script of epilepsy.

Transitional Phenomena—Winnicott

The psychiatrist most relevant to the question of how the physician should relate to Maria is Winnicott. His major insight was that there is not always a clear distinction between truth and fabrication. There is a "third space" intermediate between the psyche and the external world. This potential space is the location of play and of all cultural experience. It is the liminal space where fantasy and reality coexist and can be played with in order to figure out the relation of your own felt experience to external reality. It is where transitional objects, like Linus' blanket, or imaginary friends can be used to experiment with different ways the child can relate to the outside world.

Use of a Restricted Code—Bernstein

Some FDs can just reflect the patient's use of a *different language* in the sense described by Basil Bernstein, the pioneer of socio-linguistics.[40] His key insight was that language limits or mediates the type of thoughts we learn to have, and is itself mediated by social relations, which are more determinative of the words we use and the sentiments we express than is our individual psyche, because "our perception", he says, "is patterned sociologically", in the sense that "forms of spoken language in the process of their learning initiate, generalize and reinforce special types of relationship [to reality]"; that is, they control, define, and limit how we perceive our environment.

The problem Bernstein's research aimed to solve was the failure of public schools in England to educate working-class children as well as they educate middle-class children. His solution was the discovery that the two classes had learned and used very different "speech codes": a "restricted" versus an "elaborated" code. Since it is only the elaborated code that is used in all classrooms, it is as if the lessons were in a different, and thus incomprehensible language for the working-class children.

> Elaborated codes orient their users towards universalistic meanings, whereas restricted codes orient, sensitize their users to particularistic meanings . . . tied to local social structure. Elaborated codes, less tied to a given or local structure thus contain the potentiality of changes in principles and so can be freed from its evoking social structure.

In other words, for him, working-class children usually do not become "bilingual". Their restricted "first language" imprisons them in a rigid structure of perceiving the world. Only the upper class, trained to use reason, can be "bilingual"; by this he means that they can overthrow the restrictions that even their more open language imposes and are able to see reality from several different perspectives. So, the physician is not limited to medical jargon; if it hinders perceiving reality, he can reject it in favor of a different explanation. This is what Maria cannot do, while her neurologist can. This is similar to the ability to have "second order" desires, by which one's rationality can override one's initial primitive first desires.

Bernstein's insight about lower class language is applicable to any insular group. Modern medicine, for example, usually creates a "restricted speech code". This becomes clear from Mishler's analysis of tape recordings of the intake history taking of several doctors.[41] The patients clearly are rambling, with lots of false starts and extraneous information, but the main driver of the interviews are clearly the physicians, who constantly interrupt to guide the patient to present their stories within the framework of the biomedical facts. There is a clear struggle between the voice of the patient using language based on his lifeworld, and that of the doctor, who spoke in the language of the scientific biomedical world.

Perhaps the patient with a factitious disorder is simply trapped in that way of perceiving her vague symptoms and is incapable of even understanding the foreign language (of rationality) in which the physician tries to reframe her illness feelings.

This is also true of nonverbal languages, including the "transitional phenomena" that Maria may be performing. Barbara Montero, a dancer who recently got a PhD in philosophy, provides an interesting case from the insular community of modern dance. Some dancers, after performing a difficult, intricate set of movements to thunderous applause, have complete and sudden amnesia of what they just accomplished. To explain what is going on here, Montero hypothesizes "bodily immersion": "Dancers may focus so intently on sensations that are at least not readily verbalizable, [and] are left without a verbal memory trace, or, in the case of certain qualitative sensations, such as feeling of pain, without a memory trace entirely." In other words . . . dancers may be fully conscious of their actions while performing, yet be left with a feeling of not remembering what they had done.[42] This sounds close to what may have been going on with Maria, especially *after* her performance of her epileptic fit.

Culture-Bound Syndrome

The psychodynamic explanation that probably fits more cases of FD than any other is that it is a "culture-bound syndrome". As a society, we in the United States clearly over-value medicine. It has become an institution that provides a comprehensive set of rituals that promise health, as the Church used to promise salvation, Medicine promises a drug or procedure to cure whatever ails us. One way of recognizing the constructed nature of this phenomenon is to notice that there are many symptoms similar to factitious disorders that our society chooses *not* to classify as factitious. For example, 95% of people who show up in ERs with chest pain turn out not to have had a heart attack, yet most are given a full and expensive workup, and told they "did the right thing" to come in, or indeed are chided for being irresponsible if they waited too long for coming in. Clearly, heart disease, as the leading cause of death in the United States, occupies a special position. It is the site of admirable heroics: CPR, that is, resuscitation with a jolt of electricity, transplants, pacemakers, and clean and easily measured treatments that work to lower blood pressure. In Australia, melanoma occupies a similar privileged position, and so performing/over-diagnosing melanoma is accepted.

Anthropologists have described how most cultures have developed their own rituals for giving permission to people whose anxieties have reached a boiling point to ask for help or release the tension, by performing socially sanctioned rituals. Probably the most common is some form of the devil or spirit possession: Zar spirits in Ethiopia, voodoo in Haiti, witches and demonic possession in the Christian world, other cultures have running amok [committing bloody violence followed by complete amnesia] in Malaysia, Piblokto [women running naked through the snow, followed by amnesia] among the Inuit, fear of shrinking penis in India. The members of each culture learn the appropriate actions, and so, when they suffer anxieties or need to express negative emotions, they will be able to perform them appropriately. When one of the Taita in Kenya needs to restore peace with a neighbor, the appropriate ceremony to cast out the spirit that caused you to insult your neighbor is to sit in front of the man drinking beer and orating about his feelings, while spitting out the beer.[43] The possessed man acts differently in Haiti than in Europe. The specificity of these actions shows that they are constructed, not just eruptions of emotion.

A close analogy is body language, like the raised middle finger, or the hand chopped into the elbow to show contempt. More elaborate is the "victory dance" in tennis. When Rafael Nadal won the Grand Slam in Melbourne, "Suddenly, Nadal punched the air like a prizefighter, flexing his arms like a bodybuilder, pumping his fists overhead and then dropping to his knees as tears flowed".[44] For the past two decades, *all* tennis players have performed the exact same dance; no one thinks they have practiced the choreography; rather, they all subconsciously learned the "proper" way of showing joy at winning. The fact that it is a totally artificial and learned performance does not make it any less genuine. Similarly, Maria's enactment of her anxieties by repeating the body language of her previous seizures (which had always brought her reassuring hugs from others) was no less genuine for being totally choreographed.

Seeking medical care by imitating precisely the signs of some appropriate disease is the culture-bound way of acceptably expressing anxiety and asking for help in the United States and United Kingdom and that was what Maria was performing. Her act was no more of a lie than the tennis player's pose after winning.

Conclusions

Why Do They Do That

There are many other valid understandings of what is going on in people who have factitious disorders; that is what one would expect given that there are an enormous variety of such behaviors. And since there are almost always multiple interacting factors producing the symptoms, the patient's imaginative inventions being only one of them. Also, it is not just the trio implied by the label "bio-psycho-social", for each of those parts has multiple working parts that themselves interact. An example on the biological level would be the common interaction of new viruses with old viruses, old antibodies, current immune response, genetic peculiarities, hormones, and proteins produced by the gut microbiome. Since the classic interactive problem that is unsolvable is the "three body problem"—to predict the future location of three bodies like the Earth, sun, and moon, where each one's gravity is changing the movement of the other two—it is clear that all diseases present multi-body interactions that are even harder to predict.

That is why the key takeaway from my proposed mechanisms is the mere fact that there *are* clear explanations of what would seem to be inexplicable behaviors. (Both Gavin and Asher found them inexplicable.) Most neuroses are *not* hard for the rest of us to understand; but most psychoses seem so different and irrational to the "normals", that it is hard to be sympathetic. To the rest of us, the psychopath seems like he comes from a different planet, and so does the patient like Maria. We are like Thomas Nagel, who wonders what it is like to be a bat.[45] Its way of "hearing" and "seeing" by echolocation has no equivalent in our bodies. This is a problem in the medical context because doctors have a duty to respect their patients, just as all citizens in a decent society have a duty to respect each other.

The philosopher Jeanette Kennett has presented a defense of that obligation. She claims that an important ground for that duty of respect is the fact that even psychotics are "striving to make sense of their experience" of the world, and thus, they are acting for reasons or out of emotions that are "in principle accessible to us". She explains how this works: We all have experienced the disorientation of unintelligibility: We wake up in a hotel room having briefly forgotten that we are on vacation, and then sigh in relief at the realization that *that* explains how we got in this strange bed. Or we get off the wrong exit of the train station and don't know which way to turn to get to the office. We become paralyzed by the questions "Where am I? and What am I doing here?" and, until we fit our current circumstances into a meaningful context, don't know what to do. So we can put ourselves into the mind of the paranoid, who notices a strange car parked across the street from his house; he wonders "am I being spied upon? . . . then, no matter how strange and unlikely . . . it may satisfy the need for intelligibility" to interpret the car as evidence that he is. Furthermore, it might even be evidence that you are an active agent worth spying upon, rather than a faulty or unimportant object,[46] Certainly, for the patient with factitious symptoms, the plausible story may be more important than the correct diagnosis.

Implications: New Diseases Require a New "Ecological" Style of Medicine

There is a steady stream of illness narratives of chronic illnesses that were originally medically unexplained, and whose legitimacy is still controversial.

The most recent is typical: Meghan O'Rourke's *The Invisible Kingdom. Reimagining Chronic Illness* (NY, March 2022). For a decade, she has suffered from debilitating fatigue and headaches with flare-ups of neurological and paralytic symptoms. It took years for her to finally be diagnosed with chronic relapsing Lyme disease plus various autoimmune disorders, with each exacerbating the other. She summarizes her condition: "I live with Ehlers-Danlos syndrome, POTS, and the positive autoimmune antibodies. I have ongoing fatigue, brain fog and neurological and connective tissue problems. They are mostly manageable". But her general statement of the lesson to be learned is: autoimmunity, CFS, and long COVID are the "diseases of our era, conditions that illuminate the need for a shift in medical thinking, from the model of the specific disease entity with a clear-cut solution to the messy reality shaped by both infection and our whole social history, a reality that no one yet fully understands". This sounds like a call for a recommitment to the biopsychosocial approach, but in fact it implies a much more radical change, which I call an "ecological" approach to disease, that will assist in analyzing patient symptoms in general and will, in the process, eliminate the problem of "factitious disorders".

Ecology is the study of the interactions of organisms and their living and nonliving environments. It assumes that everything in the world we live in is interconnected at many levels. So, individuals interact with other individuals, while groups of them interact with other groups and species and environments. Everything exists in constant relationships with smaller and larger biomes and ecosystems. No living thing exists only as an individual, and so can be understood only as embedded in complex relationships in a "web of life". It was Darwin who invented this academic field with his theory of evolutionary change caused by natural selection in a struggle for existence that pitted each against the other. He and most of his readers saw this as proving that competition was the normal and thus desirable way of behaving (an unsurprising reflection of the nineteenth-century British imperialist–capitalist structure of society). And so, when bacteriology was soon discovered, a "war paradigm", which saw bacteria as enemies and parasites to be killed, was unthinkingly adopted to explain our newfound relationship with microbes. It is only in the past two decades that we have begun to realize that almost all microbes are symbiotes, living commensally with other organisms, and are not inherently pathogens or parasites.

The main example of this insight—that the often unseen cooperation of different species is both beneficial and necessary for the flourishing of each—is the discovery of the human microbiome. Each normal human's body hosts hundreds of colonies of bacteria, viruses, and fungi. The largest is in our gut—thousands of species, trillions of individuals. These produce hundreds of complex molecules, many mimicking our hormones, proteins, and signaling chemicals. They mediate many of our normal body functions, including our moods; many communicate directly through the vagus nerve with our brain. There are more of these microbial cells than human cells in our body. Ingesting an antibiotic, we inadvertently kill many of them, disrupting our normal immune system, which is why sometimes the best cure for a disease is to reintroduce them to restore our ecological balance, the homeostasis that equals "health". One of the lessons of ecology is to beware of the unintended consequences of disrupting the biomes. Like a clock, everything is interconnected, there are no "unimportant" parts.

One area where we already act like this is dentistry. Tooth decay ("caries") is caused by several bacteria that form colonies of biofilms in which they break down the enamel. No dentist thinks that the cure is to kill these bacteria, which are a part of the normal mouth microbiome; rather, we strengthen the enamel with fluoride, slow the overgrowth by reducing sugars in the mouth, and scrape off the biofilm by daily brushing. Preventing cavities is accomplished without even knowing about, much less removing, the actual cause. Similarly with stomach ulcers, where, even after we discovered the bacteria that cause them, we did not prophylactically kill it; *Heliobacter pylori* are part of the normal ecosystem of most people's stomachs, so we only remove it when it actually causes an ulcer. We reduce the appearance of the disease by reducing its other causes, like stress.

The two most ambitious suggestions for introducing an ecological paradigm into medicine are Barabasi's heavily biological "network medicine", which is a modernization of Engel's biopsychosocial approach, and Stephen Mumford's very philosophical/theoretical holism that he calls "dispositionalism". Both originate as attempts to solve the problems and paradoxes I have raised about unexplained and factitious diseases. Our experience with long COVID since 2020 has made us all familiar with the ubiquity of the type of problems visible in chronic fatigue, fibromyalgia, PTSD, lower back pain, irritable bowel syndrome, autoimmune diseases, etc.: (1) unknown mechanism, unknown cause, no organic pathology, (2) too many variations in how it manifests in different individuals, with only some of those differences having a biological rationale; the bon mot "if you've seen one case of long COVID, you've seen [only] one" is a good summary; and 3) many complex interactions with genetics, and wide regional variations in reaction.

Barabasi, a network physicist, applied his network model to medicine at the invitation of the *New England Journal of Medicine*, which asked him to comment[47] on Christakis's paper claiming that obesity is "contagious", in that it spreads through social ties in social networks. Christakis analyzed 30 years of data on the same five thousand people in the Framingham Heart Study. He found that if John's best friend Nick becomes obese, John is 57% more likely to become obese, and 171% more likely if they were such good friends that Nick had also named John as his best friend;

while if his brother or wife became obese, he was only 40% more likely to follow suit—so genetics or physical proximity were less important than friendship. Christakis had no idea why this should be, or what mechanism could be involved, but he said that was not important. If you are interested in changing a whole population and making a public health intervention, you don't need proof of causality or even knowledge of the mechanism. Barabasi's commentary generalized this. Traditional medicine insisted on asking "why?" and "how?" When you see connections in a network, the important question is rather "what is connected"; that knowledge will tell you where to intervene to change the outcome. And you will discover many surprising connections. So, at the disease level, diabetes, say, is linked to obesity, asthma, and glioblastoma. Lyme disease is linked to an overactive immune response, so patients' symptoms can come and go as the two diseases exacerbate each other. At a metabolic level, genes, proteins, hormones, gut bacteria, and local pollution interact to moderate or exacerbate symptoms. And at a social level, Christakis's social links, family ties, and stresses at work all interact with complex and often unpredictable outcomes. Each of the three levels (disease, molecular–metabolic, social–environmental) reacts with the other levels and with myriad factors within its own level.

Barabasi's model predicts that many diseases will be "unexplained" at some level because all humans live in three enormously complex environments—molecular, individual body, and society. Each has a complex ecology, and the three systems create a super-ecology with their own interactions. Multifactorial causation among billions of individuals is the rule In a sense, every individual is his own environment, and so should have many unique responses. to the environment. Personalized medicine or population-wide interventions that are statistically effective are the two medical possibilities that work. Our present system, of creating diagnostic categories and fitting each individual patient into one of them, is doomed to failure, certainly in all of the "new" diseases.

Mumford[48] sees similar problems in all medicine, of which MUS are simply the most visible cases. When there are no known mechanisms behind the symptoms, there can be no clear-cut classification, especially when the individual variation in symptoms is so great. But scientific medicine is based on the assumption of regularities, that the same cause will produce the same effect. Mumford then suggests a new paradigm that better fits the new type of multi-causal, chronic, heterogenic presentation of most of the MUS: He calls it "dispositionalism." It is very Aristotelian, based on the idea that all things have certain intrinsic basic properties, predispositions, potentialities. It is senseless, a category mistake, to ask "why"—they just do.

And all dispositions can exist in an unmanifested way. A woman can be fertile without ever getting pregnant, and a person could have a gene that usually causes disease without ever developing it. A disposition will usually manifest only through interaction with other dispositions; it is rare for one to be both necessary and sufficient for a certain outcome. And the interactions are not always linear and additive. Complexity, multifactorialism, and holism are the norm. Don't say that your eye "sees"; without a brain to interpret and a heart to pump blood, seeing would not occur. Same for your brain "thinking". Don't say that the virus gives you the flu; what happens after the virus enters your blood depends on whether a vaccine produced antibodies, how strong your immune system is, and many other factors. "Dispositionalism allows us to embrace the characteristic features of MUS: causal complexity, individual variety, context sensitivity, and real emergence. It also allows for a more person-centered medicine". It applies not only to MUS but also to "illnesses that we typically take to be medically explained, such as heart disease".

Summary

The rather rare phenomenon of "factitious disorders" is problematic for several reasons. It is almost impossible to distinguish it from related somatic symptom disorders that are several magnitudes more prevalent. The clinician must rely on identifying consciousness or intentionality, since by definition there is no physical sign to justify the alleged symptom. And so-called factitious disorders overlap substantially with the enormous number of simply "unexplained" but real complaints. The attempt to distinguish the two undermines the trusting/caring relationship between doctor and patient, and the benefit of succeeding is minimal. So, along with medically unexplained symptoms, factitious disorders are at the borders of our modern biomedical paradigm. In this, they are similar to placebo and nocebo effects, whose existence and strength have been strongly verified, They, too, produce striking physical symptoms greatly in excess of the known power of their physical cause, yet no one thinks the patient is faking the result. The main importance of MUS and FD phenomena is as a spur to recognize the weaknesses of biomedicine and to correcting them. I suggest a few ways of changing that paradigm, basically modifying Engel's biopsychosocial paradigm in light of recent insights into epigenetics and other network phenomena in medicine. At the least, this will encourage doctors to remember that their patients are complex bundles of often inexplicable interactions, but still humans who are in distress, and have come to them for some alleviation, which their profession obligates them to provide.

Notes

1 Thomas Sydenham, *Observationes medicae circa morborum acutorum historiam et curationem* (London: G. Kettilby, 1676); R. G. Latham, trans., *Medical*

Observations Concerning the History and the Cure of Acute Diseases (Birmingham, AL: Classics of Medicine Society for the Sydenham Society, 1848–50), 14. See also: G. G. Meynell, "John Locke and the Preface to Thomas Sydenham's *Observations Medicae*," *Medical History* 50, no. 1 (January 1, 2006): 93–110, doi: 10.1017/s0025727300009467.

2 Franz Kafka, *The Metamorphosis,* as found in *Franz Kafka: The Complete Stories,* ed. Nahum N. Glatzer (New York: Schocken Books, 1971), 89.

3 William Shakespeare, Sonnet 138. For an online copy of the text, which is widely available, see the Folger Shakespeare Library: https://shakespeare.folger.edu/shakespeares-works/shakespeares-sonnets/sonnet-138/.

4 Edward Snow, "Loves of Comfort and Despair: A Reading of Shakespeare's Sonnet 138," *ELH* 40 (1982): 462–83.

5 I am making reference to Claude Levi-Strauss's contribution to the 1970's debate on the existence of cannibalism. ["We are all cannibals," 1993, English translation in his *We Are All Cannibals* (New York: Columbia University Press, 2016), 88.] Some young anthropologists claimed that there never were any primitive tribes that practiced cannibalism and that gullible nineteenth-century anthropologists took as literally true their informants' tall tales because they fit in and justified the European imperialists' myth that their conquest of the third world was justified as a civilizing mission, whose necessity was proven by the natives' disgustingly immoral practices like cannibalism. Levi-Strauss agrees that the extreme cases were not well documented and vanishingly rare (e.g., we know of no tribe of Hannibal Lector's who found human flesh a culinary delicacy, or tribes who would just as likely get food by killing a human in the neighboring village as a deer in the neighboring forest). But Levi-Strauss is convinced by the widespread reports of ritual cannibalism—eating parts of your dead relatives as signs of respect (which spread kuru in New Guinea) or your enemy's heart to help win the next battle. He then notes that this is not significantly different from our own practices of incorporating dead body parts into our bodies by organ transplants, or injections of pituitary cells (which spread Creutzfeldt–Jakob prions in England in 1990). Defined that broadly, "we are all cannibals" and so it is not a disgusting practice limited to primitive people but a universal of human behavior. My chapter will show that inventing or exaggerating physical symptoms is commonly done by all of us, if only because all illnesses (and thus all diseases) have psychosocial in addition to biological causes. This was the insight of George Engel, "The Need for a New Medical Model: A Challenge for Biomedicine," *Science* 196 (4286) (April 8, 1977): 129–36, which is still considered controversial. Engel's own BPS model was really more of a slogan to attack crude biological reductionism; it is no accident that he wrote at the beginning of the simultaneous attack on paternalism in medicine; both movements were more a plea for eclecticism and open-mindedness (not to mention a recognition of the centrality of the patient's actual experience of his illness) than a denial that most diseases *were* mainly biological, and most doctors *did* know best. A good survey is S. Nassir Ghaemi, *The Rise and Fall of the Biopsychosocial Model, Reconciling Art and Science in Psychiatry* (Baltimore: The Johns Hopkins University Press, 2010); he concludes his sympathetic, but devastating critique by saying: the model is "not completely wrong," it was "an advance [. . .] over biological and psychiatric dogmatisms, but a temporary advance, not a final solution" (p. 214).

6 Richard Asher, "Munchausen's Syndrome," *The Lancet* (February 10, 1951): 339ff, https://doi.org/10.1016/S0140-6736(51)92313-6. The statistics on FD

and related MUS are notoriously inaccurate. The most believable are the ones that measure *every* patient over several years in a large and sable group. The most recent are from France and Norway.

7 Between 1995 and 2019, ten million patients were seen at the largest hospital in Rennes, a city of 200,000. Only 49 of them were diagnosed with FD; that is about 5 in a million. In Norway, which has national health insurance and a computerized health registry, in 2018, among the four million total population of Norway, 40 were FD—that is about 10 per million. If the United States is comparable, that is about three thousand people. The most convincing US survey, which Kaplan and Sadock rely on, is the 2013 study of 3.8 million consecutive patients listed in the National Hospital Discharge Survey, which found only 380 FDs, which equals about 30,000 in the whole United States.

8 One assumes that official lists of diseases represent a consensus of the experts, but the story of how FD became an officially recognized disease in the DSM is shocking. The editor, Robert Spitzer, had read a single paper suggesting that FD be included, so he visited the authors and discussed the paper for 45 minutes, after which he asked for a typewriter, and on the spot composed the entry and criteria for FD that were then included verbatim in the final draft. No expert committee, no consultation for a major change in the definition of psychopathology. Alix Spiegel, "The Dictionary of Disorder. How One Man Revolutionized Psychiatry," *The New Yorker*, January 3, 2005, https://www.newyorker.com/magazine/2005/01/03/the-dictionary-of-disorder. See also the DSM-III.

9 American Psychiatric Association, *Diagnostic and Statistical Manual: Mental Disorders* (Washington, DC: Mental Hospital Service, 1952).

10 The DSM-II was published by the APA—American Psychiatric Association, *Diagnostic and Statistical Manual of Mental Disorders*, 2nd ed. (Washington, DC: American Psychiatric Association, 1968)—as were DSM-III (1980), DSM-IV (1994), and DSM-5 (2013) when they switched from Roman numerals to Arabic numbers.

11 The ICD is the International Classification of Diseases put out by the World Health Organization. Every disease is given a numeric code that identifies that particular derivation of the disease. The current version is ICD-11 (2022). ICD-9 was used from 1979 to 1994. ICD-10 was in use from 1994 to 2021.

12 I ignore the obvious main purpose for creating new categories: to rationalize the billing and payment process of insurance companies and national health services. The diagnostic categories of DSM-I and DSM-II (*Diagnostic and Statistical Manual of Mental Disorders*, versions 1 and 2) were ignored by most psychiatrists, and the books sold few copies; only when insurance companies insisted on requiring billing codes did DSM-II come into widespread use and, to everyone's surprise, become a best seller and the major source of income for the APA (American Psychiatric Association).

13 The most widely used is in neurology; see Elisabeth Sherman, Daniel Slick, and Grant Iverson, "Multidimensional Malingering Criteria for Neuropsychological Assessment: A 20-Year Update of the Malingered Neuropsychological Dysfunction Criteria," *Archives of Clinical Neuropsychology* 35 (2020): 735–64. They are open about the overlap of malingering with factitious disorders (and so of the importance of listening to the self-reported symptoms of even the malingerer)—as well they should be, given the extraordinarily high percentage their test identifies as malingerers: 50% of claimants in military or penal settings, pain clinics, and college students asking for ADHD accommodations. A positive interpretation of Symptom Validity and Performance Validity Tests

because they "allow for the development of probabilistic diagnostic criteria" is given by Michael Chafetz, "The Other Face of Illness-Deception: Diagnostic Criteria for Factitious Disorder with Proposed Standards for Clinical Practice and Research," *Clinical Neuropsychologist* 34, no. 3 (2020): 454–76.

14 This turns the physician into an adversary, thus undermining trust. "Even if malingerers did, in fact, outnumber truth tellers in the patient population, their existence should not condemn truth-tellers to being treated as deranged, or as lying until proven otherwise, as the associated costs are simply too high," L. W. Ekstrom, "Liars, Medicine and Compassion," *Journal of Medicine and Philosophy* 37 (2012): 159–80.

15 Kerr White, "The Ecology of Medical Care," *New England Journal of Medicine (NEJM)* 265 (1961): 285; L. A. Green et al., "The Ecology of Medical Care Revisited," *NEJM* 344 (2001): 2021–25. The most recent study is by N. Steinbrecher et al., "The Prevalence of Medically Unexplained Symptoms in Primary Care," *Psychosomatics* 52, no. 3 (2011): 263–71, who claims about 40% of physical complaints presented to a GP are unexplained. One of the few studies that followed up on such patients for a few years is R. C. Smith et al., "Minor Acute Illness: A Preliminary Research Report on the Worried Well," *Journal of Family Practice* 51, no. 1 (2002): 24–29; he followed 833 "frequent users" for whom no physical findings were found initially. Two years later, 35% turned out to have had some organic disease, 51% had a minor acute illness, and only 14% still had no physical signs that might explain the illness and so met the criteria for "somatization disorder".

16 John Fry, Donald Light, and Robert M. Lawrence, *Reviving Primary Care. A US-UK Comparison* (Abingdon-on-Thames: Routledge, 1995). Divides the disease seen in a typical private practice in the UK as 46% minor ailments that are benign and self-limiting (such as upper respiratory infections, skin disorders, emotional problems, and gastrointestinal problems); 40% = chronic mental and physical disorders (such as arthritis, psychiatric, blood pressure, obesity), and only 14% are major diseases (such as heart attack, stroke, cancer, accidents, major infections).

17 Michel Foucault, *Birth of the Clinic: An Archaeology of Medical Perception*, transl. A. M. Sheridan (Abingdon-on-Thames: Routledge, 1973). See also the works of Bruno Latour, including *Reassembling the Social: An Introduction to Actor-Network-Theory* (Oxford: Oxford University Press, 2007).

18 Kelly A. Joyce, *Magnetic Appeal: MRI and the Myth of Transparency* (Ithaca: Cornell University Press, 2010) is surprised at how quickly doctors accepted the idea that the images generated by a computer algorithm "alone offers the truth about a patient's condition." He calls the "high status as evidence . . . of these mechanically produced images . . . thought to provide an unmediated slice of the world . . . the myth of photographic proof." This "attribution of precision . . . produces a halo of certainty" for the machine image, and thus a claim for it to be superior to the old-fashioned physical exam, much less the patients' oral testimony" (pp. 48–55).

19 Symbolized by the amount of time the typical internist allows his patient to answer his opening question: "what brings you here today?". . . eighteen seconds before he interrupts.

20 The model of this view of the superiority of the photographic image goes back to the beginning of photography. The common mid-nineteenth century metaphor for the photograph was "nature drawing her own picture," for example, an unmediated (and therefore closer to "true") self-generated representation,

which could "stand in for and even replace the scientific specimen rather than merely representing it." So the camera for the scientist was like eyeglasses for the nearsighted, enhancing and correcting perception, not just reflecting what one would otherwise incorrectly think was there. Corey Keller, *Brought to Light: Photography and the Invisible 1840–1900* (New Haven: Yale University Press, 2008), 24. See more generally Lorraine Daston, "The Image of objectivity," *Representations* 40 (Fall 1992): 81–128.

21 Emma Weisblatt, Peter Hindley, and Charlotte Ulrikka Rask, "Medically Unexplained Symptoms in Children and Adolescents," chapter 7, pp. 158–74, in *Medically Unexplained Symptoms, Somatization and Bodily Distress. Developing Better Clinical Services*, eds. Francis Creed, Peter Henningsen, and Per Fink (Cambridge: Cambridge University Press, 2011), quote at p. 159. Weisblatt notes that older textbooks of child psychiatry *did* consider migraine and asthma as "psychosomatic disorders."

22 Erik B. Rasmussen, "Making and Managing Medical Anomalies: Exploring the Classification of 'Medically Unexplained Symptoms'," *Social Studies of Science* 50, no. 6 (2020): 901–31, at p. 902.

23 Mark Nichter, "The Mission Within the Madness: Self-Initiated Medicalization as Expression of Agency," chapter 14 in *Pragmatic women and body politics*, ed. Margaret Lock, Cambridge Studies in Medical Anthropology, 5 (Cambridge: Cambridge University Press, 1998) at p. 329.

24 NIH figures, cited by Diane O'Leary, "Why Bioethics Should Be Concerned with Medically Unexplained Symptoms," *American Journal of Bioethics* 18, no. 5 (2018): 6–15, at p. 11. I always round off such numbers, since they are obviously inexact estimates, usually projections of probabilities from a smaller sample. To cite an exact figure is to imply a false accuracy. Modesty is especially appropriate for our topic, which is precisely defined by lies, exaggerations, and uncertainties about what it even is that you are measuring.

25 My suggestion for an acronym.

26 One of the first attempts to generalize this to a critique of the increasing medicalization of normality like PMS and IBS was T. Quill, M. Lipkin, and P. Greenland, "The Medicalization of Normal Variants: The Case of Mitral Valve Prolapse," *Journal of General Internal Medicine* 3, no. 3 (1988): 267–76, which tells of the recent conversion into a pathology of a trivial but measurable variation (a mid-systolic "click") in a heart valve, because it was associated with "a remarkable potpourri of common phenomena including 'atypical' chest pain, dyspnea, fatigue, dizziness, palpitations, anxiety [no doubt caused by the diagnosis itself] and arrhythmias."

27 Robert Swerlick, "Melanoma Screening—Intuition and Hope Are Not Enough," Editorial Comment on the *JAMA Network, JAMA Dermatology* (April 6, 2022) in reaction to Martha Matsumoto, Sarah Wack, Martin A. Weinstock et al., "Five-Year Outcomes of a Melanoma Screening Initiative in a Large Health Care System," *JAMA Dermatology* 158, no. 2 (2022): 504–12, doi:10.1001/jamadermatol.2022.0253.

28 Emily Wong, "It Is Time to Focus on Asymptomatic Tuberculosis," *Clinical Infectious Diseases* 72, no. 12 (2021): e1044–46; Q. A. ten Bosch, "Contributions from the Silent Majority Dominate Dengue Virus Transmission," *PLOS Pathogens* 14, no. 5 (2018): e1006965. It has long been known that over 95% of people infected with poliovirus remain asymptomatic. The recent discovery that gastric ulcers were a bacterial infection has been widely misunderstood: Half the world has *Helicobacter pylori* in their stomach, yet only in a few

does this infection produce an ulcer; the bacteria is necessary but not sufficient to cause the disease: M. Go, "The Natural History and Epidemiology of *Helicobacter pylori* infection," *Alimentary Pharmacology and Therapeutics* 16 (2002): 3–15. See my concluding comments on Rom Harre's concept of "dispositionalism", which I take as a solution to the problem of just *what* FDs and MUSs are, which is also a good explanation of such common anomalies of "medically *explained*" disease.

29 Gyorgi Buzsaki, *The Brain from inside out* (Oxford: Oxford University Press, 2019), should be read with David Poeppel's critique: "Against the Epistemological Primacy of the Hardware: The Brain from Inside Out, Turned Upside Down," *eNeuro* 7, no. 4 (July 2020): 1–8. See also Mark J. Edwards, Rick A. Adams, Harriet Brown et al., "A Bayesian Account of 'Hysteria'," *Brain* 135 (2012): 3495–512; P. R. Corlett et al., "Toward a Neurobiology of Delusions," *Progress in Neurobiology* 92, no. 3 (2010): 345–69. Corlett's summary is accurate for all of the above: "delusions result from aberrations in how brain circuits . . . respond to prediction errors" by overriding perceptions, memory, and bodily agency.
Buzsaki talks of the "good-enough brain . . . fast and efficient, but not particularly precise." To an outsider like me, the general argument seems to combine elements of Tversky and Kahneman's reactions to uncertainty, (Charles) Pierce's abductive inferences, and Winnicott's "good enough" mothers. Amos Tversky and Daniel Kahneman, "Judgement Under Uncertainty: Heuristics and Biases: Biases in Judgments Reveal Some Heuristics of Thinking Under Uncertainty," *Science* 185, no. 4157 (September 27, 1974): 1124–131, doi:10.1126/science.185.4157.1124; Tomis Kapitan, "Pierce and the Autonomy of Abductive Reasoning," *Erkenntnis* 37, no. 1 (July 1992): 1–26; D. W. Winnicott, *Playing and Reality* (Abingdon-on-Thames: Routledge, 1991).

30 Lisa Bortolotti, *The Epistemic Innocence of Irrational Beliefs* (Oxford: Oxford University Press, 2020), 45–50, citing Nisbett's article from 1977 and Haidt's from 2001. Richard E. Nisbett and Timothy DeCamp Wilson, "The Halo Effect: Evidence for Unconscious Alteration of Judgments," *Journal of Personality and Social Psychology* 35, no. 4 (1977): 250–56; Jonathan Haidt, "The Emotional Dog and Its Rational Tail: A Social Intuitionist Approach to Moral Judgment," *Psychological Review* 108, no. 4 (October 2001): 814–34. See also Tahir Rahman, J. Reid Meloy, and Robert Bauer, "Extreme Overvalued Belief and the Legacy of Carl Wernicke," *Journal of American Academic Psychiatry and Law* 47, no. 2 (June 2019): 180–87.

31 Kafka, always the perceptive analyst of bureaucracy's inherent injustice, shows how both doctor and patient unthinkingly accept the normality of this suspicion, as seen in my epigraph from *The Metamorphosis*, note 2.

32 Hector Gavin, *Prize Essay for Military Surgery* (Edinburgh: University of Edinburgh, 1835–6), 11, my emphasis; the eleventh category is slaves, who used to be frequent feigners, but, in the post-abolition British colonies, the "sanatory effects of freedom . . . have shown in the moral regeneration that they no longer feign disease," (p. 12).

33 Both essays are reprinted in Francis Avery Jones, *Richard Asher Talking Sense* (London: Pitman Medical, 1972).

34 Robert Thomas, *The Modern Practice of Physic, Exhibiting the Character, Causes, Symptoms, Prognostics, Morbid Appearances and Improved Method of Treating the Diseases of All Climates*, 8th ed. (New York: Longman, etc., 1825), 381, 388.

35 Ernst H. Gombrich, *Meditations on a Hobby Horse, and Other Essays on the Theory of Art* (London: Phaidon, 1971).

36 Arthur Barsky, "Forgetting, Fabricating and Telescoping. The Instability of the Medical History," *Archives of Internal Medicine* 162, no. 9 (2002): 981–84. If this is true of "normal" patients, how much more so of those suspected of being factitious. His patients "falsely recall medical events and symptoms that did not in fact occur. Their unreliability of recall is affected by personality . . . anxiety, depression, and pain or bodily distress."

37 Sebastian Gardner, *Irrationality and the Philosophy of Psychoanalysis* (Cambridge: Cambridge University Press, 1993), 17–18.

38 Catherine Z. Elgin, *True Enough* (Cambridge, MA: MIT Press, 2017), quotes on pp. 1–3, 30.

39 Jean-Paul Sartre, *Being and Nothingness* (New York: Philosophical Library, 1956), 47ff.

40 Basil Bernstein, *Class, Codes and Control. Vol 1: Theoretical Studies Towards a Sociology of Language* (Abingdon: Routledge, 1971), passages quoted on pp. 27, 76, 176. See especially chapter 1: "Sociological determinants of perception." This seems similar to the later American movement to recognize "ebonics" and "black English" as second languages in ghetto schools.

41 Elliot G. Mishler, *The Discourse of Medicine: Dialectics of Medical Interviews* (New York: Ablex, 1984). Thirty years after Mishler, the situation seems much better, at least among European physicians—they seem explicitly aware that there are two linguistic worlds at play, based on "differing knowledge domains" and seem to be walking on eggs to validate the patients' experience of his unexplained symptoms by translating their jargon. Inge Stortenbeker, Wyke Stommel, Sandra van Dulmen et al., "Linguistic and Interactional Aspects That Characterize Consultations About Medically Unexplained Symptoms: A Systematic Review," *Journal of Psychosomatic Research* 132 (May 2020): 109994.

42 Barbara Gail Montero, "The Paradox of Post-Performance Amnesia," *Midwest Studies in Philosophy* 44 (2019): 38–47.

43 Grace Harris, *Casting Out Anger. Religion Among the Taita of Kenya* (Cambridge: Cambridge University Press, 1978).

44 Christopher Clarey, "Rafael Nadal Wins the Australian Open, His 21st Grand Slam Title," *New York Times*, January 30, 2022, https://www.nytimes.com/2022/01/30/sports/tennis/nadal-medvedev-australian-open.html.

45 Thomas Nagel, "What Is It Like to Be a Bat?—Panpsychism," chapter 12 in *Mortal Questions* (Cambridge: Cambridge University Press, 1979).

46 Jeanette Kennett, "Striving to Make Sense. The Duty of Respect for Persons With Psychosis," *Philosophy, Psychiatry & Psychology* 28, no. 3 (2021): 231–33.

47 Albert-Laszlo Barabasi, "Network Medicine—From Obesity to the 'Diseasome'," *New England Journal of Medicine* 357, no. 4 (June 26, 2007): 404–7.

48 Thor Eriksen, Roger Kerry, Stephen Mumford et al., "At the Borders of Medical Reasoning: Aetiological and Ontological Challenges of Medically Unexplained Symptoms," *Philosophy, Ethics and Humanities in Medicine* 8 (2013): 11.

Reference List

Asher, Richard. *Richard Asher Talking Sense*. Edited by Francis Avery Jones. London: Pitman Medical, 1972.

Barabasi, Albert-Laszlo. "Network Medicine—from Obesity to the 'Diseasome'." *New England Journal of Medicine* 357., no. 4 (June 26, 2007): 404–7.

Barsky, Arthur. "Forgetting, Fabricating and Telescoping. The Instability of the Medical History." *Archives of Internal Medicine* 162, no. 9 (2002): 981–84.

Bernstein, Basil. *Class, Codes and Control. Vol 1: Theoretical Studies Towards a Sociology of Language.* Abingdon: Routledge, 1971.

Bortolotti, Lisa. *The Epistemic Innocence of Irrational Beliefs.* Oxford: Oxford University Press, 2020.

Buzsaki, Gyorgi. *The Brain From Inside Out.* Oxford: Oxford University Press, 2019.

Chafetz, Michael. "The Other Face of Illness-Deception: Diagnostic Criteria for Factitious Disorder With Proposed Standards for Clinical Practice and Research." *Clinical Neuropsychologist* 34, no. 3 (2020): 454–76.

Clarey, Christopher. "Rafael Nadal Wins the Australian Open, His 21st Grand Slam Title." *New York Times*, January 30, 2022. https://www.nytimes.com/2022/01/30/sports/tennis/nadal-medvedev-australian-open.html.

Corlett, P. R., J. R. Taylor, X.-J. Wang, P. C. Fletcher, and J. H. Krystal. "Toward a Neurobiology of Delusions." *Progress in Neurobiology* 92, no. 3 (November 2010): 345–69. doi:10.1016/j.pneurobio.2010.06.007.

Daston, Lorraine. "The Image of Objectivity." *Representations* 40 (Fall 1992): 81–128.

Diagnostic and Statistical Manual: Mental Disorders (aka: DSM, DSM-I). Washington, DC: American Psychiatric Association, Mental Hospital Service, 1952.

Diagnostic and Statistical Manual of Mental Disorders. 2nd ed. (DSM-II). Washington, DC: American Psychiatric Association, 1968.

Diagnostic and Statistical Manual of Mental Disorders. 3rd ed. (DSM-III). Washington, DC: American Psychiatric Association, 1980.

Edwards, Mark J., Rick A. Adams, Harriet Brown, Isabel Pareés, and Karl J. Friston. "A Bayesian Account of 'Hysteria'." *Brain* 135 (2012): 3495–512. doi:10.1093/brain/aws129.

Ekstrom, L. W. "Liars, Medicine and Compassion." *Journal of Medicine and Philosophy* 37 (2012): 159–80.

Elgin, Catherine Z. *True Enough.* Cambridge, MA: MIT Press, 2017.

Engel, George. "The Need for a New Medical Model: A Challenge for Biomedicine." *Science* 196, no. 4286 (April 8, 1977): 129–36.

Eriksen, Thor, Roger Kerry, Stephen Mumford, Svein Anders Noer Lie, and Rani Lill Anjum. "At the Borders of Medical Reasoning: Aetiological and Ontological Challenges of Medically Unexplained Symptoms." *Philosophy, Ethics and Humanities in Medicine* 8 (2013): 11.

Foucault, Michel. *Birth of the Clinic: An Archaeology of Medical Perception.* Translated by A. M. Sheridan. Abingdon-on-Thames: Routledge, 1973.

Fry, John, Donald Light, and Robert M. Lawrence, *Reviving Primary Care. A US-UK Comparison.* Abingdon-on-Thames: Routledge, 1995.

Gardner, Sebastian. *Irrationality and the Philosophy of Psychoanalysis.* Cambridge: Cambridge University Press, 1993.

Gavin, Hector. "On Feigned and Factitious Diseases, Chiefly of Soldiers and Seaman, on the Means Used to Simulate or Produce Them, and on the Best Modes of Discovering Impostors." Prize Essay for Military Surgery. University of Edinburgh, 1835–6. https://wellcomecollection.org/works/z27advzh/items?canvas=11.

Ghaemi, S. Nassir. *The Rise and Fall of the Biopsychosocial Model, Reconciling Art and Science in Psychiatry*. Baltimore: Johns Hopkins University Press, 2010.

Go, M. "The Natural History and Epidemiology of *Helicobacter pylori* Infection." *Alimentary Pharmacology and Therapeutics* 16 (2002): 3–15.

Gombrich, Ernst H. *Meditations on a Hobby Horse, and Other Essays on the Theory of Art*. London: Phaidon, 1971.

Green, L. A., G. E. Fryer Jr., B. P. Yawn, D. Lanier, and S. M. Dovey. "The Ecology of Medical Care Revisited." *New England Journal of Medicine* 344, no. 26 (2001): 2021–25. doi:10.1056/NEJM200106283442611.

Haidt, Jonathan. "The Emotional Dog and Its Rational Tail: A Social Intuitionist Approach to Moral Judgment." *Psychological Review* 108, no. 4 (October 2001): 814–34.

Harris, Grace. *Casting Out Anger. Religion Among the Taita of Kenya*. Cambridge: Cambridge University Press, 1978.

Joyce, Kelly A. *Magnetic Appeal: MRI and the Myth of Transparency*. Ithaca: Cornell University Press, 2010.

Kafka, Franz. "The Metamorphosis." In *Franz Kafka: The Complete Stories*, edited by Nahum N. Glatzer. New York: Schocken Books, 1971.

Kapitan, Tomis. "Pierce and the Autonomy of Abductive Reasoning." *Erkenntnis* 37, no. 1 (July 1992): 1–26.

Keller, Corey. *Brought to Light: Photography and the Invisible 1840–1900*. New Haven: Yale University Press, 2008.

Kennett, Jeanette. "Striving to Make Sense. The Duty of Respect for Persons With Psychosis." *Philosophy, Psychiatr & Psychology* 28, no. 3 (2021): 231–33.

Latour, Bruno. *Reassembling the Social: An Introduction to Actor-Network-Theory*. Oxford: Oxford University Press, 2007.

Levi-Strauss, Claude. *We Are All Cannibals*. New York: Columbia University Press, 2016.

Matsumoto, Martha, Sarah Wack, Martin A. Weinstock, et al. "Five-Year Outcomes of a Melanoma Screening Initiative in a Large Health Care System." *JAMA Dermatology* 158, no. 2 (2022): 504–12. doi:10.1001/jamadermatol.2022.0253.

Meynell, G. G. "John Locke and the Preface to Thomas Sydenham's *Observations Medicae*." *Medical History* 50, no. 1 (January 1, 2006): 93–110. doi:10.1017/s0025727300009467.

Mishler, Elliot G. *The Discourse of Medicine: Dialectics of Medical Interviews*. New York: Ablex, 1984.

Montero, Barbara Gail. "The Paradox of Post-Performance Amnesia." *Midwest Studies in Philosophy* 44 (2019): 38–47.

Nagel, Thomas. *Mortal Questions*. Cambridge: Cambridge University Press, 1979.

Nichter, Mark. "The Mission Within the Madness: Self-Initiated Medicalization as Expression of Agency," chapter 14. In *Pragmatic Women and Body Politics*, edited by Margaret Lock, Cambridge Studies in Medical Anthropology, 5. Cambridge: Cambridge University Press, 1998.

Nisbett, Richard E., and Timothy DeCamp Wilson. "The Halo Effect: Evidence for Unconscious Alteration of Judgments." *Journal of Personality and Social Psychology* 35, no. 4 (1977): 250–56.

O'Leary, Diane. "Why Bioethics Should Be Concerned With Medically Unexplained Symptoms." *American Journal of Bioethics* 18, no. 5 (2018): 6–15.

Poeppel, David. "Against the Epistemological Primacy of the Hardware: The Brain From Inside Out, Turned Upside Down." *eNeuro* 7, no. 4 (July 2020): 1–8.

Prentice, Melissa. "Prosecuting Mothers Who Maim and Kill: The Profile of Munchausen Syndrome by Proxy Litigation in the Late 1990s." *American Journal of Criminal Law* 28 (2001): 373–411.

Quill, T., M. Lipkin, and P. Greenland. "The Medicalization of Normal Variants: The Case of Mitral Valve Prolapse." *Journal of General Internal Medicine* 3, no. 3 (1988): 267–76.

Rahman, Tahir, J. Reid Meloy, and Robert Bauer. "Extreme Overvalued Belief and the Legacy of Carl Wernicke." *Journal of American Academic Psychiatry and Law* 47, no. 2 (June 2019): 180–87. doi:10.29158/JAAPL.003847-19.

Rasmussen, Erik B. "Making and Managing Medical Anomalies: Exploring the Classification of 'Medically Unexplained Symptoms'." *Social Studies of Science* 50, no. 6 (2020): 901–31.

Sartre, Jean-Paul. *Being and Nothingness.* New York: Philosophical Library, 1956.

Sherman, Elisabeth, Daniel Slick, and Grant Iverson. "Multidimensional Malingering Criteria for Neuropsychological Assessment: A 20-Year Update of the Malingered Neuropsychological Dysfunction Criteria." *Archives of Clinical Neuropsychology* 35 (2020): 735–64.

Smith, R. C., et al. "Minor Acute Illness: A Preliminary Research Report on the Worried Well." *Journal of Family Practice* 51, no. 1 (2002): 24–29.

Snow, Edward. "Loves of Comfort and Despair: A Reading of Shakespeare's Sonnet 138." *ELH* 40 (1982): 462–83.

Spiegel, Alix. "The Dictionary of Disorder. How One Man Revolutionized Psychiatry." *The New Yorker*, January 3, 2005. https://www.newyorker.com/magazine/2005/01/03/the-dictionary-of-disorder.

Steinbrecher, N., S. Koerber, D. Frieser, and W. Hiller. "The Prevalence of Medically Unexplained Symptoms in Primary Care." *Psychosomatics* 52, no. 3 (2011): 263–71. doi:10.1016/j.psym.2011.01.007.

Stortenbeker, Inge, Wyke Stommel, Sandra van Dulmen, et al. "Linguistic and Interactional Aspects That Characterize Consultations About Medically Unexplained Symptoms: A Systematic Review." *Journal of Psychosomatic Research* 132 (May 2020): 109994.

Swerlick, Robert. Editorial Comment: "Melanoma Screening—Intuition and Hope Are Not Enough." *JAMA Network, JAMA Dermatology* (April 6, 2022) in reaction to Martha Matsumoto, Sarah Wack, Martin A. Weinstock, et al., "Five-Year Outcomes of a Melanoma Screening Initiative in a Large Health Care System." *JAMA Dermatology* 158, no. 2 (2022): 504–12. doi:10.1001/jamadermatol.2022.0253.

Sydenham, Thomas. *Observationes medicae circa morborum acutorum historiam et curationem.* London: G. Kettilby, 1676.

Sydemham, Thomas, and R. G. Latham, trans. *Medical Observations Concerning the History and the Cure of Acute Diseases.* Birmingham, AL: Classics of Medicine Society for the Sydenham Society, 1848–50.

ten Bosch, Q. A., H. E. Clapham, L. Lambrechts, V. Duong, P. Buchy, B. M. Althouse, et al. "Contributions From the Silent Majority Dominate Dengue Virus Transmission." *PLoS Pathogens* 14, no. 5 (2018): e1006965. https://doi.org/10.1371/journal. ppat.1006965.

Thomas, Robert. *The Modern Practice of Physic, Exhibiting the Character, Causes, Symptoms, Prognostics, Morbid Appearances and Improved Method of Treating the Diseases of All Climates.* 8th ed. New York: Longman, etc., 1825.

Tversky, Amos, and Daniel Kahneman. "Judgement Under Uncertainty: Heuristics and Biases: Biases in Judgments Reveal Some Heuristics of Thinking Under Uncertainty." *Science* 185, no. 4157 (September 27, 1974): 1124–31. doi:10.1126/science.185.4157.1124.

Weisblatt, Emma, Peter Hindley, and Charlotte Ulrikka Rask. "Medically Unexplained Symptoms in Children and Adolescents." In *Medically Unexplained Symptoms, Somatisation and Bodily Distress. Developing Better Clinical Services*, edited by Francis Creed, Peter Henningsen, and Per Fink, 158–74. Cambridge: Cambridge University Press, 2011.

White, Kerr. "The Ecology of Medical Care." *New England Journal of Medicine* 265 (1961): 285.

Winnicott, D. W. *Playing and Reality.* Abingdon-on-Thames: Routledge, 1991.

Wong, Emily. "It Is Time to Focus on Asymptomatic Tuberculosis." *Clinical Infectious Diseases* 72, no. 12 (2021): e1044–46.

Part II

Historic Cases of Malingering

5 'Because She Pretended to Be Pregnant and Was Not'

Fake Royal Pregnancies in Medieval Scotland

Emma Trivett

Due to medieval understanding of the reproductive process and the absence of modern medical technologies like ultrasound, pregnancy lent itself to being faked in the Middle Ages. There are accounts which claim that two different medieval queens of Scotland pretended to be pregnant. The *Chronicle of Lanercost* declares that Yolande de Dreux, second queen of Alexander III (r. 1249–86), faked a pregnancy and tried to substitute an heir to secure her position in Scotland after the king's death, while the *Liber Pluscardensis* states that David II (r. 1329–71) and Queen Margaret Logie's marriage ended because Margaret pretended to be pregnant. According to the *Lanercost* and the *Liber*, respectively, Yolande and Margaret faked pregnancies at pivotal moments of uncertainty for the Scottish succession—in 1286, after the unexpected death of Alexander III, and during the reign of David II, whose first marriage of several decades had been childless. When David and Margaret were married in 1364, David was still without (and increasingly eager for) a biological Bruce heir. Both accounts of fake pregnancies are unique, and neither is included in any other medieval chronicle, so it is unlikely that either woman really faked a pregnancy, but it is remarkable that such accusations were made against the queens. It is the chroniclers' use of fake pregnancies to malign, discredit and blame the queens, rather than the matter of the accounts' truthfulness which is the focus of this chapter. Ultimately, the chronicles illustrate the ambiguity around reproduction and knowing about pregnancy in the Middle Ages, and they demonstrate how this uncertainty could be negotiated by queens and weaponized against them by others.

Faking Pregnancy

Before we look at the chronicle claims about the Scottish queens, it is worthwhile considering the specific implications incited by a claim of fake pregnancy and how it might have differed from other claims made against medieval queens such as, for instance, an accusation of adultery. It is also

DOI: 10.4324/9781003452324-8

important to establish the significance of pregnancy as a narrative device in medieval chronicles. Indeed, chronicler comments about other medieval queens of the British Isles, such as Isabella of France, Joan Plantagenet and Marie de Coucy, imply that queens were associated with their reproductive role, at least by the chroniclers. In other words, a queen's life could be summed up in a chronicle with a report on her fertile successes or failures and chroniclers describe pregnancy and fertility to demonstrate good queenship and portray a queen's success. Therefore, it follows that emphasising a queen's reproductive failure with an accusation of a fake pregnancy could be used to vilify or malign a queen too.

Fake pregnancy is mentioned in medieval legal sources from England and France. Fiona Harris-Stoertz argues that the attention to fake pregnancy in medieval law was a response to fears about inheritance.[1] There was societal concern about what women might do to manipulate the reproductive process, whether mothers themselves or the midwives and women who attended births, and this is reflected in the emergence of laws relating to pregnant women and childbirth from the twelfth and thirteenth centuries.[2] The legal requirement of hearing the infant cry from the birthing chamber was established in England during Edward I's reign to combat the fear that a false heir might be smuggled in when the men were not looking.[3] There is also a protocol in *Bracton,* a twelfth-century codification of English law, for determining whether a woman was faking pregnancy: the woman was to 'be examined by responsible matrons, by feeling her breasts and abdomen, in order to discover the truth'. If the woman was thought to be pregnant after this humiliating and invasive examination, or even if there was some uncertainty about her condition, she was to be confined in the king's castle until she gave birth, or until she could be shown to have been faking pregnancy.[4] While confined, she was to be kept away from any pregnant maids and potential collaborators.[5] Such procedures indicate the risk associated with faking a pregnancy as well as fear about women substituting heirs; women's bodies were subject to intense scrutiny and invasive examination by 'honest women' as part of the legal protocol for determining pregnancy. The emergence of legislation to protect against women substituting heirs, even though men might have been just as motivated to present a false or illegitimate heir, is particularly striking because it makes supplying a fake heir a uniquely gendered crime.[6]

In another example from English common law, a pregnancy offered a woman some control over her future. 'Pleading the belly', or declaring a pregnancy, was a legal recourse which could give a woman a reprieve or even pardon from an execution sentence.[7] Faced with a desperate situation, women who pleaded the belly were able to use their reproductive bodies as a way to leverage some control over their fate.[8] Holly Barbaccia, Bethany Packard and Jane Wanninger suggest that the medieval and early modern practice of pleading the belly is representative of the 'broader network of ways in which women work[ed] to author their futures'.[9] Faking pregnancy and pleading the belly are alike in the sense that they were both cases where a woman could harness some authority or control over her (usually dire) circumstances using her reproductive role. The process for determining pregnancy when a woman pleaded the belly was the same as that used to determine whether a woman was pretending to be pregnant in inheritance disputes, and she was subject to examination by experienced matrons or 'honest women'.[10] This protocol demonstrates that women who tried to claim influence by citing pregnancy were treated with suspicion and subjected to physical examination to determine if they were trying to deceptively exploit the unique authority of pregnancy for personal advantage.

Although accusations of faked pregnancies appear in contemporary legal disputes, adultery was a more common accusation against medieval queens.[11] For instance, the eleventh-century *Encomium Emmae Reginae* commissioned by Emma of Normandy, claims that Harold, son of Emma's husband Cnut and his first wife, Ælfgifu of Northampton, was fathered by a priest.[12] In a later-medieval example, it was rumoured that Margaret of Anjou's son was not fathered by Henry VI.[13] These claims, made by rival claimants to the throne, use adultery to discredit a royal heir and open up the succession for another—in Queen Emma's case, her own son, and in Margaret's, the Yorkist faction in the fifteenth century. The adulterous queen character is also a recognisable trope in medieval French romance literature. Peggy McCracken argues that the adulterous queen's body was split between two men (the king and the lover), which challenged contemporary ideas about property and proper succession in medieval France. Notably, the adulterous queen character is always remarkably childless and, therefore, is a careful disassociation of reproduction from sexual (mis) conduct. This conflicts with the reality of a queen's body, in which her female sexuality and the political future of the realm were intertwined.[14] McCracken argues that the character of the adulterous queen existed in the context of courtly love literature, but it developed from deeper societal worry about dynastic reproduction, inheritance and succession which were threatened by a sexually transgressive female body.[15] There is some similarity between adultery and faking pregnancy, as a faked pregnancy also implies that the queen jeopardised the legitimate succession and exploited her reproductive role for personal prestige.

There are significant differences between adultery and pretending to be pregnant, however. First, there is no sexual transgression involved in a fake pregnancy. In the models of historic and romantic queens accused of adultery, the legitimate inheritance was threatened by the woman's sexual exploits and her attempt to cover them up. In the examples of Ælfgifu of Northampton and Margaret of Anjou, their adultery is implied by suggesting that their sons were fathered by someone other than the king. In contrast, the claims that Yolande de Dreux and Margaret Logie pretended to be pregnant highlight that neither queen produced a child; there is no insinuation that they were genuinely pregnant but with someone else's child, so they are not accused by the chroniclers of a sexual transgression. A fake pregnancy hinges on the absence of children, rather than the need to pass off a lover's child as the king's heir. The charges against the two Scottish queens are rooted in their childlessness, not sexual misconduct.

Accounts about fake pregnancies are unusual, but royal births are regularly mentioned in medieval chronicles from England and Scotland. Indeed, there is some sense that chroniclers used fertility to communicate a queen's success. For instance, the continuation of the *Flores Historiarum* chronicle—a fourteenth-century source from England—draws attention to the queen of England, Isabella of France's production of two sons to demonstrate her success as a young queen. The *Flores* writer declares that:

> at Eltham in Kent on the 15 August, Lady Isabella the queen was adorned with a double blossom when she gave birth to the lord king's second son. . . . In light of giving birth to these noble offspring, the said queen was famous for her fertility.[16]

Married to Edward II of England, Isabella of France is infamous for the role she played, along with her eldest son (future Edward III), in the deposition of her husband in 1327. Edward II and Isabella were married in 1308, but the queen was overshadowed by her husband's favourite, Piers Gaveston, for the first years of her tenure as queen.[17] A chronicle from St Albans Abbey mentions Isabella's sorrow due to Edward's neglect when he chose to flee from his nobles with Gaveston instead of staying with his 'then pregnant' queen.[18] This episode preserves contemporary perceptions of Edward's unmanly and un-kingly behaviour; the chronicler uses Isabella's pregnancy to highlight the king and queen's contrasting fulfilment (or, in Edward's case, neglect) of their gendered roles within the mediaeval monarchy. The chroniclers' emphasis on Isabella's fertility juxtaposes her good queenship with her husband's inappropriate actions, highlighting his flawed kingship. It shows the resentment that existed in the 1310s towards the king, based largely on his preference for his favourite, and the sympathy this inspired for his queen, Isabella.[19] In short, her pregnancy and maternity are used to demonstrate Isabella's success as a queen in chronicle narratives.

Chroniclers certainly used queenly pregnancy 'for dramatic effect' in other instances, too.[20] An oft-cited example is that of the Flemish chronicler Jean Froissart's account of Queen Philippa of Hainault's intercession with her husband, Edward III of England, to spare six burghers of Calais in

1347.[21] John Carmi Parsons has argued that Philippa probably was pregnant in 1347, but she would still have been in the very early weeks of her pregnancy and would not have been visibly pregnant when she interceded with her husband on behalf of the burghers.[22] However, according to Froissart, the queen was heavily pregnant when she pleaded at the king's feet to spare the men of Calais.[23] Froissart's exaggeration of Philippa's pregnancy serves to strengthen her influence and the appeal to her husband; Lisa Benz-St John describes how Froissart's enhanced depiction of Philippa's pregnancy 'gave her a symbolic capital that she could "spend" to give weight to her act of intercession'.[24]

Generally, chroniclers tend to associate queens with fertility and reproduction. For instance, the two queens of Alexander II of Scotland—Joan Plantagenet and Marie de Coucy—are both hardly mentioned by chroniclers; when they are, it is to report on their reproductivity. Alexander II and Joan were married for 17 years, but they were still childless in 1238 when Joan died prematurely at the age of 27.[25] Joan is barely mentioned in the contemporary chronicles that survive for thirteenth-century Scotland—namely, the *Chronicle of Melrose*, *Chronicle of Lanercost,* and the later medieval sources known as John of Fordun's *Chronica gentis scotorum*, Walter Bower's *Scotichronicon* and Andrew of Wyntoun's *Orygynale Cronykil* which preserve earlier, lost accounts from the thirteenth century.[26] For instance, Andrew of Wyntoun covered Alexander and Joan's life together in just a few lines, writing that after their wedding in England in 1221, Alexander brought Joan back to his own country, but 'he had no children with that lady. For she died after that'.[27] Scholars have previously supposed that the relative silence about Joan's queenship in the contemporary narrative sources was due to her childlessness; Jessica Nelson posited that Joan was unable to achieve influence or exercise authority in Scotland because of her failed fertility.[28] In contrast to Joan, Alexander II's second queen, Marie de Coucy, produced the longed-for son and heir within the first 2 years of her marriage to the king. However, the references to Joan and Marie in the chronicles do not clearly present one failed and one successful queen: Marie is mentioned as infrequently as Joan despite having successfully provided the king with an heir. Indeed, Andrew of Wyntoun's passages about the two queens are strikingly similar in structure and content: directly following the passage about Joan's death, Wyntoun recorded that Alexander 'took as his wife Dame Mary, Sir Ingram de Courcy's daughter. She gave him Alexander the Third, who was the next king after [Alexander II]'.[29] Whether they were childless or mothers to heirs, queens could be diminished in their reproductive achievements by chroniclers.

Theresa Earenfight writes that 'pregnancy, in and of itself, was a powerful way for a queen to establish legitimacy'.[30] Indeed, there seems to have been at least one historical medieval queen who does genuinely seem to have invented a pregnancy to maintain her authority; Violant de Bar, a late medieval queen of Aragon, pretended to be pregnant after her husband died so that she could keep her position and prevent rivals from taking power.[31] Pregnancy was significant in medieval chronicles too, and the comments about Isabella of France, Joan Plantagenet, Marie de Coucy, and Philippa of Hainault demonstrate how chroniclers drew attention to fertility and emphasised queenly pregnancies to reflect or model ideal queenship. Even in more subtle examples like that of Scottish queens Joan Plantagenet and Marie de Coucy, chroniclers discuss queens in relation to their reproductive roles. Rooted in this context, we must consider an accusation that a queen pretended to be pregnant to be a specific charge with narrative significance. The attention to fake pregnancies in medieval law sheds some light on what this significance was: legal recourse for fake pregnancies originated from gendered fear about women's ability to exploit and manipulate legitimate succession. Women could exert some control over their fate in a moment of desperation by 'pleading the belly' and the invasive examination to which they were subject in order to determine pregnancy demonstrates the societal fear that women performed pregnancy to leverage control and influence. Finally, faking a pregnancy to supply a false heir was a uniquely gendered crime which derived from the state of childlessness rather than the act of adultery; this is important for understanding the significance of the chroniclers' accusations against the two Scottish queens.

The Queens' Fake Pregnancies in Chronicles

Yolande de Dreux was Alexander III of Scotland's second wife and queen. Alexander had been married to Margaret Plantagenet for 25 years, and the couple had produced three children—two sons and a daughter—together. However, Queen Margaret died in 1275 and by 1284, all three of the couple's adult children had also died.[32] Alexander III's only surviving biological heir was his granddaughter, the daughter of the king of Norway and Alexander's daughter, Margaret.[33] The Scottish crown did have a history of passing to a brother rather than a son, like in the case of Alexander III's own grandfather, William the Lion who inherited the throne from his brother, Malcolm IV, but Alexander III had no siblings. All three of his paternal aunts had also died by 1259, and only one had produced a child, a daughter, who had died in 1237.[34] The situation facing the Scottish succession in 1284 was therefore dire, and Alexander III likely felt tremendous pressure to remarry and produce an heir to whom he could leave his throne. In order to secure the succession, in November 1285, at the age of 43, Alexander married Yolande de Dreux, the daughter of a French nobleman.[35]

Eighty years, a succession crisis and the Wars of Independence later, David II (the second Bruce king) married Margaret Logie in 1364. Like Alexander III, David had been married to an English princess for decades, but unlike his thirteenth-century predecessor, David had not produced any biological heirs with his first queen, Joan of the Tower.[36] Margaret Logie was not another foreign bride nor great diplomatic match, but a Scottish noblewoman who had been married once before and had a son with her first husband.[37] Scholars have suggested that Margaret was probably David's mistress prior to 1364, when the couple married.[38] Sir Thomas Gray, an English knight who had been imprisoned in Edinburgh in the 1350s and wrote a chronicle, reports that 'David took to wife Margaret de Logie, a lady who had been married already, and who had lived with him for some time. This marriage was made solely on account of love, which conquers all things'.[39] The Scottish chronicler Walter Bower claims that David married Margaret for lust, writing that:

> with the aim therefore of providing for the succession to the kingdom from the fruit of her womb (if God granted it), King David chose a most beautiful lady, Margaret Logie, the widow of John Logie, perhaps not so much for the excellence of her character as a woman as for the pleasure he took in her desirable appearance.[40]

Like Yolande and Alexander III's union, there was particular pressure for David and Margaret to produce an heir when they married. David II was the only living son of Robert 'the Bruce' I, and he was increasingly intent on producing his own biological heir in the 1360s.[41] Unlike Alexander III, David II had a capable heir-presumptive to whom he could leave his throne in the form of his adult nephew, Robert the Steward, son of David's elder half-sister. He was 9 years older than David, battled-hardened and with four adult sons of his own. The power struggle between David and his nephew dominated domestic politics in Scotland in the 1360s and would have decisively swung in David's favour if he had produced his own Bruce heir. The chronicler reports about fake pregnancies must be read with these succession contexts in mind, when there was exceptionally immense pressure on both Yolande and Margaret to provide heirs.

Yolande and Alexander III's marriage was short and mainly a footnote at the end of Alexander's reign, a brief episode preceding the succession crisis of the 1290s. As such, it is not unexpected that Yolande features so little in contemporary sources. The *Chronicle of Lanercost*, however, mentions Yolande de Dreux far more than in any other contemporary account. The writer recounts how Alexander III repeatedly ignored good advice to wait out a storm late one night in 1286 because he was determined to travel across the Forth from Edinburgh to be reunited with his new wife, Yolande, who was staying in Kinghorn in Fife.[42] Alexander made it safely to the town of Inverkeithing in Fife and was again advised to delay his late-night onward journey to Kinghorn because of the bad weather but he refused, and during the ride along the shore from Inverkeithing, he fell from his horse and died.[43] Before this description of the events that led to Alexander's death, the *Lanercost* chronicler claimed that Alexander's marriage to Yolande was 'to his own sadness, and to the everlasting damage of the whole kingdom'.[44] This line is followed with a description of the changeable, ambitious nature of Yolande: allegedly many people declared that before her marriage, she had pledged to become a nun but then changed her mind, 'with the readiness of a woman's heart and with ambition for a kingdom'.[45] These comments precede the description of Alexander's death, so the reader is primed to see Yolande as an unpredictable, wily and ambitious woman even before learning that Alexander III would surely have still lived if he had not been so determined to reach his wife. The chronicler implicitly blames Yolande and her womanly wiles for Alexander's untimely death, for she was the reason he was so set on making the dangerous late-night journey in the storm.

The *Lanercost* chronicler then describes that after Alexander's death, in the absence of an obvious and mature heir, his kingdom was ruled by a group of guardians. These magnates administered the kingdom and granted Yolande her rightful dower lands as Alexander's widow.[46] Yet despite this just treatment, the widowed queen,

> resorting to feminine cunning, was pretending to be pregnant, so that the guardians would postpone their decision [about who was to be Alexander's heir] and she might more easily acquire favourable public opinion for herself. But, in the way that women's craft always turns out terribly in the end, with her deceit she disturbed the land from the day of the king's death until the Feast of the Purification [Alexander died on 19 March 1286, and the Feast of the Purification was 2 February 1287], and would not allow honest women to examine her condition. And so that she could discredit those from whom she had received reverence and honour, she decided to delude the nation forever by substituting the child of another.[47]

As part of her elaborate plan, Yolande apparently arranged for a baby boy to be brought to her so she could pass him off as her own; a white marble font was made for the infant's baptism and nobles and dignitaries gathered at Stirling where Yolande was confined before the birth in a lying-in of her own arranging.[48] Thankfully (indicated by the tone of the chronicler), Yolande's trickery was uncovered by William of Buchan who revealed her scheme to all those assembled and awaiting the birth. And so 'she departed from the land with shame, first attracted by the promise of wealth from across the sea and united in marriage with a king. This is what I have to say on the fidelity of a woman'.[49] The implication from the *Lanercost* account is that producing an heir was critical for the queen to maintain influence in the wake of Alexander's unexpected death and so she invented a pregnancy in an effort to secure her otherwise uncertain future as a new, foreign, widowed queen.

Offering a different description of events than the *Chronicle of Lanercost*, other contemporary accounts suggest that the queen might really have been pregnant in 1286. A chronicle from Osney Abbey records that there was some delay in determining Alexander III's heir after his death because Yolande 'seemed to be pregnant'.[50] Walter Bower also mentions that 'it was then being said [after Alexander's death] that [Queen Yolande] was pregnant' and the Scottish magnates congregated together at Clackmannan eight months later to await the birth but the labour 'failed to take place or else there was a stillbirth'.[51] Nelson suggests that there was perhaps a real pregnancy in 1286 because there was an uprising by the Bruce family against the Balliols (two families with claims to the Scottish throne) that might imply a royal pregnancy had ended in miscarriage or stillbirth, 'throwing plans for the succession into jeopardy'.[52] Ultimately, there seems to have been contemporary confusion and uncertainty about Yolande's possible pregnancy.

In comparison with *Lanercost's* account about Yolande pretending to be pregnant, the late fifteenth-century *Liber Pluscardensis* has much less to say about Margaret Logie's fake pregnancy:

> King David set about espousing Margaret Logie, daughter of Sir Malcolm Drummond, a noble and most beautiful lady, at Inchmurthow; and he raised her to the throne with great magnificence as queen. He did not stay very long with her before again getting a divorce, because she pretended to be pregnant and was not. This was about the Feast of Fasten-Even in the year 1369.[53]

The passage follows an account of David's proposed plan to admit a son of the English king, Edward III, into the Scottish succession as his heir and his secret relief when the Scottish magnates refused to accept the deal (supposedly, he had only originally agreed to the plan because he had been Edward III's prisoner).[54] The *Liber* then praises David's kingly mercy in his treatment of nobles who rebelled against him in 1364 over his succession proposal.[55] This is immediately followed by a few lines about David and Margaret's marriage in 1364 and then the faked pregnancy and their resulting 'divorce'. The *Liber* chronicler claims that Margaret went to Rome to contest the divorce and had plans to marry the king of England (another sign of her treachery to David and Scotland) before she died in 1369. Finally, the writer of the *Liber* concludes the whole account by claiming that David had imprisoned Robert the Steward's sons because Margaret wished it, but that he quickly righted this wrong once he was free from her influence. The *Liber* declares that 'after this king David ruled his kingdom admirably' until his death in 1371.[56]

In contrast to the length and detail of the *Lanercost* comments about Yolande, the *Liber's* passage about Margaret's fake pregnancy and the end of the marriage is short and blunt. However, situated in the narrative as it is, it forms part of the juxtaposition of the characters, actions and roles of Margaret and David, which ultimately attributes the failures of David's reign to his second queen. The *Liber Pluscardensis* is a late fifteenth-century account from Pluscarden Abbey, near Elgin in north-east Scotland. The narrative is primarily an abridgement of Walter Bower's *Scotichronicon*, but the *Liber's* writer diverges from or embellishes Bower's history at several points.[57] Queen Margaret's fake pregnancy is only mentioned by the *Liber* writer and does not appear in Bower. Instead, Bower's claim that David II married Margaret for her beauty rather than her character is followed by six and a half chapters about the folly of choosing a wife for lust and how to pick a good wife, illustrating all the ways that David went wrong.[58] Bower finishes the lesson by stating that '[David] lived with [Margaret] for a short time, [but following animosity that arose between them] he divorced her about the beginning of Lent 1369'.[59] Working from Bower's narrative, the *Liber* author's account of fake pregnancy reinforces Margaret's unsuitability as both wife and queen and achieves the same outcome as Bower's wordy condemnation of marriages based on lust. The *Liber* lumps the blame for the king's imprisonment of Robert the Steward's sons *and* the royal marriage's failure on Margaret. The *Liber's* claim that Margaret pretended to be pregnant attributes the breakdown of the royal marriage (recorded by Bower too) to Margaret's reproductive failure and exclusively places the blame on the queen by accusing her of trying to substitute a false heir.

It is worth noting the singularity of both the chronicle accounts about fake pregnancies. Yolande's fake pregnancy is only mentioned by the *Lanercost* chronicle, and just the *Liber Pluscardensis* declares that Margaret and David II's marriage ended because Margaret pretended to be pregnant. The *Lanercost* chronicler was writing in the late thirteenth/early fourteenth century, and the *Liber* was composed at the end of the fifteenth century, so it could be that the later *Liber Pluscardensis* chronicler confused and misattributed the fake pregnancy from the *Lanercost* narrative to the wrong queen.[60] However, the significant difference in the texture of the accounts suggests otherwise.[61] The *Lanercost* chronicler describes

Yolande's deception in lengthy detail. He carefully works to establish her ambitious and changeable nature and her pivotal role in causing Alexander's premature death, before describing her attempt to manipulate the legitimate succession by faking a pregnancy. In contrast, the *Liber Pluscardensis* passage about fake pregnancy is short, just one line, and we are given no details beyond the fact that Margaret pretended to be pregnant and her marriage to David ended as a result. The writer of the *Liber* does not develop Margaret's sinful character in the course of the narrative and her fake pregnancy serves a very different purpose in the *Liber Pluscardensis* than the *Lanercost's* claim about Yolande. Margaret's fake pregnancy ended the royal marriage, while Yolande's pregnancy is her ultimate, immoral, and self-serving response to the instability that followed Alexander III's unexpected death in the *Lanercost* account. The marked differences between how the fake pregnancies are worked into the chronicle narratives indicate that the two accounts are distinct and intentional, rather than the result of confusion over queens by the later *Liber Pluscardensis* chronicler.

Interpreting the Fake Pregnancy Accusations

The difficulty determining pregnancy in the early stages and the imprecise understandings of the reproductive process created a unique time during pregnancy when a queen (and woman) could leverage a kind of influence using the potential of her reproductive body. Just Yolande's *declaration* that she was pregnant after Alexander III died supposedly bought her a year of influence with and support from the Scottish magnates. The desire for a Bruce heir also seems to have given Margaret Logie considerable political influence throughout the 1360s. In 1368 she confronted the Earl of Ross in Inverness over a dispute about a land grant and arranged for his arrest and the seizure of his lands.[62] Michael Penman notes that such political actions were not unusual for Margaret during her tenure as queen, and he argues that her power derived from her ability to exert pressure as 'the woman who might give [David II] a child'.[63] Societal suspicion that women could leverage pregnancy, or the potential for pregnancy, is demonstrated in the accusations of fake pregnancies in the chronicle accounts. In the narratives, the queens are portrayed as trying to exploit the power of pregnancy by faking pregnancies to control their futures in times of incredible uncertainty. There is a second layer to the chronicle accusations too: the chroniclers weaponised the power of pregnancy to blame and discredit Yolande and Margaret by claiming that both women pretended to be pregnant to secure their positions. Underpinning these accounts is the reality of diagnosing pre-modern pregnancy, especially early pregnancy, and the ambiguity and uncertainties around the possible but ultimately unknowable status of reproduction until a healthy child was born.

The *Chronicle of Lanercost* presents Yolande's calculated attempt to control her fate after Alexander's death as an unjust and ruthless response to the situation. In the narrative, not only does Yolande upset the reproductive process by failing to have a child and trying to substitute another baby as Alexander's, but she also disturbs the legal recourse for determining whether a woman was pregnant. Outlined earlier, *Bracton's* protocol for establishing if a woman was faking pregnancy required an examination by lawful, or wise and trustworthy women.[64] The *Lanercost* author explicitly mentions that Yolande would 'not allow honest women to examine her condition'.[65] The chronicle condemns Yolande not only for her plotting but also for her refusal to follow the correct legal process (which would have exposed her 'pregnancy' as a lie).

The *Lanercost's* reference to the feast of Purification adds another layer of intent to Yolande's supposed actions. The Feast of Purification was an important feast day in the medieval calendar. Falling 40 days after Christmas, it marked the purification of the Virgin Mary after Jesus's birth.[66] Like Jesus's mother, medieval women celebrated their own rite of purification, or Churching, four to six weeks after giving birth; the ritual simultaneously marked the cleansing of the sin of the female body following childbirth and celebrated maternity.[67] Importantly, the Churching, or purification ceremony, signalled a woman's reintegration into the Christian community and Church.[68] The rite was therefore a highly performative ritual which celebrated a woman's motherhood but also emphasised the liminal, outsider status of a woman before she was readmitted into her community after childbirth.[69] In the *Chronicle of Lanercost*, the discovery of Yolande's deception on the Feast of Purification seems to be a comment about her out-sider status as a new, French-born and widowed queen who concocted an elaborate scheme to gain admittance into the community and secure her position as mother of the Scottish king. Reminiscent of *Lanercost's* reference to the Feast of Purification, the *Liber Pluscardensis* also declares that Margaret Logie's attempt to pass off a fake pregnancy was discovered around the time of the Feast of Fasten-Even. Fasten-Even was a Scottish feast, also known as Beef-Brose (or broth) day, which was celebrated on Shrove Tuesday and was associated with confession and the absolution of sin in preparation for Lent.[70] The mention of it by the *Liber* seems intended to further imply the sinfulness of Margaret's deceit when she pretended to be pregnant.

The queen's sinful character is highlighted in the *Chronicle of Lanercost's* narrative too. The chronicler's emphasis of Yolande's sinfulness hinges on the medieval understanding that sin was a cause of infertility in order to blame the queen for the succession crisis. The chronicler portrays Yolande's moral failing by mentioning that she had abandoned her commitment to become a nun because of her ambition for a kingdom. He also implies that it was her sexual allure which drove Alexander to risk and lose his life by travelling late at night through a storm to reach her. These depictions of her sinful, feminine character explain why Yolande and Alexander did not produce an heir (incidentally, absolving Alexander III of any responsibility for leaving Scotland in such a situation), and thus, the narrative of faked pregnancy and queenly treachery is not only a way to illustrate the unhappy state of Scotland in 1286, but it blames Yolande personally for the lack of heir because of her innate, sinful character.

It *is* possible that the *Lanercost* chronicler was simply confused about the details of a royal pregnancy in 1286. Fiona Harris-Stoertz investigated the 'somewhat shaky notions' about the length of the gestational period in twelfth- and thirteenth-century legal sources.[71] *Bracton* concluded that an infant should be deemed illegitimate if the husband was dead, away or somehow incapacitated as much as a year before the child's birth, thus making the gestational period 52 weeks.[72] Another legal text advises a more realistic 40-week wait for a birth after a husband's death before declaring the child to be illegitimate.[73] According to the *Lanercost* chronicler, Yolande was 'pregnant' from before 19 March 1286 (the day that Alexander III died, so they could have not been together for at least a day or two before that while the king was in Edinburgh), until the Feast of Purification (2 February 1287), when her deception was uncovered before all the court assembled at Stirling. Remarkably, after 54 weeks of 'pregnancy', it was only the discerning William of Buchan—a member of the (male) Scottish elite—rather than the length of her pregnancy which alerted the gathered nobles to Yolande's plot in the *Lanercost's* account.[74] While there were varied understandings about the length of gestation, Yolande's 'pregnancy' seems incredibly long, even by *Bracton's* standard of 52 weeks. Rather than a reflection of the *Lanercost's* confusion about a royal pregnancy, the chronicler's report of Yolande's fake pregnancy is a crafted narrative which utilises concern about women's ability to manipulate the legitimate succession, derived from the actual uncertainty about pregnancy in the medieval world, to blame the isolated and foreign dowager queen for the succession crisis that would continue to plague Scotland for much of the fourteenth century.

While Yolande de Dreux might have genuinely been pregnant in 1286, the *Chronicle of Lanercost* employed the uncertainty about the queen's possible pregnancy to accuse her of exploiting (and causing) the instability that settled over Scotland in the wake of Alexander III's unexpected death. Barbaccia *et al* contend that characters in medieval and early modern literature who raised the unprovable possibility of pregnancy 'disrupt[ed] the passage of time, assumptions of inheritance, and the supposedly inevitable advance from one phase of life to the next'.[75] Yolande's fake pregnancy in the *Chronicle of Lanercost* represents the complete breakdown of order in Scotland; her transgressive actions as a woman and queen demonstrate the chaotic state of Scotland in 1286, left without a clear or able heir after Alexander's unexpected death. The description of Yolande's performance of pregnancy and the plot to substitute another baby indicate the gravity of Alexander's unexpected death without an heir. Yolande manipulated her natural reproductive role and duty as queen—to provide a legitimate heir to the throne—by pretending to be pregnant and arranging for another's child to inherit the crown of Scotland. The *Lanercost* chronicler parallels Yolande's unnatural actions with the unsettled state of Scotland, left without an heir, and rationalises the situation by blaming the deplorable character and behaviour of the queen.

According to the *Liber Pluscardensis* writer, Margaret Logie's attempt to fake a pregnancy was the reason for the breakdown of the royal marriage. We know that around 1369–70 David II seems to have been pursuing another (younger) Scottish noblewoman, Agnes Dunbar, whom he hoped to marry.[76] There is no evidence that David and Margaret Logie were actually granted a divorce (and infertility was not legal grounds for divorce in the fourteenth century), but David was increasingly concerned about producing a biological heir and his interest in Agnes Dunbar does indicate that he had given up hope of producing an heir with his second queen, Margaret, by the end of the 1360s. We have no way of knowing what caused that decision, but the *Liber* author explains it by blaming Margaret for faking a pregnancy. Pretending to be pregnant is something only a queen who believed she would never conceive an heir would attempt and Margaret's supposed fake pregnancy in the *Liber* represents this real point of change in the royal marriage, from a time of possibility and potential when there was hope for an heir and Margaret was able to exercise considerable political influence as David's consort, to the point when the marriage ended because of continued childlessness.

Significantly, a claim of fake pregnancy was a particularly gendered condemnation of the queen and her fertility which left the king's masculinity completely untarnished. Accusing a queen of adultery implicated the king's masculinity because it implied that he was beaten by another man and unable to maintain control of his wife. However, a king's manhood was not at stake if a queen pretended to be pregnant and he is left blameless in her manipulation of her reproductive role and dynastic duty to provide a legitimate heir. This is a significant part of the chronicles' comments about both Yolande and Margaret's fake pregnancies. The *Lanercost* chronicler blames the chaotic state of Scotland in 1286 specifically on Yolande but is careful not to blacken Alexander III's image. In the *Liber Pluscardensis* too, the writer depicts the failings of David II's kingship in the 1360s as Queen Margaret's fault, particularly the imprisonment of Robert the Steward's sons. Like the *Lanercost's* account about Yolande, the *Liber's* assertion that Margaret pretended to be pregnant also places the blame for childlessness solely and squarely on the queen, while at the same time redeeming David II's character and absolving him of all responsibility for bad kingship *or* the end of the marriage because of reproductive failure.

In both chronicles, the fake pregnancy serves an important narrative purpose as it communicates the treacherous nature of the queen and justifies her loss of position. Margaret's deception explains David II's real desire to end the royal marriage and marry someone else, while Yolande's selfish manipulation of her reproductive role is a gendered anecdote which illustrates the disorder in Scotland after Alexander III's death without a capable heir in 1286 and cathartically lays the blame for the situation on the new foreign queen. The fake pregnancy narratives are remarkable because they illustrate how queens could harness authority and influence from the possibility of pregnancy due to the uncertainties around knowing about pregnancy and childbirth in the Middle Ages. The chronicle accounts weaponise this influence to condemn Yolande and Margaret by accusing them of attempting to use the leverage that came from pregnancy for personal gain and to the detriment of the legitimate Scottish succession.

Conclusion

It was possible to pretend to be pregnant in the Middle Ages because of uncertainty around the reproductive process and the fact that the chroniclers make such claims against the two queens highlights the reality of discerning pregnancy—especially early pregnancy—in the Middle Ages. The risk associated with faking pregnancy and being discovered also demonstrates how difficult determining pregnancy truly was in the thirteenth and fourteenth centuries, for who would have reasonably pretended to be pregnant if there was such a great chance of losing everything if you were found out (as Yolande and Margaret's cases indicate). We can see the ambiguous understandings of reproduction in the claims of fake pregnancies, particularly in the fact that the impossibly long gestation of Yolande's 'pregnancy' did not raise any alarm bells for the Scottish magnates. Ultimately, the chroniclers' accusations against queens Yolande and Margaret preserve the suspicion that women could and would manipulate the uncertainty and ambiguities of pregnancy to serve their own purposes, to the detriment of rightful inheritance, legitimate succession and legal process.

Whether or not Yolande or Margaret really pretended to be pregnant in order to provide an heir and maintain their positions at the centre of the Scottish court, the chroniclers thought it was acceptable to make these claims about the queens. As part of their didactic purpose as historical accounts, medieval chronicle records needed to be trusted by medieval audiences.[77] As such, chroniclers took care to assure their audience of their reliability and the sources for their information.[78] Accounts like the histories kept by the *Lanercost* and *Liber* writers were only useful if they were close enough to the 'facts'. Therefore, they could only describe what might *reasonably* have happened, as far as it fell within what could be accepted as the truth by their audiences. In this respect, chronicles are particularly valuable as sources, not for their 'facts', but for their preservation and testimony of contemporary perceptions and understanding.[79] In this light, the use of fake pregnancies to explain the events of 1286 and 1369, respectively, must have been believable to medieval audiences. The chronicles do more than preserve the contemporary suspicion about women's manipulation of the reproductive process, however; the *Lanercost* and *Liber* writers demonstrate how fear about the queen's influence from her reproductive potential could be weaponised to blame and vilify a queen by accusing her of trying to leverage pregnancy.

There is an important parallel between Yolande de Dreux in 1286 and Margaret Logie in the late 1360s which underpins the chroniclers' accusations that the queens attempted to perform pregnancy for personal gain. Yolande was the last queen of Scotland before the succession crisis in the 1290s and the Wars of Independence, which devastated Scotland and saw the Bruce family ascend to the throne. At the other end of the time spectrum, the Wars of Independence ended in David II's reign, and he died in 1371 without ever producing a Bruce heir; his crown passed to the Stewarts, through Robert 'the Bruce' I's eldest daughter's line. In this case, David's second queen, Margaret Logie, was the last queen in a period when the Scottish succession had been especially precarious. Failures of royal fertility bookended this period of deep upheaval in Scottish history, and the specific implications of a fake pregnancy—a uniquely gendered crime by a queen who manipulated the legitimate succession because she had failed to produce a rightful royal heir— highlight the heightened fear, instability and hope, which existed around the succession in Scotland in the fourteenth century. This uncertainty about royal inheritance and real nervousness about the succession is representative of Scottish history between 1286 and the late fourteenth century; this is captured and productively employed by the chroniclers in their accounts about the first and last queens of this period pretending to be pregnant.

Notes

1 Fiona Harris-Stoertz, "Pregnancy and Childbirth in Twelfth- and Thirteenth-Century French and English Law," *Journal of the History of Sexuality* 21, no. 2 (May 2012): 263–81. However, there is no mention of fake pregnancy in the *Regiam Majestatem*, the medieval compendium of Scots law; see Thomas Cooper, ed., *Regiam Majestatem and Quaniam Attachiamenta: Based on the Text of Sir John Skene* (Edinburgh: Stair Society, 1947).

2 Harris-Stoertz, "Pregnancy and Childbirth," 266. This distrust of mothers appears in laws concerning abortions and infanticide and in the emergence of legislation that addressed substituted children and faked pregnancies.

3 Hearing the heir cry is also cited in the *Regiam Majestatem*, Book II, cap. 58, no. 1, p. 168: '*si ex eadem haeredem habuerit auditum, vel brayantem inter quatuor parietes*' ('if by her he has an heir who lives long enough to be heard crying within four walls'). On hearing the infant cry, see Gwen Seabourne, "It Is Necessary That the Issue Be Heard to Cry or Squall Within the Four [Walls]: Qualifying for Tenancy by the Curtesy of England in the Reign of Edward I," *The Journal of Legal History* 40, no. 1 (2019): 44–68.

4 *Bracton* does not make a distinction, but this level of scrutiny and the resulting legal protocol were likely reserved for higher status women because of concerns about rightful inheritance in the Middle Ages.

5 *Bracton*, vol. 2, 201–4. Harris-Stoertz adds that if it was found that the woman was not pregnant, she would be imprisoned or fined, Harris-Stoertz, "Pregnancy and Childbirth," 277.

6 Harris-Stoertz, "Pregnancy and Childbirth," 277, notes that men had equal reason to wish to substitute fake heirs.

7 Sara M. Butler, "More Than Mothers: Juries of Matrons and Pleas of the Belly in Medieval England," *Law and History Review* 37, no. 2 (May 2019): 353–96.

8 Holly Barbaccia, Bethany Packard, and Jane Wanninger, "Maybe Baby: Pregnant Possibilities in Medieval and Early Modern Literature," in *Gendered Temporalities in the Early Modern World*, ed. M. E. Wiesner-Hanks (Amsterdam: Amsterdam University Press, 2018), 216; 231–32.

9 Barbaccia et al., "Maybe Baby," 216.

10 Butler, "More Than Mothers," 364–68.

11 Harris-Stoertz, "Pregnancy and Childbirth," 277.

12 Pauline Stafford, "Ælfgifu of Northampton," *ODNB*, published September 23, 2004. Harris-Stoertz, "Pregnancy and Childbirth," 278. There is a visual reference to this in the Bayeux Tapestry. See Patricia Stephenson, "Where a Cleric and Ælfgyva . . .," in *The Bayeux Tapestry: New Approaches: Proceedings of a Conference at the British Museum*, eds. Michael J. Lewis et al. (Oxford: Oxbow Books, 2011), 71–74.

13 Diana E. S. Dunn, "Margaret of Anjou," *ODNB*, published September 23, 2004; Kristen Geaman, "A Bastard and a Changeling? England's Edward of Westminster and Delayed Childbirth," in *Unexpected Heirs in Early Modern Europe: Potential Kings and Queens*, ed. Valerie Schutte (Basingstoke: Palgrave McMillan, 2017), 15–17.

14 Peggy McCracken, "The Body Politic and the Queen's Adulterous Body in French Romance," in *Feminist Approaches to the Body in Medieval Literature*, eds. Linda Lomperis and Sarah Stanbury (Philadelphia: University of Pennsylvania Press, 1993), 44.

15 McCracken, "The Body politic," 46–47.

16 *Flores Historiarum*, ed. Henry R. Luard (London: Rolls Series, 1890), iii, 176: '*domina Isabella regina, gemino flore decorate, apud Eltham in Cantia, quinto decimo die mensis Augusti, domino regi filium peperit secundum, . . . Ante ortum hujus regalis propaginis, qua dicta regina nobiliter exstitit prole foecunda*'.

17 Lisa Benz St John, *Three Medieval Queens: Queenship and the Crown in Fourteenth-Century England* (New York: Palgrave Macmillan, 2012), 2–3.

18 'Johannis de Trokelowe Annales," in *Johannis de Trokelowe et Henrici de Blaneforde chronica et annales*, ed. Henry Thomas Riley (London: Rolls Series,

1866), 75, claims that the king decided to go to Newcastle, not thinking of the risk, 'nor the weeping queen, then pregnant' (*'nec fletibus Reginae, tunc praegnantis'*) so that he could be with Piers Gaveston. The author of these annals (spanning 1307–1327) is now thought to be William Rishanger, and Trokelowe his scribe.

19 Emma Trivett, "It Was Greatly Feared That the Queen Was Barren': Perceptions and Management of Royal Fertility in Thirteenth- and Fourteenth-Century England and Scotland" (unpublished, Ph.D. thesis, University of Edinburgh, 2021), 50–56.

20 Theresa Earenfight, *Queenship in Medieval Europe* (London: Palgrave McMillan, 2013), 7.

21 Jean Froissart, *Oeuvres de Froissart*, ed. Kervyn de Lettenhove (Brussels, 1867–1877), vol. 5, 215.

22 John Carmi Parsons, "The Pregnant Queen as Counsellor and the Medieval Construction of Motherhood," in *Medieval Mothering*, eds. John Carmi Parsons and Bonnie Wheeler (New York: Garland Publishing, 1996), 40–41. See also Paul Strohm, "Queens as Intercessors," in *Hochon's Arrow: The Social Imagination of Fourteenth-Century Texts* (Princeton: Princeton University Press, 1992), 102–3.

23 *Froissart*, vol. 5, 215.

24 Benz St John, *Three Medieval Queens*, 54.

25 Jessica Nelson, "Queens and Queenship in Scotland, Circa 1067–1286" (unpublished, Ph.D. thesis, King's College University of London, 2006), 182.

26 Trivett, "It Was Greatly Feared That the Queen Was Barren," 56–60.

27 Andrew of Wyntoun, *The orygynale cronykil of Scotland*, ed. David Laing (Edinburgh: Edmonston and Douglas, 1872–79), ii, 238: 'on that lady na barne he gate./Fra scho ded wes, efftyre that.' Wyntoun does mention Joan again, briefly. He describes that Alexander and Joan's union brought stability to Scotland, stating that 'all was quiet, settled, and peaceful. For [Henry III and Alexander] were two kings of peace.' Joan was crucial in maintaining this peaceful relationship: 'there was the Queen, this Alexander's wife, this Henry's sister: without her, strife.' See *Wyntoun*, ii, 239, 243.

28 Nelson, "Queens and Queenship," 164–89.

29 *Wyntoun*, ii, 238: 'To wyff he weddyt Dame Mary, Schyr Ingramys dowchtyr de Cowcy. Alysandyr the thryd on hyr he gat, nest hym that Kyng wes efftyr that.'

30 Earenfight, *Queenship*, 7.

31 Ibid.

32 Norman Reid, *Alexander III, 1249–1286: First Among Equals* (Edinburgh: John Donald, 2019), 340–41.

33 Ibid.

34 Richard Oram, *Alexander II: King of Scots, 1214–1249* (Edinburgh: Birlinn, 2012), 152, 216.

35 Nelson, "Queens and Queenship," 254.

36 Michael Penman, *David II, 1329–71* (East Linton: Tuckwell, 2004), 204.

37 Penman, *David II*, 247–48.

38 Ibid., 269.

39 *Sir Thomas Gray's Scalacronica*, ed., Maxwell, 174.

40 Walter Bower, *Scotichronicon*, ed. D. E. R. Watt (Aberdeen: Aberdeen University Press,1987–1998), vii, 332: *Volens igitur rex David previdere pro successione regni de fructu ventris sui, si Deus dederit, elegit unam speciossimam*

dominam, Margaritam Logy relictam [Johannis Logy], forte non tam bonitate virtutis feminee quam voluptate forme appertitive;' [. . .].

41 Trivett, "It Was Greatly Feared That the Queen Was Barren," 91–101.

42 *Chronicon de Lanercost*, ed. Joseph Stevenson (Edinburgh: Bannatyne Club, 1839), 116–17.

43 Ibid., 116.

44 Ibid., 114: *'sibi in dolerem et toti provinciae in damnum perpetuum'*.

45 *Chronicon de Lanercost*, 116: *'sed facilitate cordis feminei et ambitu regni retro respexisse'*.

46 *Chronicon de Lanercost*, 117: *'dominae reginae, relictae Alexandri, pro sua tertia protionem assignantes.'*

47 *Chronicon de Lanercost*, 117–18: *'At illa, astu femineo usa, impregnatam esse mentiebatur, ut suspensos animo redderet patriotas, et sibi favorem populi procliviorem faceret. Sed, quoniam semper mulieris versutia miserum vertit in exitum, cum solitasset terram suis simulationibus a die mortis regis usque ad festum Purificationis [Fe. 2, 1287], nec matronas admitteret honestas ad discernendum suum statum, ut ignominiam retribueret his a quibus receperat reverentiam et honorem, statuit perpetuo deludere populum supponendo sibi partum alienum.'*

48 *Chronicon de Lanercost*, 118: *'Fontem novum extrui fecit de marmore candido'* ('a new font was made of white marble').

49 *Chronicon de Lanercost*, 118, *'Sic recessit a terra cum verecundia, qui prius intuitu tantum eleemosinae de transmarinis adducta et associata est regi copulae. Hoc dixerim pro fide feminarum. . .'*

50 "Annales Monasterii de Osenia," in *Annales Monastici*, ed. Henry R. Luard (1869), vol. 4, 306; Nelson, "Queens and Queenship," 258.

51 Bower, *Scotichronicon*, vi, 10–11. *'Quo die ibidem congregabantur custodes regni quia eo tunc dicebatur reginam. Joletam sive Jolandam impregnasse, ad cuius fetum producendum et visendum expectabant.'*

52 Nelson, "Queens and Queenship," 259. Nelson relies on A.A.M. Duncan for this suggestion: A. A. M. Duncan, *The Kingship of the Scots, 842–1292: Succession and Independence* (Edinburgh: Edinburgh University Press, 2002), 178.

53 *Liber Pluscardensis*, ed. Frederick Skene (1877), i, 307: *'Hiis itaque stabilitis, disposuit se rex David ad disponsandum Margaretam de Logi, filiam domini Malcolmi de Drummond, nobilem [et] pulcerrimam dominam, apud Enchemarthow; et in reginam magnifice exaltavit. Sed cum ea non tempore multo perduravit quin iterum divorcium celebravit, eo quod ipsa impregnatam finxit et non fuit; et hoc circa festum Carnis Brevii, anno Domini M.CC.LXIX.'* English translation by Skene, *Liber Pluscardensis*, ii, 233.

54 *Liber Pluscardensis*, i, 305–6.

55 Ibid., 306: *'Sed tamen, considerate causa, propter distruccionem patriae et alias multas inconveniencias et dampna sequenda, rex, qui clemens et misericors erat, micius cum eis agendo, eidem hac vice misericorditer remisit, attendens quod magnae nobilitatis est regi miserere cum ulcisci poterit.'* ('But, thinking over the matter, and because of the destruction of the country and many other troubles and losses that would follow, the king, who was kind and merciful, dealt with them mildly, mercifully giving them this time, thinking that it is more noble for a king to have mercy when he could have revenge.')

56 *Liber Pluscardensis*, i, 307, *'Post hoc autem rex David regnum suum optime rexit'*.

57 On the fourteenth- and fifteenth-century Scottish chronicles and their connections, see Marjorie Drexler, "The Extant Abridgements of Walter Bower's 'Scotichronicon'," *The Scottish Historical Review* 61, no. 171 (1982): 63–64; Sally Mapstone, "Older Scots Literature and the Court," in *The Edinburgh History of Scottish Literature: From Columba to the Union (Until 1707)*, eds. Ian Brown et al. (Edinburgh: Edinburgh University Press, 2007), 273–85.

58 Bower, *Scotichronicon*, vii, 332–59.

59 Ibid., 358: "*cum qua parvo tempore habitavit, et [sed propter quasdam simultates inter eos conceptas] divorcium celebravit.*" The inserted section is only included in one extant manuscript.

60 It is worth noting that there are no indications that the *Chronicle of Lanercost* was known to the later writer of the *Liber Pluscardensis*. On the composition of the chronicles, see Christine McGladdery, "Liber Pluscardensis," in *Encyclopedia of the Medieval Chronicle*, eds. Graeme Dunphy and Cristian Bratu (Leiden: Brill, 2010). Antonia Gransden, *Historical Writing in England: c. 550 to c. 1307* (London: Routledge & Kegan Paul, 1974), 494–501.

61 There is also no evidence that the Pluscarden author knew of or consulted the *Chronicle of Lanercost*.

62 Penman, *David II*, 364.

63 Ibid.

64 Although Yolande was Queen of Scotland, the *Chronicle of Lanercost* was a northern English chronicle, hence the use of *Bracton* for this analysis. The practices involving examination by honest women outlined in *Bracton* were also used in other countries in the Middle Ages. See Butler, "More than Mothers," 356–61. Similar language also appears in a miracle of St Margaret of Scotland: A women's long-dead fetus was delivered with the help of the saint and 'devout and respectable women'. See Robert Bartlett, ed. and trans., *Miracles of Saint Æbbe of Coldingham and Saint Margaret of Scotland* (Oxford: Clarendon Press, 2003), 80–83; Harris-Stoerz, "Pregnancy and Childbirth," 277: This practice is also mentioned in the *Britton* and the *Fleta* law books and was standard protocol for establishing things like whether a woman had sexual intercourse, or whether a man was impotent.

65 *Chronicon de Lanercost*, 118: '*nec matronas admitteret honestas ad discernendum suum statum.*'

66 Roberta Gilchrist, *Medieval Life: Archaeology and the Life Course* (Woodbridge: Boydell & Brewer, 2012), 171. Gail McMurray Gibson, "Blessings From Sun and Moon: Churching as Women's Theatre," in *Bodies and Disciplines: Intersections of Literature and History in Fifteenth-Century England*, eds., Barbara Hanawalt and David Wallace (Minneapolis, MN, 1996), 139–54.

67 Gilchrist, *Medieval Life*, 182.

68 Ibid.

69 Ibid., 182–84. My thanks to Dr Rachel M. Davis for highlighting the significance of this feast in the *Lanercost* narrative.

70 See *Dictionaries of the Scots Language*, accessed November 11, 2021, https://www.dsl.ac.uk/entry/snd/beef.

71 Harris-Stoerz, "Pregnancy and Childbirth," 270, the thirteenth-century text *Britton* was based on *Bracton*, as was the *Fleta*, which was also from the thirteenth century but a less popular text than *Britton*.

72 Harris-Stoerz, "Pregnancy and Childbirth," 280.

73 *Britton*, see Harris-Stoertz, "Pregnancy and Childbirth," 280.
74 It is also interesting to note that 'William of Buchan' is either a confusion for the contemporary earl of Buchan, named Alexander, or a fictional character invented by the *Lanercost* chronicler. See Nelson, "Queens and Queenship," 260 for the suggestion that 'William' was confused with 'Alexander'.
75 Barbaccia et al., "Maybe Baby," 232.
76 Penman, *David II*, 271, 373–74, for David's plans to marry Agnes Dunbar in 1369.
77 Chris Given-Wilson, *Chronicles: The Writing of History in Medieval England* (London: Bloomsbury, 2007), 65–78.
78 Elisabeth Van Houts, *Memory and Gender in Medieval Europe, 900–1200* (Basingstoke: MacMillan, 1999), 21; Given-Wilson, *Chronicles*, 1–20.
79 Strohm, *Hochon's Arrow*, 4.

Reference List

Primary Sources

"Annales Monasterii de Osenia." In *Annales Monastici*, edited by Henry R. Luard, vol. 4. London: Longman, Green, Longman, Roberts and Green, 1869.
Bower, Walter. *Scotichronicon*. 9 vols. Edited by D. E. R. Watt. Aberdeen: Aberdeen University Press, 1987–98.
Bracton, H. *On the Laws and Customs of England*. Edited by George Woodbine and Translated by Samuel E. Thorne. 4 vols. Cambridge, MA: Belknap Press, 1968.
Chronicon de Lanercost. Edited by Joseph Stevenson. Edinburgh: Bannatyne Club, 1839.
Cooper, Thomas. *Regiam Majestatem and quoniam attachiamenta*. Edinburgh: Stair Society, 1947.
Flores Historiarum. Edited by Henry R. Luard. 3 vols. London: Rolls Series, 1890.
Froissart, Jean. *Oeuvres de Froissart*. 24 vols. Edited by Kervyn de Lettenhove. Brussels: V. Devaux, 1867–1877.
"Johannis de Trokelowe Annales." In *Johannis de Trokelowe et Henrici de Blaneforde chronica et annales*. Edited by Henry Thomas Riley. London: Rolls Series, 1866.
Liber Pluscardensis. Edited by Frederick Skene. 2 vols. Edinburgh: William Paterson, 1877–1880.
Maxwell, Herbert. *Sir Thomas Gray's Scalacronica*. Glasgow: MacLehose & Sons, 1907.
Wyntoun, Andrew of. *The orygynale cronykil of Scotland*. Edited by David Laing. 3 vols. Edinburgh: Edmonston and Douglas, 1872–79.

Secondary sources

Barbaccia, Holly, Bethany Packard, and Jane Wanninger. "Maybe Baby: Pregnant Possibilities in Medieval and Early Modern Literature." In *Gendered Temporalities in the Early Modern World*, edited by M. E. Wiesner-Hanks, 213–34. Amsterdam: Amsterdam University Press, 2018.

Bartlett, Robert, ed. and transl. *Miracles of Saint Æbbe of Coldingham and Saint Margaret of Scotland*. Oxford: Clarendon Press, 2003.

Benz St John, Lisa. *Three Medieval Queens: Queenship and the Crown in Fourteenth-Century England*. New York: Palgrave MacMillan, 2012.

Butler, Sara M. "More Than Mothers: Juries of Matrons and Pleas of the Belly in Medieval England." *Law and History Review* 37, no. 2 (May 2019): 353–96.

Drexler, Marjorie. "The Extant Abridgements of Walter Bower's 'Scotichronicon'." *The Scottish Historical Review* 61, no. 171 (1982): 62–67.

Duncan, A. A. M. *The Kingship of the Scots, 842–1292: Succession and Independence*. Edinburgh: Edinburgh University Press, 2002.

Earenfight, Theresa. *Queenship in Medieval Europe*. London: Palgrave McMillan, 2013.

Geaman, Kristen. "A Bastard and a Changeling? England's Edward of Westminster and Delayed Childbirth." In *Unexpected Heirs in Early Modern Europe: Potential Kings and Queens,* edited by Valerie Schutte, 11–33. Basingstoke: Palgrave Macmillan, 2017.

Gibson, Gail McMurray. "Blessings From Sun and Moon: Churchings as Women's Theatre." In *Bodies and Disciplines: Intersections of Literature and History in Fifteenth-Century England,* edited by Barbara Hanawalt and David Wallace, 139–54. Minneapolis: University of Minnesota Press, 1996.

Gilchrist, Roberta. *Medieval Life: Archaeology and the Life Course*. Woodbridge: Boydell & Brewer, 2012.

Given-Wilson, Chris. *Chronicles: The Writing of History in Medieval England*. London: Bloomsbury, 2007.

Gransden, Antonia. *Historical Writing in England: c. 550 to c. 1307*. London: Routledge & Kegan Paul, 1974.

Harris-Stoertz, Fiona. "Pregnancy and Childbirth in Twelfth and Thirteenth-Century French and English Law." *Journal of the History of Sexuality* 21, no. 2 (May 2012): 263–81.

Mapstone, Sally. "Older Scots Literature and the Court." In *The Edinburgh History of Scottish Literature: From Columba to the Union (Until 1707),* edited by Ian Brown, Thomas Clancy, Susan Manning, and Murray Pittock, 273–85. Edinburgh: Edinburgh University Press, 2007.

McCracken, Peggy. "The Body Politic and the Queen's Adulterous Body in French Romance." *Feminist Approaches to the Body in Medieval Literature,* edited by Linda Lomperis and Sarah Stanbury, 38–64. Philadelphia: University of Pennsylvania Press, 1993.

McGladdery, Christine. "Liber Pluscardensis." In *Encyclopedia of the Medieval Chronicle,* edited by Graeme Dunphy and Cristian Bratu. Leiden: Brill, 2010.

Nelson, Jessica. "Queens and Queenship in Scotland, Circa 1067–1286." Ph.D. thesis, King's College University of London, 2006.

Oram, Richard. *Alexander II: King of Scots, 1214–1249*. Edinburgh: Birlinn, 2012.

Parsons, John Carmi. "The Pregnant Queen as Counsellor and the Medieval Construction of Motherhood." In *Medieval Mothering,* edited by John Carmi Parsons and Bonnie Wheeler. New York: Garland Publishing, 1996.

Penman, Michael. *David II, 1329–71*. East Linton: Tuckwell, 2004.

Reid, Norman. *Alexander III, 1249–1286: First Among Equals*. Edinburgh: John Donald, 2019.

Seabourne, Gwen. "It Is Necessary That the Issue Be Heard to Cry or Squall Within the Four [Walls]': Qualifying for Tenancy by the Curtesy of England in the Reign of Edward I." *The Journal of Legal History* 40, no. 1 (2019): 44–68.

Stephenson, Patricia. "Where a Cleric and Ælfgyva . . ." In *The Bayeux Tapestry: New Approaches: Proceedings of a Conference at the British Museum*, edited by Michael J. Lewis, Gale R. Owen-Crocker, and Dan Terkla, 71–74. Oxford: Oxbow Books, 2011.

Strohm, Paul. *Hochon's Arrow: The Social Imagination of Fourteenth-Century Texts*. Princeton: Princeton University Press, 1992.

Trivett, Emma. "'It Was Greatly Feared That the Queen Was Barren': Perceptions and Management of Royal Fertility in Thirteenth- and Fourteenth-century England and Scotland." Ph.D. thesis, University of Edinburgh, 2021.

Van Houts, Elisabeth. *Memory and Gender in Medieval Europe, 900–1200*. Basingstoke: MacMillan, 1999.

6 Feigning Madness
The Case of William Hawkyns, 1552 London

Wendy J. Turner

In 1996, I found a curious reference in the *Calendar of State Papers: Domestic* for Edward VI that referenced a man who "feigned himself mad". The communication was about a man of no historic consequence, William Hawkyns, who might have concocted madness-like symptoms to avoid the death penalty for treason—or so it seemed. There was a strange item near the end in what the editors called a "holograph", which normally indicates a note added after the signature in the handwriting of the author of the letter rather than in the scribe's hand. When I examined the actual letter, the whole was in the handwriting of the Duke of Northumberland, John Dudley, the king's regent, and the note was a comment he added as a hastily written postscript.[1] Astonishingly both to contemporaries and to me, William Hawkyns, pretended to be *"frenticus"*, a frantic, and was subsequently committed to the Tower. How does one pretend for a year or more, to have uncontrolled physical motions as well as mental health symptoms? Why would he do such a thing? Or was he actually mentally ill? These are likely unanswerable questions, but this chapter explores the story of William Hawkyns, the charges against him, whether he might have been mentally ill, and the relationship of his actions to the socio-political climate of London at the time.

There is a temptation to confuse William Hawkyns with another of the same name, the father of John Hawkins, who became a hero in the battle against the Spanish Armada. This other Hawkyns family, however, is from Plymouth, not London. The Plymouth William Hawkyns was named in records associated with former monastic lands doled out by Henry VIII to William FitzWilliam, the Lord Keeper of the Privy Seal.[2] And, while those Hawkynses were not yet gentry or nobility in society, they did benefit indirectly alongside several other families from these former monastic lands. The London William Hawkyns of the present study, though, was a schoolteacher, residing somewhere near Fleet Street, likely east of the Fleet River inside the old city walls.

DOI: 10.4324/9781003452324-9

William "Kept A Schole"

Among the State Papers is the letter mentioned earlier from John Dudley, Duke of Northumberland (recently named Regent), to Sir William Cecil dated 27 October 1552. It concerns William Hawkyns, who "kept a school about St. Bartholomew's",[3] providing a clue as to where he may have resided or where he worked. St Bartholomew "the Great" is most likely *the* St Bartholomew meant here since no other could have been referenced without an epithet ("the Less" or "by the Exchange"). Several schools were in the area around St Bartholomew's Church, which, with its surrounding support buildings including its own medieval foundation cathedral school, bordered "Schmyt Fyeld" (Smithfield).

It is not likely that Hawkyns worked at the cathedral, or the record would have stated he worked "at" instead of *near* ("about") St Bartholomew's. There were, however, other educational institutions in the area at that time, only streets away, including several charity schools, all still small and quite unorganized at this time: St Bride Fleet Street School,[4] St Andrew Holborn School, St Giles-Cripplegate School (which later would be called St Giles "without" Cripplegate),[5] St Sepulchre Holborn School,[6] and Christ's Hospital (school), which was in the old Greyfriars monastery.[7]

This last school, and several of the others, have foundation dates of a year or two *after* Hawkyns was arrested, but they may have begun earlier with less formality. Greyfriars Monastery in Farringdon on Newgate Street, dissolved in 1538, was used for a variety of purposes until it was given to the city of London at the end of 1547 following the death of Henry VIII. In 1553, London made it a charity school for "orphans", children without fathers or without either parent, and changed the name to Christ's Hospital. Christ's Hospital was one of the original "Blue Coat Schools", so named since all the children wore blue robes (later blue coats). Hawkyns could have been on the teaching staff there before the name change. St Giles Cripplegate School—later "-without-Cripplegate" and now inside the Barbican—dates from 1527. It was not far from St Bartholomew's, much like St Sepulchre Holborn Charity School, which sat southwest of St Bartholomew's Hospital on the north side of the Holborn Viaduct. Those lands were originally part of the Priory of St Bartholomew as early as 1137 where a pre-Norman church was founded and dedicated to St Edmund the King and Martyr.[8] If it was this school, it seems more likely the letter would have said "near Cripplegate" or "at St. Giles" since both of those landmarks were well recognized. As it is, the letter said "about St. Bartholomew's" likely meaning that Hawkyns taught at a small private school somewhere between St Sepulcher and St Bartholomew, east of the Fleet River, and in the general area of Smithfield. Most importantly, the record established him as an educated man by acknowledging him as a teacher.

The letter from Dudley to Cecil also mentions that Hawkyns brought an "idea [and] was also once before the councell for a matter at Flete Brydge".[9] This might mean that he met some of the Council members near or at the bridge about his "idea". Or it could indicate that he had ideas about the bridge, which he likely lived near, and that he had spoken to someone on the Council about his concerns, perhaps also "appearing" before the Council with his "idea" or on another matter. Concerns about the bridge are completely plausible, as the bridge needed periodic repairs or rebuilding. The Fleet Bridge, originally the Ponte de Fleete, spanned the Fleet River between Fleet Street and Ludgate Hill near Fleet Prison and seems to have been one of the locations in London where people of all levels met socially, conducted business, and discussed politics. These sorts of interactions might have provided Hawkyns the access to a member of the Council. The merchant-tailor, Henry Machyn, provides insight into interactions at the Fleet Bridge in his diary.

> The xxj day of Marche [1552,] dyd ryd thrugh Lo[ndon on horseb]ake ij yonge feylles boyth of on horse [*two young fellows, both on one horse*], and on[e of them] carehyng a spytt up ryght and a duke rostyd [*a roasted duck*], and . . . Nugatt [Newgate], and ther they alyth [left] of ther horse . . . and the duke [duck] at Nugatt, and so was led with the . . . begers thrugh Flett lane with many pepull won . . . to the Rose at the Flet bryge, the taverne wher . . . to have hetten yt [*eaten it*] there, and I left them ther, and [came to] the court to dener [*dinner*; the courtyard of Machyn's house]; one of them dwellt at the Sun.[10]

This relatively innocent meeting at the Rose Tavern near Fleet Bridge is illustrative of all the different people who gathered there—a merchant-tailor, the two young men with their horse and duck, the beggars, and many others. The bridge was also a place where people passing pushed bread and other food in through the prison bars for those inside, or where miscreants met one another unnoticed among the crowd. For example, in 1556 just 4 years after Machyn's account, William Hinnes confessed to having illicit business dealings with several men at both Fleet Bridge and Greenwich, which seems to have been connected by the Thames as a highway of information, goods, and politics. Hinnes said that he met a man named Bethell (or Bedell) "at Fleet Bridge" and at Greenwich for conversations about a man named John Benbow of Chapel Royal, who apparently stole shovels, spades, and poles as well as an 80-ton ship. Hinnes "[r]eported [the] landing of certain English gentlemen in the West of England", and also confessed to having dealings with John Dethicke, who had alchemical skill, and they planned to take foreign coins, "*ealdergylders*", and try to turn them into gold. The papers end with a confession by another man, Thomas White, who says that he introduced Dethicke to Hinnes and that they both knew about his "plot for seizing the treasure in custody of Brigham, a Teller of the Exchequer, and for killing the Queen and King".[11] If William Hawkyns had met with one or more Council members about "a matter at Flete Brydge" and been encouraged to bring other ideas, even speaking before the whole Council, perhaps he felt welcomed among a social status where he did not generally belong. Nothing more was written about Hawkyns' life or his surroundings until he tried to meet with the king in Greenwich.

The Council members were charged to protect the king at all times after a string of individuals attempted to see, accost, or even kidnap the young king. The most dramatic event was in January 1349 when Edward the young king was 11 years old. John Fowler, a member of the privy chamber, later confessed "to his being urged by the Lord Admiral [Thomas Seymour] to procure the King's opinion as to his marriage" to the king's sister, Elizabeth, and to bribing the king.[12] Thomas Seymour wanted to secure his position at court. He had married Katherine Parr, the last wife of Henry VIII, but she died on 5 September 1548. Then, on 16 January 1549, Thomas Seymour—Admiral of England, King Edward VI's uncle and brother to Edward Seymour, Duke of Northumberland and Regent—tried to kidnap Edward VI from his bedchamber. Thomas broke into the king's rooms, which alerted the dog. When the king's spaniel began barking, Thomas shot the dog.[13] The incident was reported by François van der Delft, the imperial ambassador, to his Emperor later in January 1549 as a shocking event, writing,

> the Admiral of England . . . attempted to outrage the person of the young King by night. . . . The alarm was given by the gentleman who sleeps in the King's chamber, who, awakened by the barking of the dog . . ., cried out 'Help! Murder!' Everybody rushed in.[14]

Thomas Seymour confessed to having told his plans to John Fowler, saying that:

> if he might have the king in his custodie as Mr. Pag[et] had[,] he wolde be glad, and that he thought a man might bring him through the gallery to his chamber and so to his howse, . . . meaning no hurte [to the king].[15]

Lawyers argued that this was high treason, and Thomas was executed in March 1549.

While Thomas Seymour had the power and finances to woo the king into his confidence, and he then later attempted secretly to take charge of the king's person, others without authority were rioting across England. The social unrest of 1548 led to a string of armed revolts in 1549. Religious grievances fueled these uprisings as much as economic ones. Commoners angered by landlords who flagrantly disregarded enclosure laws, using common grazing ground as if it was their property and allowing sheep to eat on other common lands or in towns, rose only to confront royal soldiers. The popular view was that Edward Seymour, Duke of Somerset, Lord Protector of the Realm, and Governor of the King's Person, sympathized with the rebels because of his sometimes-liberal sounding and often disorganized and uncoordinated proclamations concerning the Church, land, and coinage issues. He angered the gentry and his fellow magnates. The growing dissatisfaction with his leadership caused the Council to turn to Somerset's rival, John Dudley. In his scheming to regain his power base and overthrow Dudley, the Council found King Edward's uncle, Edward Seymour, guilty of treason. They removed him from office and later executed him for his crimes in January 1552, just as the new *Book of Common Prayer* and new Act of Supremacy were announced, and William Hawkyns entered recorded history.[16]

Further exacerbating this story is the spread of a new disease in 1548, the so-called Sweating Sickness, which continued until the summer of 1551. This mystery disease, likely a type of hantavirus, had symptoms that came on suddenly and many victims actually died before the day was out.[17] The English Sweat might be one reason why so few uprisings happened in 1550; people avoided going out, hoping to avoid this dreaded disease as well as plague outbreaks (Black Death) and smallpox. The spread of the "Sweat" also set the public and the Council members on edge as they tried to protect the king from risking his health at public engagements or contact with anyone outside their small circle.

Even with all his protection, the king's location was known by William Hawkyns and most other people on any given day. Henry Machyn notes the king's movements regularly, along with (helpfully) pointing out cases of the English Sweat or plague, to explain why the king leaves this location or that. For example, on July 6, 1551,

> the Kynges grace rod thrugh Grenwyche parke unto Blake heth [*Black Heath*, on the edge of Greenwich], and my lord of Darbe, and [several other people . . .] and the same night the Kyng suppyd at Depforth [*Deptford*] in a shype [*ship*] with my lord Admyral, [and the lords] of the conselle, and with many gentylmen.[18]

The very next day, Machyn writes that there:

> begane a nuw swet in London, and . . . ded [*dead*] my lord Crumwell in Leseter-shyre, and was bered [*buried*] [with a stand]ard, a baner of

armes, and cote, elmett, sword, targett, and sc[ochyons, and] harold; and the sam tyme ded my lord Powes, and the x day [at W]ollwyche, sir John Lutterell, knyght, a nobull captayne.

The Council grew concerned for the health and safety of the king, and themselves, and the court withdrew from Westminster Palace to Hampton Court on 10 July.[19] The king finally emerged from Hampton Court in August for the installation of new members to the Order of the Garter at Windsor. This is to say that 1551 and 1552 not only saw uprisings and troubles among the Council members, but there was also a resurgence of plague and the new disease of the English Sweat at the same time. The king was often kept outside of the London area in palaces and castles such as Hampton Court and Greenwich. And just like Henry Machyn, merchant-tailor, knows the king's whereabouts, so does everyone else, including William Hawkyns.

Edward VI may have been in London for Easter, 1552. His sister, Elizabeth, rode through London to the King's Palace on 17 March and was again spotted in St James' Park on 19 March.[20] Then, Edward made a public appearance on Saint George's Day (April 28) at Westminster Cathedral where he wore his robes of the Garter and proceeded inside for evensong. On April 30, though, the king left London for Greenwich early in the morning. William Hawkyns attempted to speak to the king "about Easter last or possibly after"[21] and John Dudley barred Hawkyns' entrance. The record does not say if Hawkyns was arrested on the spot, held and released and later incarcerated again, or if he was allowed to leave but was arrested and held at a later time.

William "Putt Upp A Byll to the Kinge"

In mid-April 1552, William Hawkyns attempted to speak "alone" with the 14-year-old King Edward VI on the topic of "a bill" he wished to put forward.[22] While the contents and subject matter of what Hawkyns proposed are unknown, it is likely it dealt with religion, perhaps an alternative or a dispensation for those wanting to worship in other ways. Religious tensions were high, particularly in the wake of the Act of Uniformity, which called for everyone to worship in the same way and to use the new prayer book—which was far more conservative than the church of Henry VIII.[23]

Whatever the reason, Hawkyns' need to speak to the king seems urgent from how he went about his task. Many readers will know the basics of the years preceding 1552, but it is worth recounting them as William Hawkyns might have viewed them. Henry VIII had wanted a male heir, and, to get one, procured a divorce from his first wife even as the Roman Catholic Church insisted he remain married.[24] He then disavowed the Church and started his own religion. He had this new church divest itself of many

Catholic trappings, making himself and other magnates rather wealthy in the process. He confiscated Church lands, closed monasteries and hospitals, and collected silver and gold from priests before they left the country. Henry finally got his son and brought a new form of religion to England; however, after his death in 1547, the English people had become increasingly divided along lines of religion—some wanting to return to Catholicism, others wanting to push the ideas of Protestantism further. These divisions deepened in the years leading up to 1552.

As a schoolteacher, William Hawkyns could have been on either side of the rift. He might have been in favour of a return to a Catholic mass; certainly, the church supported its cathedral schoolteachers well. Hawkyns, though, a learned man, might have read much on Luther and other Protestant reformers and sided with their "radical" beliefs. Both positions existed side by side in sixteenth-century London. Hawkyns, who could have taught at one of the local church schools, might well have taken the Oath of Supremacy required of all those serving as public or church officials. This oath, an allegiance to the king as the Supreme Governor of the Church of England, was highly controversial.[25] When Thomas Cranmer issued the (first) *Book of Common Prayer* on 15 January 1549, it was intended as a simplified version of the Catholic service for the new Church of England and its new priests. Yet its existence only further outraged a large portion of the population, many of whom were still staunch believers in Catholicism even after the Oath of Supremacy. While followers of Protestantism rejoiced, those individuals still hoping for a return to the Catholic mass became angry, as their conceptualization of religion was frustrated.

Tensions further increased in England when Cranmer, with Dudley's encouragement, issued a controversial second (new) *Book of Common Prayer*, endorsed by Parliament in January 1552 and announced the same month, only about 12 weeks before William Hawkyns attempted to speak to the king. Even some followers of Henry VIII's new church found this book to have gone too far in the direction of Luther. This release of the new *Book of Common Prayer* was followed by Dudley's enactment of a new Act of Uniformity, which, depending on the school he worked for, Hawkyns might have been forced to sign. Both of these were to begin in March. Likely, this is the impetus for Hawkyns' actions. At some point before March, possibly even before January, William Hawkyns met with someone from the Council about "a matter at Fleet Bridge", then, after the announcement in January, he got to work—with at least one other person—before attempting to see the king around the time of "Easter last or possibly after" only to be stopped by Dudley.

There are a few other topics that could have been the subject of Hawkyns' bill. As an intelligent and educated individual, he may have had thoughts on the other prominent problems of the day, such as how to resurrect the failing economy. Agricultural troubles, particularly among the wool merchants, had grown over the early years of Edward's reign, as prices dropped for English wool in Europe. The English economy was dependent on the wool trade as their most lucrative export, making up nearly four-fifths of all English exports,[26] and had been experiencing economic difficulties since the death of Henry VIII. Other possible subjects for Hawkyns' bill could have included the structure of government or the line of succession or even the saving of a religious school. The record does not say, but of these topics, only a few would rise to the attention of the crown. Hawkyns must have been powerfully motivated to undertake such a risky and foolish endeavour as attempting to speak to the king *alone*. Perhaps he thought the king might have a more lenient ear for the subject matter than, say, Dudley or Thomas Cranmer,[27] the Archbishop of Canterbury, and that the king, as head of both the church and state, could enact change without Dudley or Cranmer.

William "Was Comyttyd at Grenwich"

There is no indication of *where* Hawkyns "attempted" to see the king, only that he did. Since he was held in the porter's lodge at Greenwich Palace and he lived in London, if Dudley let him leave and arrested him later, it would be more probable that he would have initially been held at Fleet Prison or the Tower of London or even a room at Westminster Palace, not at Greenwich. And yet, Hawkyns was in custody between 17 April, Easter Day, and 9 June 1552 and held in the porter's lodge at Greenwich. The reason the end date must be 9 June or earlier is that there is a letter to the Mayor of London to move Hawkyns from the Tower dated 10 June, so Hawkyns must have been at the Tower on or before 10 June.

If the king was at Greenwich, it is strange that Dudley would hold someone in the same location as the king, especially someone who had attempted to see his Highness with an unknown purpose—possibly with the intent of harming rather than informing his majesty. Princess Elizabeth was in London from 17 March at the king's palace and many supposed that she was in London specifically to visit her brother. An attempt by Hawkyns to see the king while his sister was also in residence at the palace would be risky indeed, but since that is the month before Easter not after. Then, the king made a public appearance on 28 April, St George's Day, at Westminster Cathedral. It was not until 30 April that he left for Greenwich. If Hawkyns tried to speak to the king in Westminster, why did the letter not read, "on or about St. George's Day" and instead mentioned Easter? But it is possible that Elizabeth left before Easter and that the king, in anticipation of St George's Day, had already moved to Westminster by Easter and was approached by Hawkyns between Easter and St George's Day. Dudley writes, though, that Hawkyns was first held in the porter's lodge at Greenwich and, perhaps, Hawkyns was taken away from the scene of his crime to a known location where Dudley or others could question him.

Another piece to the puzzle of timing is that on 30 April, Parliament made a pronouncement concerning revelry on May Day. According to Henry Machyn, the king left London the same day for Greenwich at eight o'clock in the morning.[28] This timeline would also fit to have Hawkyns attempt to speak to the king the night before, on 29 April, which would prompt the king's move first thing on the morning of 30 April. Dudley might have taken Hawkyns with them or had him brought to Greenwich for his initial interrogation, away from London's prying eyes. Dudley only says that Hawkyns attempt was near or just after Easter. It seems likely that it was between 17 and 29 April, Easter to the day after St George's Day, when the king was in either Westminster or London.

Greenwich is not far from London, a little over eight miles (13 km) away but on the far side of the river. There was a royal residence in this location by at least 1300. Henry V (r. 1413–1422) gave the residence to Thomas Beaufort, Duke of Exeter, for his life. When Thomas died in 1426, Henry made the same arrangement with Humphrey, Duke of Gloucester, who improved the property and named his house "Bella Court". It again reverted to the crown when Humphrey died in 1447. Margaret of Anjou, wife of Henry VI, improved and enlarged the riverside house of Humphrey, adding piers for her friends who arrived by boat, naming the whole site *Placentia*, the "Pleasant Place". Later, it became known as the King's House at Greenwich or Greenwich Palace. Henry VIII spent a lot of time there as had his brother, Edmund. Mary, Elizabeth (I), and Edward (VI) were born there.[29] It was because of its location—near London but not too near—that it and Hampton Court Palace were favoured by so many kings and queens.

In the letter from Dudley to Cecil, Dudley writes that, William Hawkyns:

> hase now confessssyd to Sir Arthur Darcy the castinge abroud and settings upp of sedicius Bylls don by hym sielf, ... He sayth there was oon [*one*] a councell with hym, whos name by no meanes he will utter to ay[r] [*Arthur*] Darcy,[30]

John Dudley trusts William Cecil, the one-time secretary of Dudley's rival, Edward Seymour. Cecil, though, cleverly threaded the political turmoil not siding with anyone and keeping all their secrets. Dudley made him a member of the Council after the death of Seymour.[31] The order of events according to Dudley in his letter to Cecil, and there is no reason to doubt him, was that Hawkyns was arrested after Easter in late April and held for some amount of time in Greenwich, then he is transferred to the Tower of London where he was questioned by Arthur Darcy.

Darcy had been entrusted with the command of the Tower in 1551, which had been in the hands of Sir John Markham, "who had suffered the Duke [of Somerset, Edward Seymour] to walk abroad", without making any of the Council aware of his decision.[32] Twenty years earlier, in 1532, a much younger Sir Arthur Darcy had met Sir John Dudley. Darcy along with Dudley, Richard Rich, and Richard Fermor stood surety for a loan made by King Henry VIII to Sir Edward Seymour.[33] By 1552, John Dudley was running the country, and Darcy was in command of the Tower with several properties across England, including a house in Dartford where the king had dinner on a ship with the admiral; likely, it was to Darcy's house they retired after the meal.

Darcy, though, was in his role as commander of the Tower when he questioned his prisoner, William Hawkyns. Then, on 10 June 1552, the Privy Council sent a letter to the Mayor of London to take Hawkyns, "who is nowe fallen owt of his wittes", to either "Lyttle St. Barthillmewes or . . . Bethellem", by which they mean St Mary of Bethlehem Hospital, more generally now known as Bedlam or Bethlem.[34] What had happened to Hawkyns? The school teacher had not indicated any mental health condition to this point in the record; he could have had an underlying condition that was brought out given the stress of his arrest, questioning, and a general sense that he would be found guilty of treason. Edward Seymour had found himself without a head with all his money, titles, and power; what chance did William Hawkyns stand against the Council?

William "Feigned Himself to Be a Frantic"

This was the point at which, according to a document of confession a year later, Hawkyns decided to pretend to be insane so that he would be transferred to Bethlem or at least spared the gallows. According to the authors of *The History of Bethlem*, "[R]aving lunatic" was one condition that might get someone admitted to Bethlem; although, another individual was described as "distraught" in his admission papers. "Lunacy" alongside being "distraught" was named as the condition of several people admitted to Bethlem (St. Mary of Bethlehem) Hospital. These seem to be the most common conditions among those listed on the intake paperwork. For example, "Robert Heath was said to be 'now Lunaticke'" in 1575, and, "in 1598, Henry Richards was described as a 'Lunatick person'". A few, such as "the Carpenter's son" were described as 'distraught' as was the widow Hallywell of Cordwainer Street Ward, who had also "'lately become lunatic, and distraught of her wits.'"[35] These same authors point out that it was in the 1540s when Bethlem was first used as "a deliberate method of general social control".[36] For example, an unnamed man was released in 1546 when the Privy Council found that the man "committed to Bedlem for certeyne lewde words in tyme of his frenesey spoken against the Kinges Majeste, . . . in respect there appered [sic] no malice in him".[37] This was not quite the same as locking someone away as if mentally ill because they did not conform socially or politically; he was considered well now and able to return home. Yet, a few months later, the Privy Council noted another man speaking "lewde words", "Oone Richard Cheseman, of the Parish of Lye in surrey, sent hither [to Bethlem, mentioned later in the record] by Sir Mathew Browne . . . to be kepte there for that he semed to be in a freneseye".[38] This time Cheseman was not speaking against the crown, and he only "seemed" to be *frenetic*. *Frenesy* was the same condition that Hawkyns either had or faked and apparently was one that was associated with lewd vocabulary, which would be easily parroted.

Other individuals before and after William Hawkyns had feigned madness to avoid the death penalty. For example, John Croshawe, in 1609, convinced the Bridewell Governors that he was mad when he "cursed his father & rayled egregiouslie upon my lord maior Mr doctor Meddowes & others".[39] The Council were convinced that Hawkyns was mentally ill, or at least they said as much when they sent "A lettre to the Mayour of London to take ordre that Hawkins, who is nowe fallen owt of his wittes, may be bestowed either at Lyttle St. Barthillmewes or at Bethellem, where the sayd Mayour shall think metest".[40] The Bethlem Hospital had been donated by the Crown to the city of London in 1547, which was why the letter went to the mayor.[41] Whether or not Hawkyns was sent there as a political "miscreant" for disagreeing with the current political and religious climate is hard to say. At this point, all the paperwork indicates that Hawkyns had a real mental illness.

Accused of treason, Hawkyns later said that he pretended to be mentally ill to avoid standing trial. Rather than faking *idiotsy*, a condition of being intellectually disabled, or to having *fatuus*, being mentally deficient, he chose to *feign* being "frantic" or "frenetic".[42] A *freneticus* was an individual incapable of controlling his body and/or emotions. Hawkyns' education and identity as a teacher would make the claim of having an intellectual disability difficult, so it seems he opted for the more realistic possibility of a break in rationality. Whether he knew this was a good choice or not as a condition that would get him into Bethlem or another hospital is impossible to say. As early as 1550 on a case-by-case basis and certainly by 1624, Bethlem began discharging all those with intellectual disabilities, labelled as "idiot" or "simple"; however, a few were allowed to remain at the hospital who worked there.[43]

The English legal tradition, which was heavily influenced by Roman law and written in either Latin or Legal French (Norman) until the time of Hawkyns, divided individuals with mental health conditions into categories based on a combination of behaviour and intellectual ability. Roman legal tradition divided the mentally impaired into two major groups, those *non compos mentis* (without mental health) and the *furiosus* (mad-persons) but made allowances for gradations within those categories, including *non sane mentis* (without sense), *fatuus* (fatuous), and *vecors* (foolish).[44] Roman legal organization for mental health issues, although influencing, did not seem to completely settle into English law. According to Margaret Trenchard-Smith, their two-part division in the *Corpus Juris Civilis* was reflected in Byzantine practice: the *furiosus* (raving mad-man) and the *fatuus* (mentally deficient) with gradations under those two broad categories.[45] While other scholars want to see this two-part Roman division throughout Europe, the terminology in English law describes something far more nuanced that had at least a three-part division with further gradations of mental health complaints. Not only did the English describe those with maniacal episodes or with intellectual disabilities, but they also recognized those unable to distinguish right from wrong. English laws, therefore, had a three-part categorization of the mentally impaired—intellectual disability, mania, and discernment issues.

The terms for mental health came out of a long tradition in English law of terminology to designate quite specific disorders. By the end of the Middle Ages, those with intellectual impairment issues were normally either an *idiota* (idiot, quite possibly an intellectually disabled person) or a *fatuus* (a person with mental deficiency) but could also be *non intellectus* (without intelligence), *ignorans* (ignorant), *non sane memoria* (without a healthy memory), or just simply *non compos mentis* (without mental ability). The term *idiota* in earlier Latin, referred to an "uneducated and common" person. Only later did it take on the more nuanced meaning of "unaware" or even "inward looking" in medieval England.[46] Those persons without the ability to discern—who could not tell the difference either between right and wrong or between reality and fantasy—were a *demens* or *amens* (delusional person), *insanus* (lit. "without health", meaning a mentally unhealthy individual), *freneticus* (a "frenzied" or "frantic" person, meaning someone without physical control), *lunaticus* (a lunatic; an individual with "phases" like the moon, moving in and out of sanity), and someone that *sciens nec bonum nec malum* (knew neither good nor bad). Erratic and dangerous individuals with the mental affliction of *furiosus* (a mad-person suffering from *furor*, in Greek *mania*) were watched closely, often accompanied by a *custos* (keeper).[47] The mental health conditions in England, therefore, ranged from relatively passive and innocent conditions—such as being *idiota* or *fatuus*—to unpredictable behavior that might be aggressive, as was the case in late medieval records of those *furiosi*.

These distinctions are important in the case of William Hawkyns, since people considered dangerous all those who were *furiosi* (people with *mania*), and they were expected to be kept in Bethlem for life. They could not safely be pardoned for their crimes and sent home under the care of relatives; instead, they were deemed a risk to the public and kept either chained or in a locked room. The disease of *freneticus* was somewhere in the middle, possibly curable, and the person would be sent to a hospital for rest and care—not always bound in chains. If Hawkyns knew enough of law and mental health gradations to understand that concessions were made for those with mental health issues[48]—because they would not have been deemed capable of controlling their will—and that he would need to fake a condition that might allow him freedom in future, he needed to imitate an illness that was not too aggressive, such as being *freneticus*, or risk being pardoned but forever incarcerated.[49]

Hawkyns "Is Now Come to His Right Wits"

Almost a year later to the day on 15 June 1553, the Privy Council sent a letter to the Lieutenant of the Tower. The council wanted the lieutenant:

> to bring tomorrow in thafternone [sic] before the lords to the Sterre Chamber these persons: John Owen, Humfrey Holte, John Brambrough, Christopher More, Leonard Esterby, Fraunces Digbie and Mistres Hoggons, presently prisoners in the Tower, and to cause William Hawkins, also prisoner there, to be conveyed to Bedlem.[50]

The same day, the Council sent another letter to the Mayor of London stating that Hawkyns "will be received and kept in Bedlam"[51] as instructed. Why had the mayor not taken Hawkyns to Bethlem or St. Bartholomews in 1552? Did the mayor not want Hawkyns in a London hospital for some reason (a former friend, an expense for the city)? It almost looks like the mayor was sending a subtle message that royal problems should be dealt with on royal property (at the Tower), not in the city.

Hawkyns, who likely knew Sir Arthur Darcy on sight by that point, confessed to him. Dudley, in haste, scribbles at the bottom of his letter to Cecil that Hawkyns "hass byn soudery tymes exaimyd by Sir Hobby and Sirr Darcy and never wold confess. Till yester day. He fayned him self to be frantic. But he ys come now to his right wyts. As sarr Darcy sayse".[52] Sir Philip Hoby spent much of his time as an ambassador to and negotiator with various countries and cities, including the Holy Roman Emperor, France, and Flanders. He joined the Privy Council in 1552. During the King's progress in July 1552, Hoby was required to live in the Tower as the royal contact in the London area,[53] and it might be at this time or other times that Hoby questioned Hawkyns with or without Darcy's company.

The confession to Darcy only made things worse for William Hawkyns because now Darcy wanted the whole story. William said that he had been:

casting abroad and setting up seditious bills done by himself and counterfeiting the archbishop of Canterbury's hand, with intent to have stirred commotion and rebellion. He says there was one a-council with him, whose name he will by no means utter to Darcy.[54]

Clearly, this was a religious matter, otherwise why would Hawkyns have been signing the archbishop's name and forging his handwriting along with handing out leaflets against the Council and church? The rebellions were far and wide in 1551 and 1552. William Hawkyns was another version of rebellion against the government run by the Council. Why Hawkyns finally dropped the ruse of *frenesy* is a good question; likely, it was exhausting to keep it up for so long.

William Should "Disclose His Counsellors or Comforters"

Hawkyns confessed that there was "one a-council with him, whose name he will by no means utter to Darcy". It was that moment and the suggestion by Dudley in his letter and comments that followed, which opened the door to the possibility that Hawkyns might have been tortured for information. Dudley writes:

> whorse [*worse*] yt shold be well don in my opynyon that some discriet persons were forthe with appyntyd [*forthwith appointed*] to have thexaminynacon of hym and dyshor [*discover*] by fayre meanes or fouele to come hym to declarr his councellors or comfortors and this to be in the meane tyme kept verry close and secret[.][55]

Hawkyns admitted to three things: (1) casting abroad, or in other words telling everyone who would listen, his seditious plan, (2) counterfeiting the archbishop's hand, and (3) setting up seditious bills done by himself. He also says that one person assisted him, but never, so far as the records show, did Hawkyns name him.

Treason was not unheard of and, in the latter half of the fifteenth century and well into the first half of the sixteenth century, frequently pardoned. Accused persons were often taken to the Tower, which may explain why Hawkyns ended up there. For example, Thomas Yonge "was taken and imprisoned in the Tower upon suspicion of treason under articles by John Bosewell clerk declared against him by bill".[56] "High treason" was defined by Parliament in 1450 to be a crime committed by any of the "king's lieges in England, Ireland, Wales, or upon the high sea", as this was considered "nefarious audacity" repugnant to the king and his laws.[57] In other words, "high treason" was reserved for those who were supposed to lend counsel to the king, and to make and uphold laws, not break them. There was also "low treason" or minor treason—this was treason within the household. For instance, a household servant attacking the property holder was considered low treason. Or a wife committing adultery could also be considered low treason against her husband. Of course, Hawkyns was only accused of treason and this, much like today, was an attack against the sovereign (head of state) or the government. By 1552, since the church had become connected to the sovereign, as head of the church, any attack against the church, state, or king could be considered treason.

Conclusions

Edward VI was only nine when he came to the throne. In the past, many scholars assumed that because he died young, he had a weak constitution.[58] New research suggests that he was a healthy boy and only became ill in the last few years of his life.[59] Yet, because he was young (his health making no difference), he had a team of men that were to govern for him until he came of age. With hindsight, they seem more focused on making sure their own fortunes and political interests were served rather than caring particularly about Edward, except to make sure that he remained alive and safe. William Hawkyns might be just one more person the Council found to be a threat to their authority to change religion and the structure of the government and to control the king.

In 1552, Edward VI now 14 should have been able to run the country himself, except his health took a turn for the worse in 1553, and he remained under the influence of those magnates who had governed the country while he was a child. He was, however, at last able to meet the members of his Council in person and even took it upon himself, in 1552, to write up rules that might improve the efficiency of the government and his Council. Yet, sadly, he almost immediately had to return to his sick bed.

William Hawkyns tried to meet a quite healthy King Edward in April of 1552. Hawkyns then feigned madness. It would be quite difficult to keep up the appearance of being a "frenzied person" for over a year, but this seems to be what William did. His mental health does not seem good in 1553, when the Council again asks the Mayor of London to admit Hawkyns to Bethlem. On the one hand, he might have succumbed to either the strain of being rebellious or perhaps his sin of forgery and deception and had a mental breakdown of some kind. On the other hand, Hawkyns might have been tortured by Hoby and/or Darcy and a head injury led to his ruse of being mad becoming permanent. Whatever happened, the paper trail grows cold here. If Hawkyns ended up in Bethlem, he likely died there. If he "came to his senses" on his own or with time, it is possible that he was executed for treason. Then again, Mary's reign was not far off. If he spent time in Bethlem and was pronounced fit to return to society after

Mary came to the throne, perhaps Hawkyns found the answer to his bill after all.

Notes

1 D. M. Loades, *John Dudley, Duke of Northumberland, 1504–1553* (Oxford: Clarendon Press, 1996).
2 *Calendar of the Patent Rolls 1548–49* (London: HMSO, 1924), 183–84, 378–84; Sheila R. Richards, ed., *Secret Writing in the Public Records, Henry VIII-George II* (London: HMSO, 1974).
3 The National Archives (hereafter TNA) State Papers, SP 10/15, no. 34; *Calendar of State Papers: Domestic Series, Edward VI, Mary, and Elizabeth, 1547–1580*, ed. Robert Lemon (London: Longman, etc. for HMPRO, 1856) (hereafter *CSPD*), 46.
4 Jay P. Anglin, "Private-Venture Grammar Schools: An Elizabethan Alternative to the Endowed School System," *Explorations in Renaissance Culture, Memphis* 5 (January 1, 1979): 1*ff*.; Sylvia L. Thrupp, *The Merchant Class of Medieval London, 1300–1500* (Ann Arbor: University of Michigan Press, 1989), 36.
5 Barbara A. Hanawalt, *Growing Up in Medieval London: The Experience of Childhood in History* (Oxford: Oxford University Press, 1995), 30.
6 Craig Rose, "Evangelical Philanthropy and Anglican Revival: The Charity Schools of Augustan London, 1698–1740," *The London Journal: A Review of Metropolitan Society Past and Present* 16, no. 1 (1991): 35–65, https://doi.org/10.1179/ldn.1991.16.1.35.
7 Nicholas Orme, *Medieval Schools From Roman Britain to Renaissance England* (New Haven and London: Yale University Press, 2006); Carole Rawcliffe, "The Hospitals of Late Medieval London," *Medical History* 28 (1984): 1–21; John Gough Nichols, *Chronicle of the Grey Friars of London*, Camden Society v. 53 (London: J. B. Nichols & Sons, 1851), xxvi–xxvii.
8 During the crusades (1190s), the Church of St. Edmund the King and Martyr was re-dedicated to St. Edmund and the Holy Sepulchre at the same time as the building of the original round Temple Church, which held the privilege to erect a Bar to collection taxes. The Temple Church sat across the lane from St. Andrews and, when the Templars moved their church and other buildings closer to the river and near to the present location of the Temple Church, the church of St. Andrews "Holborn" opened a school near the site of the renamed Holborn Bar.
9 TNA State Papers, SP 10/15, no. 34; *CSPD*, p. 46.
10 *The Diary of Henry Machyn, Citizen and Merchant-Taylor of London, 1550–1563*, Original Camden os., pp. 13–21 (London: Camden Society, 1848) (hereafter *Machyn*), January–June 1552, British History Online, https://www.british-history.ac.uk/camden-record-soc/vol42/pp13–21.
11 *CSPD*, p. 77.
12 *CSPD*, p. 13.
13 Claire Ridgway, "16 January 1549—Thomas Seymour Tries to Kidnap Edward VI," *The Tudor Society*, January 2015, https://www.tudorsociety.com/16-february-1549-thomas-seymour-tries-to-kidnap-edward-vi/.
14 *Calendar of State Papers, Spain*, vol. 9, 1547–1549, p. 332. See also Ridgeway; and Julia Hickey, "Elizabeth and Thomas Seymour," *The History Jar: English History from 1066*, April 16, 2018, https://thehistoryjar.com/2018/04/16/elizabeth-and-thomas-seymour/#comments.

15 Chris Skidmore, *The Lost King of England* (New York: St. Martin's Press, 2007), 97–104.

16 G. J. R. Parry, "Inventing 'The Good Duke' of Somerset," *The Journal of Ecclesiastical History* 40, no. 3 (1989): 370–80, doi:10.1017/S0022046900046522.

17 Paul Heyman, Leopold Simons, and Christel Cochez, "Where the English Sweating Sickness and the Picardy Sweat Caused by Hantaviruses?" *Viruses* 6, no. 1 (January 2014): 151–71.

18 *Machyn*, July 1551.

19 Ibid.

20 *Machyn*, March 1552.

21 TNA State Papers, SP 10/15, no. 34.

22 Ibid; and *Calendar of State Papers: Domestic Series of the reign of Edward VI 1457–1553*, PRO rev., ed. C. S. Knighton (London: HMSO, 1992), 270, #746.

23 James C. Spalding, *The Reformation of the Ecclesiastical Laws of England, 1552*, Sixteenth Century Essays & Studies (Kirksville, MO: Truman State University Press, 1992); Oliver Wort, "Reception Without the Theory: On the Study of Religion in Early Modern England," *Annual Bulletin of Historical Literature* 96, no. 1 (December 2012): 8–15; Geoffrey Holt, "The Education of Catholics from the Act of Uniformity to the Catholic Relief Acts," *British Catholic History* 27, no. 3 (2005): 346–58, https://doi.org/10.1017/S0034193200031484.

24 For more information on the English Reformation, see G. W. Bernard, *The King's Reformation* (New Haven: Yale University Press, 2007); Richard Rex, *Henry VIII and the English Reformation*, British History in Perspective Series (London: Palgrave Macmillan, 2006).

25 Readers will recall that Thomas More was executed by Henry VIII for his refusal to swear. G. W. Bernard, *The King's Reformation: Henry VIII and the Remaking of the English Church* (New Haven: Yale University Press, 2007).

26 John H. Gendron, "Employment Preservation and Textile Regulation in Early Modern England, 1550–1640," *Journal of Institutional Economics* 17, no. 4 (2021): 529–43, doi:10.1017/S1744137421000187.

27 David Selwyn and Paul Ayris, eds., *Thomas Cranmer: Churchman and Scholar* (Woodbridge: Boydell, 1999); Susan Wabuda, *Thomas Cranmer* (London: Routledge, 2017).

28 *Machyn*, April 1552.

29 Like Henry VIII, James I spent time here and several of his children were also born here. Charles I built the "Queen's House" for his Queen, Henrietta Maria. Oliver Cromwell had most of the palace torn down to make way for a hospital in 1660/1. See Anniina Jokinen, "Greenwich Palace," *Luminarium: Encyclopedia Project*, August 12, 2010, http://www.luminarium.org/encyclopedia/greenwichpalace.htm.

30 TNA State Papers, SP 10/15, no. 34.

31 William Cecil continued to have good luck at staying alive by being true to his beliefs and being, quite simply, honest. He stood against Dudley and with other attorneys in opposition to changing the order of succession (Lady Jane Grey) and was also able to win favour with Queen Mary later. See Stephen Alford, *The Early Elizabethan Polity: William Cecil and the British Succession Crisis, 1558–1569* (Cambridge: Cambridge University Press, 2002); Brett Usher, *William Cecil and Episcopacy, 1559–1577* (London: Routledge, 2016); W. S. C. Copeman, "The Gout of William Cecil—First Lord Burghley (1520–98)," *Medical History* 1, no. 3 (July 1957): 262–64. Cambridge University Press, 2012, https://doi.org/10.1017/S0025727300021323.

32 Edward VI, "Diary Entry," October 31, 1551, in Patrick Fraser Tytler, *England Under the Reigns of Edward VI. And Mary* (London: Richard Bentley, 1839), 6; and Edward VI (King of England), *Literary Remains of King Edward VI: Edited From His Autograph Manuscripts, With Historical Notes and a Biographical Memoir*, vol. 2 (London: B. Franklin, 1857), 358.

33 Stanley Thomas Bindoff, *The House of Commons, 1509–1558*, D-M (London: Secker and Warburg, Parliament Trust, 1982), vol. II, 14.

34 *Acts of the Privy Council of England*, ns (1552–1554), ed. John Soche Dasent (London: HMSO, 1892), vol. IV, 72.

35 Jonathan Andrews, Asa Briggs, Roy Porter, Penny Tucker, and Keir Waddington, *The History of Bethlehem* (London: Routledge, 1997), 121. London Metropolitan Archives at the Bethlem Museum of the Mind, "Minutes of the Court of Governors," vol. 4, folio 44, "Minutes of the Court of Governors," CLC/275/MS33011/004.

36 Andrews et al., *The History of Bethlehem*, 117.

37 *Acts of the Privy Council 1542–7*, 388. See also Andrews et al., *The History of Bethlehem*, 116.

38 *Acts of the Privy Council 1542–7*, 481.

39 Andrews et al., *The History of Bethlehem*, 117. London Metropolitan Archives at the Bethlem Museum of the Mind, "Minutes of the Court of Governors," vol. 5, folio 338v, "Minutes of the Court of Governors," CLC/275/MS33011/005.

40 *Acts of the Privy Council, 1552–4*, p. 72.

41 Andrews et al., *The History of Bethlehem*, 157. In 1553, Edward VI also granted Christ's, Bridewell and St. Thomas's to the City. The Mayor, Commonality, and Citizens of London formed a corporation as the "Governors of the Possessions, Revenues and Goods of the same Hospitals." See Andrews in the same place.

42 Wendy J. Turner, "Defining Mental Afflictions in Medieval English Administrative Records," in *Disability and Medieval Law: History, Literature, Society*, ed. Cory James Rushton (Newcastle upon Tyne: Cambridge Scholars Publishing, 2013), 134–37.

43 Andrews et al., *The History of Bethlehem*, 121. At earlier times on a case-by-case basis, if an individual seemed well enough and posed no threat, they were released. See Andrews et al., *The History of Bethlehem*, 116.

44 Margaret Trenchard-Smith, "Insanity, Exculpation and Disempowerment in Byzantine Law," in *Madness in Medieval Law and Custom*, ed. Wendy J. Turner (Leiden: Brill, 2010), 41–45.

45 Ibid., 42.

46 Turner, "Defining," 135.

47 Ibid., 142.

48 Henry of Bratton, aka *Bracton*, c. 1210–68, *De legibus et consuetudinibus Angliae: On the Laws and Customs of England*, ed. G. E. Woodbine and transl. S. E. Thorne, 4 vols. (Cambridge, MA: Harvard University Press, 1968–77), vol. 2, 423; Sara M. Butler, *The Language of Abuse: Marital Violence in Later Medieval England* (Leiden: Brill, 2007), 114–16; Thomas A. Green, *Verdict According to Conscience; Perspectives on the English Criminal Trial Jury, 1200–1800* (Chicago: University of Chicago Press, 1985), 53–59; Elizabeth Papp Kamali, "*Felonia Felonice Facta*: Felony and Intentionality in Medieval England," *Criminal Law and Philosophy* 9 (2015): 397–421, see 406; Bryce Lyon, *A Constitutional and Legal History of Medieval England*, 2nd ed. (New York: Norton, 1980), 295; Wendy J. Turner, *Care and Custody of the Mentally*

Ill, Incompetent, and Disabled in Medieval England (Turnhout: Brepols, 2013), 31–62.

49 Wendy J. Turner, "Mental Health and Homicide in Medieval English Trials," *The Medieval Brain*, special issue, Deborah Thorpe, ed. *Open Library of Humanities* 4, no. 2 (2018): 11; Sara M. Butler, "Representing the Middle Ages: The Insanity Defense in Medieval England," in *The Treatment of Disabled Persons in Medieval Europe*, eds. Wendy J. Turner and Tory Vandeventer Pearman (Lewiston: Mellen, 2010); Paul Krueger et al., eds., *Corpus Iuris Civilis*, 3 vols. (Berlin: Weidmann, 1954–59), Code v.70.6, VI.22.9/Digest XXVIII. 1.2: 6–7/Institutes II. 7, § 1; Margaret Trenchard-Smith, "Perceptions of Unreason in the Byzantine Empire to the End of the First Millennium" (Ph.D. thesis, University of California, Los Angeles, 2006), 90; Margaret Trenchard-Smith, "Insanity, Exculpation and Disempowerment in Byzantine Law," in *Madness in Medieval Law and Custom*, ed. Wendy J. Turner (Leiden: Brill, 2010), 39–56. In **law**, the legal treatise titled *Leges Henrici Primi* (c. 1108–18), pp. 224–25 (L. J. Downer, ed., *Leges Henrici Primi* [Oxford: Clarendon Press, 1972]), for instance, there were provisions for the mentally incapacitated. See also: Patrick Wormald, *Making of English Law: King Alfred to the Twelfth Century, Vol. I: Legislation and Its Limits* (Hoboken, NJ: Wiley-Blackwell, 2001), 411–65.
Premodern **medicine** had a complex system of categories and terminology to describe conditions of mental health. See Wendy J. Turner, "Defining Mental Afflictions in Medieval English Administrative Records," in *Disability and Medieval Law: History, Literature, Society*, ed. Cory James Rushton (Newcastle upon Tyne: Cambridge Scholars Publishing, 2013), 134–56; Eliza Buhrer, "Law and Mental Competency in Late Medieval England," *Reading Medieval Studies* XL (2014): 82–100; H. M. Hickey, "The Lexical Prison: Impairment and Confinement in Medieval and Early Modern England," *Parergon* 34, no. 2 (November 2, 2017): 133–57.

50 *Acts of the Privy Council of England*, p. 288 (June 15, 1553).

51 See above. Andrews et al., *The History of Bethlehem*.

52 TNA State Papers, SP 10/15, no. 34.

53 P. S. Edwards, "Hoby, Sir Philip (1504/5–58) of Leominster, Herfs., Bisham, Berks. And the Blackfriars, London," in *The History of Parliament: The House of Common 1509–1558*, ed. S. T. Bindoff, https://www.historyofparliamentonline.org; Gordon Goodwin, "Hoby, Philip," in *Dictionary of National Biography*, ed. Sidney Lee (London: Smith, Elder & Col, 1891), vol. 27, 54–44.

54 TNA State Papers, SP 10/15, no. 34.

55 Ibid; see also: *CSPD*, p. 72, p. 270, p. 288.

56 *Calendar of the Close Roll, Henry VI, Vol. 6, 1454–1461* (London: HMSO, 1947), 420.

57 *Calendar of the Close Roll, Henry VI, Vol. 5, 1447–1454* (London: HMSO, 1941), 182.

58 Grace Holmes, Frederick Homes, and Julia McMorrough put forth the hypothesis that Edward might have died of tuberculosis that developed after he had childhood measles: "The Death of Young King Edward VI," *The New England Journal of Medicine* 345 (July 5, 2001): 60–62, doi:10.1056/NEJM200107053450111.

59 Diarmaid MacCulloch, *The Boy King: Edward VI and the Protestant Reformation* (Berkeley: University of California Press, 2002), 21; Jennifer Loach, *Edward VI*, ed. George Bernard and Penry Williams (New Haven: Yale University Press, 1999), 161; G. R. Elton, *Reform and Reformation* (London: Edward Arnold, 1977), 372.

Reference List

Archival

London Metropolitan Archives at the Bethlem Museum of the Mind. "Minutes of the Court of Governors." 4, folio 44, "Minutes of the Court of Governors," CLC/275/MS33011/004.
London Metropolitan Archives at the Bethlem Museum of the Mind. "Minutes of the Court of Governors." 5, folio 338v, "Minutes of the Court of Governors." CLC/275/MS33011/005.
The National Archives, SP: State Papers

Printed Primary

Acts of the Privy Council of England, ns, vol. IV (1552–1554). Edited by John Soche Dasent, 72. London: HMSO, 1892.
Calendar of State Papers: Domestic Series of the Reign of Edward VI, 1457–1553, PRO rev. ed. Edited by C. S. Knighton. London: HMSO, 1992.
Calendar of State Papers: Domestic Series, Edward VI, Mary, and Elizabeth, 1547–1580. Edited by Robert Lemon. London: Longman, etc. for HMPRO, 1856.
Calendar of State Papers, Spain, vol. 9, 1547–1549.
Calendar of the Close Roll, Henry VI, vol. 5, 1447–1454. London: HMSO, 1941.
Calendar of the Close Roll, Henry VI, vol. 6, 1454–1461. London: HMSO, 1947.
Calendar of the Patent Rolls, 1548–49. London: HMSO, 1924.
The Diary of Henry Machyn, Citizen and Merchant-Taylor of London, 1550–1563. Original published in Camden old series, pp. 13–21, London: Camden Society, 1848. British History. https://www.british-history.ac.uk/camden-record-soc/vol42/pp13-21.
Downer, L. J. *Leges Henrici Primi* (c. 1108–18). Oxford: Clarendon Press, 1972.
Edward VI (King of England). "Diary Entry," 31 October 1551. In *England Under the Reigns of Edward VI and Mary*, edited by Patrick Fraser Tytler. London: Richard Bentley, 1839.
Edward VI (King of England). *Literary Remains of King Edward VI: Edited From His Autograph Manuscripts, With Historical Notes and a Biographical Memoir*. Vol. 2. London: B. Franklin, 1857.
Henry of Bratton, aka *Bracton*, c. 1210–68, *De legibus et consuetudinibus Angliae: On the Laws and Customs of England*. Edited by G. E. Woodbine. Translated by S. E. Thorne. 4 vols. Cambridge, MA: Harvard University Press, 1968–77.
Krueger, Paul, et al. *Corpus Iuris Civilis*. 3 vols. Berlin: Weidmann, 1954–59.
Richards, Sheila R., ed. *Secret Writing in the Public Records, Henry VIII-George II*. London: HMSO, 1974.

Secondary

Alford, Stephen. *The Early Elizabethan Polity: William Cecil and the British Succession Crisis, 1558–1569*. Cambridge: Cambridge University Press, 2002.
Andrews, Jonathan, Asa Briggs, Roy Porter, Penny Tucker, and Keir Waddington. *The History of Bethlem*. Reprint: 2013. London: Routledge, 1997.

Anglin, Jay P. "Private-Venture Grammar Schools: An Elizabethan Alternative to the Endowed School System." *Explorations in Renaissance Culture* 5 (January 1, 1979): 1ff.

Bernard, G. W. *The King's Reformation: Henry VIII and the Remaking of the English Church.* New Haven: Yale University Press, 2007.

Bindoff, Stanley Thomas. *The House of Commons, 1509–1558.* Vol. II, D-M. London: Secker and Warburg, Parliament Trust, 1982.

Buhrer, Eliza. "Law and Mental Competency in Late Medieval England." *Reading Medieval Studies* XL (2014): 82–100.

Butler, Sara M. *The Language of Abuse: Marital Violence in Later Medieval England.* Leiden: Brill, 2007.

———. "Representing the Middle Ages: The Insanity Defense in Medieval England." *The Treatment of Disabled Persons in Medieval Europe*, edited by Wendy J. Turner and Tory Vandeventer Pearman. Lewiston: Mellen, 2010.

Copeman, W. S. C. "The Gout of William Cecil—First Lord Burghley (1520–98)." *Medical History* 1, no. 3 (July 1957): 262–64. Cambridge University Press, 2012. https://doi.org/10.1017/S0025727300021323.

Edwards, P. S. "Hoby, Sir Philip (1504/5–58) of Leominster, Herfs., Bisham, Berks. And the Blackfriars, London." In *The History of Parliament: The House of Common 1509–1558*, edited by S. T. Bindoff. https://www.historyofparliamentonline.org.

Elton, G. R. *Reform and Reformation.* London: Edward Arnold, 1977.

Gendron, John H. "Employment Preservation and Textile Regulation in Early Modern England, 1550–1640." *Journal of Institutional Economics* 17, no. 4 (2021): 529–43. doi:10.1017/S1744137421000187.

Goodwin, Gordon. "Hoby, Philip." In *Dictionary of National Biography*, edited by Sidney Lee, vol. 27, 54–44. London: Smith, Elder & Col, 1891.

Grace Holmes, Frederick Homes, and Julia McMorrough. "The Death of Young King Edward VI." *The New England Journal of Medicine* 345 (July 5, 2001): 60–62. doi:10.1056/NEJM200107053450111.

Green, Thomas A. *Verdict According to Conscience; Perspectives on the English Criminal Trial Jury, 1200–1800.* Chicago: University of Chicago Press, 1985.

Hanawalt, Barbara A. *Growing Up in Medieval London: The Experience of Childhood in History.* Oxford: Oxford University Press, 1995.

Heyman, Paul, Leopold Simons, and Christel Cochez. "Where the English Sweating Sickness and the Picardy Sweat Caused by Hantaviruses?" *Viruses* 6, no. 1 (January 2014): 151–71.

Hickey, H. M. "The Lexical Prison: Impairment and Confinement in Medieval and Early Modern England." *Parergon* 34, no. 2 (November 2, 2017): 133–57.

Hickey, Julia. "Elizabeth and Thomas Seymour." *The History Jar: English History From 1066*, April 16, 2018. https://thehistoryjar.com/2018/04/16/elizabeth-and-thomas-seymour/#comments.

Holt, Geoffrey. "The Education of Catholics from the Act of Uniformity to the Catholic Relief Acts." *British Catholic History* 27, no. 3 (2005): 346–58. https://doi.org/10.1017/S0034193200031484.

Jokinen, Anniina. "Greenwich Palace." *Luminarium: Encyclopedia Project*, August 12, 2010. http://www.luminarium.org/encyclopedia/greenwichpalace.htm.

Kamali, Elizabeth Papp. "*Felonia Felonice Facta*: Felony and Intentionality in Medieval England." *Criminal Law and Philosophy* 9 (2015): 397–421.

Loach, Jennifer. *Edward VI*. Edited by George Bernard and Penry Williams. New Haven: Yale University Press, 1999.

Loades, D. M. *John Dudley, Duke of Northumberland, 1504–1553*. Oxford: Clarendon Press, 1996.

Lyon, Bryce. *A Constitutional and Legal History of Medieval England*. 2nd ed. New York: Norton, 1980.

MacCulloch, Diarmaid. *The Boy King: Edward VI and the Protestant Reformation*. Berkeley: University of California Press, 2002.

Nichols, John Gough. *Chronicle of the Grey Friars of London*. Camden Society, 53. London: J.B. Nichols & Sons, 1851.

Orme. *Medieval Schools From Roman Britain to Renaissance England*. New Haven and London: Yale University Press, 2006.

Parry, G. J. R. "Inventing 'The Good Duke' of Somerset." *The Journal of Ecclesiastical History*, 40, no. 3 (1989): 370–80. doi:10.1017/S0022046900046522.

Rawcliffe, Carole. "The Hospitals of Late Medieval London." *Medical History* 28 (1984): 1–21.

Rex, Richard. *Henry VIII and the English Reformation*. British History in Perspective Series. London: Palgrave Macmillan, 2006.

Ridgway, Claire. "16 January 1549—Thomas Seymour tries to kidnap Edward VI." *The Tudor Society* (January 2015). https://www.tudorsociety.com/16-february-1549-thomas-seymour-tries-to-kidnap-edward-vi/.

Rose, Craig. "Evangelical Philanthropy and Anglican Revival: The Charity Schools of Augustan London, 1698–1740." *The London Journal: A Review of Metropolitan Society Past and Present* 16, no. 1 (1991): 35–65. https://doi.org/10.1179/ldn.1991.16.1.35.

Selwyn, David, and Paul Ayris, eds. *Thomas Cranmer: Churchman and Scholar*. Woodbridge: Boydell, 1999.

Skidmore, Chris. *The Lost King of England*. New York: St. Martin's Press, 2007.

Spalding, James C. *The Reformation of the Ecclesiastical Laws of England, 1552*. Sixteenth Century Essays & Studies. Kirksville, MO: Truman State University Press, 1992.

Thrupp, Sylvia L. *The Merchant Class of Medieval London, 1300–1500*. Ann Arbor: University of Michigan Press, 1989.

Trenchard-Smith, Margaret. "Insanity, Exculpation and Disempowerment in Byzantine Law." In *Madness in Medieval Law and Custom*, edited by Wendy J. Turner. Leiden: Brill, 2010.

———. "Perceptions of Unreason in the Byzantine Empire to the End of the First Millennium." Ph.D. thesis. University of California, Los Angeles, 2006.

Turner, Wendy J. *Care and Custody of the Mentally Ill, Incompetent, and Disabled in Medieval England*. Turnhout: Brepols, 2013.

———. "Defining Mental Afflictions in Medieval English Administrative Records." In *Disability and Medieval Law: History, Literature, Society*, edited by Cory James Rushton. Newcastle upon Tyne: Cambridge Scholars Publishing, 2013.

———. "Mental Health and Homicide in Medieval English Trials." *The Medieval Brain*, special issue, Deborah Thorpe, ed. *Open Library of Humanities* 4, no. 2 (2018): 11.

Usher, Brett. *William Cecil and Episcopacy, 1559–1577*. London: Routledge, 2016.

Wabuda, Susan. *Thomas Cranmer*. London: Routledge, 2017.

Wormald, Patrick. *Making of English Law: King Alfred to the Twelfth Century, Vol. I: Legislation and Its Limits*. Hoboken, NJ: Wiley-Blackwell, 2001.

Wort, Oliver. "Reception Without the Theory: On the Study of Religion in Early Modern England." *Annual Bulletin of Historical Literature* 96, no. 1 (December 2012): 8–15.

7 "A Decietfull Gypsay [sic]".[1] Malingering, Performance and Princess Sophia's "Fitts"

Carolyn A. Day

Illness and scandal plagued the royal family during the eighteenth century, with the most obvious being George III's madness. The scandals attached to the sons and the King's brothers are well-known and several of the daughters also became embroiled in untoward activities, some of which intersected with their health. For instance, the youngest daughter Princess Amelia died after a long struggle with consumption and an equally long clandestine relationship with General Charles Fitzroy. Princess Augusta engaged in an affair as did Princess Sophia; however, in her case there was a connection between her behaviour and the performance of ill health. Her established health problems, including her stomach cramps and pains in her side, were used as a cover for the possible birth of an illegitimate child in 1800.[2] Even more surprisingly, there were questions surrounding her early bouts of illness in 1793. A couple of months into the episode Princess Elizabeth wrote that Sophia was:

> making us all very uneasy, though we are assured she is not in the least shadow of danger. . . . You know well enough how many unhappy hours that makes me pass in every sense of the word. But at Court, one learns deceit.[3]

This mention of deceit in navigating the court and performing the appropriate response to illness provides a glimpse into one of the ways deception, performance, court intrigue and illness intermingled for the Royal Family, particularly in the case of Princess Sophia's fits.

Blue-eyed and fair-haired, Princess Sophia was born in 1777 as the twelfth child of King George III and Queen Charlotte, and their fifth daughter. Her elder sisters (Royal, Augusta and Elizabeth) formed one unit, were educated separately and lived away from the three younger daughters, Mary, Sophia and Amelia. These women had a different experience than their older sisters, in part due to the impact of George III's illness which began in October 1788. During the King's mental derangement, the younger

DOI: 10.4324/9781003452324-10

princesses lived separately under the watchful care of Lady Charlotte Finch (who had first been appointed governess to the royal children in 1762) and a number of sub-governesses including Miss Martha Gouldsworthy (nicknamed Gouly or Gooly), Mlle de Montmollin and Miss Gomm, an arrangement that continued in the years that followed.[4] After their father's first bout with mental instability, his physicians and those charged with running the state applied pressure on the Queen to focus her attention less on her children and more on maintaining her husband's health.[5] Charlotte was keenly aware this would have serious implications for Mary, Sophia and Amelia, stating "I pity my three younger daughters, whose education I can no longer attend to".[6]

Although the king recovered by March 1789, the die was cast, and the young princesses had a very different childhood from that of their elder sisters. Lacking the Queen's careful oversight, the younger daughters lived primarily under the watchful gaze of a number of governesses at the Lower Lodge at Windsor. While the elder princesses had undergone a challenging academic upbringing tempered with strong moral training, the junior princesses' education reflected the Queen's new priorities.[7] Mrs Papendiek was quick to assert of their education that "I believe we must all admit that it fell short of that of the three elder Princesses", whom she styled as "very clever women" and "thoroughly useful members of society".[8] The younger girls' knowledge in botany, geography and history was limited, and their musical and artistic training was less robust than that of their sisters. Instead, their instruction was more heavily focused on the textile arts and they were proficient in embroidery, lacemaking and the like.[9]

Despite this inauspicious upbringing, as a young child Princess Sophia won the affection and approbation of her governesses and was often mentioned as the favourite. This was particularly the case for Marianne Moula and Mary Hamilton, who styled her a "Sweet, engaging child".[10] In 1789, Fanny Burney acknowledged she was the Duke of Clarence's "professed favorite",[11] and a number of years later, her brother Edward also called her "that clever little thing and my first favourite, Sophy".[12] Sophia was intelligent, but a bit shy and self-conscious; particularly as she was very nearsighted and embarrassed by her condition, preferring to watch the world through a blurry film than to publicly wear her spectacles. As she grew up, the "little favourite" became "increasingly withdrawn", as she was often uncomfortable with the rigours of public life, but her fragile appearance disguised a sharp tongue.[13]

Sophia had been considered delicate from an early age with the fault believed to be her abrupt weaning as a baby.[14] Mademoiselle Moula identified Sophia's "tendency to 'nervous irritation', thought her cruelly 'subject to low spirits'" and stated her possessed of "more sensibility than all the others put together".[15] This excessive sensibility was connected to the functioning of the nervous system and health, and as such increased concerns she might suffer from the "family disease". This hereditary weakness of scrofulous origin was believed to be a legacy from Saxe-Gotha, introduced by the Dowager Princess of Wales, and one thought responsible for the untimely deaths of the young princes Alfred (1780–1782) and Octavius (1779–1783).[16] "Little" or "Poor" Sophy's nervous disposition manifested in serious, if mysterious, health issues beginning in the summer of 1793 at the age of 16.

The timeline for Sophia's illness is unclear. Flora Fraser mentions she had a bad bout of chickenpox, likely in April of 1793. She then developed what was described as "a bad swallow", followed by months marked by repeated faintings.[17] However, this assertion may be a function of the timing of Sophia's symptoms and a conflating of her distinct illness with that of her sisters. The surviving letters make no mention of Sophia and only speak of Augusta and Elizabeth suffering from chickenpox. Then in April, Sophia even wrote to her brother about their symptoms but made no mention of herself having any.[18] The Queen did write in May of 1793 that Sophia had been in bed for 3 weeks but did not mention any details.[19]

Lucy Kennedy provides the most comprehensive description of Sophia's illness and stated that her disorder originated with her brother's departure for the continental war, writing:

> Princess Sophia . . . has been afflicted with a violent nervous Disorder the whole summer, She went with the Family to Greenwich to see her Brother, the Duke of York . . . Embark for Germany . . . it affected P.S. So much, that she Fell into Fits, which have Encreased, and Continued Ever Since.[20]

The embarkation occurred at the end of February, months before the purported chickenpox episode, and although all six princesses were present, it was the Queen and Princess Elizabeth who "could not refrain from dropping a tear of sympathy".[21] Sophia's illness is not really mentioned until May of 1793, when there are reports of her recovery. On 6 May, the newspapers stated "Princess Sophia is much Recovered from her late Indisposition",[22] and two days later, the Queen reported that "the Physicians think Sophia also mending".[23] These assertions were premature, as in June the papers once again stated she was "much indisposed".[24] By the end of July, there were even alarmed reports that her "indisposition . . . was . . . so much increased, as to cause apprehensions of danger".[25] Sophia was certainly having difficulty when she wrote the Prince of Wales' birthday felicitations at the end of the month in a very shaky hand, though this is the only letter that bears any material imprint of her illness.

Not only is the timeline unclear, so too is the illness described by Lucy Kennedy who wrote Sophia:

> takes from 50, to 80 [fitts], in ye 24 Hours, Falls Back in her Chair, more or Less Convulsed, Recovers Soon does Not Complein[sic] of Pain, and goes on with her Work, or Book as if nothing had happened, until she Sink again.[26]

This description was echoed by the royal apothecary Robert Battiscombe who stated "Prs Sophia has had Hysteric faintings for weeks . . . from 60 to 100 faintings every day".[27] These fits were accompanied by difficulty in swallowing, which in some cases brought on fainting.[28]

After months of treatment, Sophia was moved to Kew at the end of July.[29] Princess Mary was sent to keep her company, and she was also attended by her governess Miss Goldsworthy, her nurse Mrs. Chevely and Lady Charlotte Bruce (the daughter of the Countess of Elgin who was treated as an adopted member of the family).[30] Here, she spent 6 weeks under the care of the rather demanding Sir Lucas Pepys (1742–1830), physician-in-ordinary to George III, whom William Munk described as "a person of great firmness and determination, somewhat dictatorial in his bearing, and formed to command".[31] Pepys was assisted by another physician-in-ordinary the "charming", Cambridge educated—but as Princess Sophia called him "simple"—Dr Thomas Gisborne.[32]

She was also under the careful eye of Mrs. Chevely, who spent her nights sleeping in the princess's room watching over the invalid.[33] Sophia was not isolated at Kew, but received visits from various family members during her stay, including the Prince of Wales, the Duke of Clarence and the Duchess of York.[34] Despite every effort, the reports on her health were mixed. Lady Elizabeth Cathcart, who had replaced Lady Charlotte Finch as a governess, received a rather alarming report from Princess Mary:[35]

> I cannot say our dear Sophia passed a good day yesterday as she had many faintings & was very uncomfortable, she went out in the carriage in the evening & had four faintings during the time she was out, she had a better night then [sic] the night before but thinks herself much the same this morning and the faintings are much the same.[36]

By August however, Sophia was writing to her father that:

> I can with truth say my swallow has improved within these last few days though not yet arrived to perfection however I am quite satisfied as I ought to be very thankful to be so well as I am after so long and tedious an illness.[37]

The papers also rejoiced at her improvement stating she was "now nearly recovered",[38] and, although she was "Rather better"[39] on her return to Windsor, by 18 September Sir Lucas Pepys determined a visit to Tunbridge Wells was "highly necessary".[40]

Sophia's physician was a firm believer in the medicinal properties of mineral water, having run a medical practice at the sea resort of Brighton early in his career. Furthermore, his grandfather had written a prominent work on the benefits of seawater for glandular disorders.[41] Pepys and Gisborne had already tried "all kinds of Nervous Medicines wth out eff-cat [sic]" on Princess Sophia, but her "Hysteric faintings"[42] continued. Chalybeate waters were often prescribed for "Hypochondriac and Hysteric Affections",[43] and Pepys investigated the idea of using "Sunning Hill Water"[44] as a treatment. This chalybeate water, from a spring in Berkshire, was thought to have "great benefit" and to aid in "recovery from dangerous Disease".[45] Pepys, however, discounted its use, believing it was "too cold".[46] Fortunately, these waters were similar to those at Tunbridge Wells,[47] which were "a light pure chalybeate" capable of warming and invigorating "the relaxed constitution", and restoring "tone and elasticity" to "the weakened fibres". Making it ideal for treating "most cold chronical disorders, lowness of spirit, weak digestions, and nervous complaints".[48] It was also accorded the ability to strengthen "the brain and origin of the nerves", making it particularly effective "in hypochondriacal disorders".[49]

Although Sophia was aware for weeks that she would be travelling, the particulars had been kept from her. The Queen, in consultation with Dr Pepys, had decided this was necessary for therapeutic reasons. On 6 October, the Queen told only Lady Elizabeth Cathcart and Mrs Chevley of the plan, and on the following morning, she ushered the rest of the Royal Family, who were also unaware, to Frogmore after breakfast. Charlotte did not even say goodbye to her daughter for fear of tipping her off.[50] This extreme secrecy was, in part, to forestall what Queen Charlotte styled "private bemoanings",[51] but the ambush was also intentional on medical grounds. Lucy Kennedy describes the scene:

> she was not told of it, until the Coach Drove to the Door, in hopes the flurry of Spirits, & agitation would make her weep, which it did violently which [sic] Relief; made her Perform her Journey better than they Could have Expected.[52]

The shock was intended to cause her to cry, and insight into this plan comes from an account in July stating that Sophia "had a flood of Tears for two hours", and afterward, she "had no more faintings that day or difficulty of swallowing which before could not be done without fainting".[53] The belief that crying relieved her nervous symptoms, and the associated swallow was used to good effect and Lady Cathcart reported on her arrival in Tunbridge Wells that Princess Sophia "was quite Chearfull and the spasms she had were shorter and quieter than any I ever saw her have".[54]

The first week at Tunbridge seems to have gone well, and Lady Cathcart worked in unison with the Queen to mitigate any new emotional distress originating from within the royal family. As Sophia's condition was of a nervous origin, Charlotte was very concerned about the effect the behaviours of the royal siblings might have on her daughter, going so far as to instruct Lady Cathcart not to leave the room should Sophia receive a visit from the Prince of Wales, writing, "I am sure a Tete a Tete will do neither of them good".[55]

Even more problematic was Princess Mary's behaviour. She had not handled the separation from her sister at all well and when she returned from Frogmore to find Sophia gone, wept profusely.[56] Queen Charlotte wrote the following day that "Mary says her heart is broke & a jumping up & down within Her . . . & I believe without Naming any body else, my Conduct by Old & Young much Criticised".[57] The Queen attempted to channel Mary's emotions, instructing her "not dwell too much in Her letters upon Her Separation from Her Sister" and "obtained Her promise for doing so".[58] Sadly Queen Charlotte's attempts were in vain, and Lady Cathcart grew increasingly concerned over the damage Sophia's siblings were doing to her charge, writing candidly to her husband, "the Volumes she receives certainly do her much Harm". This was especially true of the letters from Mary which she stated were "the most cruel and childish you can possibly imagine".[59] Sophia was "gay happy and contended" until "these abominable Letters either arrive, or are to be answered".[60]

Princess Mary was the worst offender and her letters were filled with:

> volumes of all their nonscense[sic] and Her fine feelings and distress, which if she had one Hundredth part of the love for her sister she professes, she would keep to herself, or if she really wished to have her at home again. God knows I am almost distracted to see every thing undone as fast as it is doing.[61]

Fortunately, Lady Cathcart had an ally in Princess Augusta, who wrote "proper" letters that "delighted" Sophia. Her relief and thanks were profuse when she told her husband to "tell Her if I was within reach I should fall down at her Feet and kiss Her hands and worship her for the charming Letter she writ".[62] Augusta's letter was supportive and encouraging and Lady Cathcart wished the other family members would cease "torment[ing] her [Princess Sophia] with Conversations, dispatches, makings up and all the tittle tattle and nonsense that worrys Her to Death".[63] The Royal siblings were not the only problem, as the longer they were at Tunbridge, the more convinced Lady Cathcart became that not was all as it seemed. Just a week after their arrival she wrote "I am much afraid she [Princess Sophia] writes very differently from what she says to us of herself".[64]

A dual picture of Sophia emerges from Tunbridge. On the one hand, she was an invalid undergoing treatment and partaking of the waters and entertainments, and on the other, as time elapsed, her attendants grew increasingly suspicious of her illness. Upon their arrival, the princess's party took up residence on the salubrious hill of Mount Pleasant with views of the surrounding valley and breezes coming in from the Sussex coast.[65] Below the hill lay the Queen's Well, the baths, and taverns, like the Sussex (where Princess Sophia's servants were lodged). There were also assembly rooms, a chapel, and the famous walks known as the pantiles.[66] Sir Lucas Pepys instructed Sophia to take the waters, which she began almost immediately.[67] She was also prescribed a variety of medicines to combat the swallow and steady her nerves including Tincture of Cardamoms, Lavender, Rhubarb, Peppermint water, and Magnesia.[68] Rhubarb, lavender, and chalybeate waters were all utilized in "Hypochondriac and Hysteric Affections".[69] Rhubarb was also though effective against heartburn and was used to treat stomach ailments, as was peppermint and tincture of cardamom (which was a warming cordial).[70] Magnesia was employed against heartburn and as a "useful and safe antacid purge".[71]

In addition to her medicines, Sophia took long walks that seemed to revive her spirits and although the spasms continued they diminished in number. Lady Cathcart provides insight into the rhythm of her time at Tunbridge. On "a good day" she "went to the Well at eight, drank the Water", afterward she walked the Pantiles, doing the walks three and a half times, before taking breakfast. Sophia then went out on horseback for 45 minutes "without being fatigued" and then walked again.[72] At noon, she returned for a second dose of the waters before taking an airing in the coach and "was in such good spirits and so much amused that . . . [she] desire[d] them to drive on a little longer".[73] Upon returning to Mount Pleasant, "she went immediately to the Piano Forte and played and sung till the Sandwiches came, when she eat some, and then went on playing".[74] On this day, she only had three slight spasms, one at 11 o'clock, one at 2:30 and again another while dressing for the evening, and Lady Cathcart reported that "[s]he has not any now with sallowing [sic]. . . . I am sure you will easily believe that this rapid progress of amendment relieves my Mind of a great weight and gives me great happiness".[75]

These "good accounts" also relieved the Queen's anxiety, and she hoped Sophia would "think of Nothing else but of Dr Horse & Air which will be the most Pleasing companions to procure Health & Strengths".[76] "Dr Horse" was indeed a companion to the Princess, as this form of gentle

exercise was accorded restorative properties, and Sophia took daily air-
ings by coach and on horseback. She even hired a local, Adam Webb, to
serve as a guide in the coach and to ride in front of her.[77] On October 22,
she was out on horseback and then in the coach covering seven miles after
spending the previous night dancing country dances and Scotch reels.[78]
Below the surface of these convivial experiences, the relationship between
Princess Sophia and her companions was rapidly souring and they and her
physicians became increasingly convinced there was something disingenu-
ous about her spasms.

The Queen continued trying to manage her daughter from afar, as Lady
Cathcart had suggested Sophia write her mother "a Full account of Her
Grievances"[79] Queen Charlotte stated these were the result of "mistakes"
and "from wont of giving Herself Time to reflect".[80] She felt strongly that
her daughter was trying to circumvent her doctor's advice, and just a few
days after her arrival wrote, "I am extremely Curious to know how S. is
pleased with Sr. Lucas Conversation or is she so Close[d] that Nothing has
transpired".[81] Eight days later she wrote again:

> I do most Earnestly wish that Sr Lucas should have another Conversa-
> tion with Her & insist upon her fulfilling every advice He gives without
> the Smallest deviation & that He would be kind enough to lay such a
> stress upon what he says that she may be brought to fear the Conse-
> quences of not following him. . . . As I fear without His preaching all
> other maxims when my Back is turned will be in vain.[82]

The very same day Lady Cathcart wrote to her husband of her own exhaustion, brought on by managing the Princess's illness, her spirits, and most
of all her attempts to keep the 16-year-old amused to prevent her "from
returning to the old way of musing".[83] Despite her fatigue, Cathcart felt she
would be "well repaid for every thing if I can see her restor'd to Her Family
in Health again".[84] However, just a day later something drastically shifted.

On 20 October, Lady Cathcart, Lady Charlotte Bruce, and Mrs Chevely
staged an intervention and "had a very serious and open conversation in
which she [Sophia] promised us not to have any more returns of Her illness".[85] This led to a remarkable piece of theater that Lady Cathcart labelled
as "too ridiculous".[86] The following morning Sophia decided she should
drown her fitts in the Well. In the coach on the way Lady Cathcart produced
a piece of paper, then Lady Charlotte Bruce "pretended to magnetise" Princess Sophia "to draw out the spasms", they then wrapped the spasms "carefully in the Paper". When the well attendant "dipped the Glass in Ly C said
once, twice, thrice & threw the Paper upon which P.S. said begone forever".[87]

Two days later, Lady Cathcart wrote "the little Gypsey" had three spasms,
which she thought performative and an attempt "to amuse the Duke of

Clarence" who was visiting.[88] This incident prompted a stern mediation from her physician and Sophia promised Sir Lucas "never after her return to Windsor to have another spasm".[89] There were no more nods to the former favourite as "poor Sophy" and instead Lady Cathcart provided a scathing commentary both on her illness and the role played by those outside forces that she and the Queen had worked so hard to mitigate, stating,

> [T]here is no trusting her and I do not think Sir Lucas has a notion how perverted her mind is and what wickedness She is returning to. . . . I own I dread this Hypocrsy and tho she has most solemnly sworn . . . to have no relapse I much fear Her Word will go for nothing when she gets back among those wicked artfull People who will support her and whose interest it is to keep her ill, but enough of this odious subject I heartily wish I had never known anything of it as to wounds me to the Soul to see such a deceit and perversion in so Young a Mind.[90]

So who were these "artfull People" who thought it was in their interest to keep her ill? Beyond the performance for her brothers, a few glimpses emerge, perhaps as part of the shifting dynamics of the Royal nursery.

In 1792 Lady Charlotte Finch finally resigned from her post due to age and infirmity, eventually being replaced by Lady Elizabeth Cathcart, and there were jealous tensions particularly between Miss Jane Gomme and Miss Planta, rival English teachers whom Miss Burney stated, "humiliate, dislike and distrust each other".[91] Even the faithful Gooly seems to have been extraordinarily involved. She had long been trusted to care for the princesses while ill; for instance, in 1786 she was charged with attending Elizabeth during her long illness at Kew, and the princess wrote of her tender care.

> She never was away from me any part of the day and she was so very good as to have a chaise longue brought into the room that she might sleep by me. I always loved her extremely, but my illnesses have made me love her and esteem her ten times more.[92]

Despite her faithful service and the high praise of her charges, Gouldsworthy seems to have been excluded from directly caring for Sophia. Once the Tunbridge plan had been decided, Queen Charlotte even tried to limit access to the princess; however, she admitted to Lady Cathcart her difficulty in politely excluding Miss Gouldsworthy:

> You must have been much surprized when all was settled between me & the Dr about Sophia's not seeing any body but Yr self, to see Miss G. come up to Dinner. The Truth is, that she asked leave to go up stairs in such a manner that I could not refuse it without offending her.[93]

The following morning when Gooly returned with the Royal family from Frogmore and found Sophia gone, her reaction mimicked Princess Mary's as she "got an Histeric Fit".[94] Although she was left behind, Martha Gouldsworthy kept up correspondence both with Sir Lucas Pepys and with Princess Sophia.[95] On 15 October, Princess Sophia communicated Mrs. Chevely, Gooly's assessment of her departure and its impact upon her health prospects. An appalled Lady Cathcart relayed the exchange writing,

> She said to Mrs Chevly to day that 'Gooly is very right in what she tells Her that tho' Her journey here being contrived and carried into execution as it was certainly has saved her many painfull [sic] moments yet Her Nerves were so shook she never will recover it'.[96]

Lady Cathcart placed the blame squarely upon Gooly's shoulders; "I am very sure this is quite a new idea that never would have entered into her Head if it had not been put there can you imagine any thing so wicked".[97] Lady Cathcart extended the blame for Sophia's conduct to her siblings whom she labelled "a parcel of Ungratefull People",[98] and to both Gooly and Miss Gomme whom she believed were manipulating Princess Mary's behavior as well as Sophia's. She labelled "Gooly and Miss Gomme. . . . Her [Sophia's] destroyers and Prs M their Dupe".[99]

Lady Cathcart was not the only one with reservations, and by this point, Princess Sophia's attendants were firmly convinced her spasms were attention seeking and that she was untrustworthy. She was perfectly fine the whole day while accompanied by Lady Cathcart or Lady Charlotte Bruce but in ten minutes she was out of their sight she treated Mrs Byerly (her dresser) to "a short one".[100] Lady Cathcart was disgusted and Sophia's defiance was treated with disdain. Her attendants "treated her so coolly after it all the Evening and were so grave that she appeared quite ashamed and has not had once since [. . . and has] been twenty seven hours without one and seems quite well".[101] Sophia seems to have tried to smooth over the anger, writing Lady Cathcart a letter "full of affection which" she "answered immediately".[102] Despite these overtures, the damage was done and Sophia's attendants now saw her as unfeeling and selfish, opinions reinforced by her lack of reaction to the execution of Marie Antoinette, which occurred while she was at Tunbridge. The event was the subject of conversation on many occasions, but the Princess's lack of feeling was repeatedly remarked upon:

> The Q of Frances Death horrid as it was affected her no more than it did your Horse. She danced Reels, Slept like a Pig and no feeling whatever. . . . There has been no more spasms since Thursday and is perfectly well.[103]

The very next day, Lady Cathcart and her charge returned to Windsor with the Princess "much recovered from her late indisposition".[104] Although Sophia seems to have taken Marie Antoinette's death in stride, it greatly affected the Royal Family. The Queen had been planning a ball scheduled for 25 October to celebrate the anniversary of her husband's accession to the throne, one which from the beginning of her sojourn at Tunbridge, had been the target for Princess Sophia's return.[105] However, as both Lucy Kennedy and the *Times* reported, "On account of the execution of the Queen of France, the grand entertainment which was to have been given by the Queen on this occasion, at Frogmore Lodge, was put off".[106] The new date was planned for "ye 8th of Novembr, Princess Sophia's Birth Day".[107]

Although Sophia's stay at Tunbridge was beneficial, Lady Cathcart was not the only individual whose attitudes toward her changed after this experience. In the next year, there are glimpses of fractured relationships produced by her illness episode. Afterward, the princess's rapport with Lady Charlotte Bruce, who had been seen as a sister and who had attended her at Tunbridge, cooled, and Sophia now described it as "civil, but very distant".[108] More striking was a shift in the Queen's attitude, one other members of the family found curious and confusing. In October of 1794, Prince Adolphus wrote to the Princes of Wales that he was:

> very sorry to hear the ill humour of a certain person [The Queen], (you know who I mean,) continues so bad: particularly her behavior towards dear Mary & Sophia is so singular, as they certainly by no means deserve it. What can possess her to be so odd, & why make her life so wretched when she could have it just the reverse?[109]

Although Flora Fraser argued the coolness was due to the Queen's inability to shake off her concerns and anxiety over "the King's illness and the fate of the French royal family",[110] the timing does not fit, nor does the choice of only two daughters to bear her ire. Lady Cathcart's reports of Sophia, coupled with the Queen's own assessments of Mary's behavior during Sophia's illness, suggest a different reading of this dynamic. There was a new coolness between Sophia and her former companions, Lady Cathcart and Lady Bruce that accompanied the Queen's singular behavior toward both Sophia and Mary (who had certainly behaved in a way contrary to her brother's assessment of her as "the sweetest tempered girls I ever saw").[111] The family was completely befuddled by Charlotte's attitude, which suggests the Queen might be reacting to behaviors unknown to the rest of her family. By the end of her bout with this illness Princess Sophia had been transformed in the minds of some from "Poor Sophy" to "a decietfull gypsay [sic]".[112]

Notes

1 "Letter from Lady Cathcart to Lord Cathcart, Tunbridge, 24 Oct. 1793," Acc. 12686, National Library of Scotland, UK.
2 The Royal family had travelled to Weymouth arriving on 31 July 1800. Here, Sophia was attended by Sir Francis Milman, who was promoted to baronet for his services in October of that year. It is generally accepted it was during this period she delivered an illegitimate child, imputed to be the son of General Garth. Lord Glenbervie mentioned the circumstances surrounding these events stating:

> I heard yesterday a recapitulation of many of the circumstances of the princess Sophia's extraordinary illness last autumn at Weymouth, from the most authentic information. They are too delicate a nature for me to choose to commit them (at least according to my present feeling) even to this safe repository. But they are such as leave scarce a doubt in my mind.

"25 March 1801," in Francis Bickley, ed., *The Diaries of Sylvester Douglas, Lord Glenbervie* (London: Constable & Co., Ltd, 1928), vol. I, 203–4; John Wardrober, *Wicked Ernest* (London: Shelfmark Books, 2002), 11–12.
3 "Letter Princess Elizabeth to Elizabeth, Lady Harcourt, 8 July 1793," Harcourt MSS, as quoted in Flora Fraser, *Princesses: The Six Daughters of George III* (London: Bloomsbury, 2004), 147.
4 Fraser, *Princesses*, 112 & 144.
5 Janice Hadlow, *A Royal Experiment: The Private Life of King George III* (New York: Henry Holt and Company, 2014), 192 & 473.
6 Charlotte Louise Henrietta Papendiek, *Court and Private Life in the Time of Queen Charlotte: Being the Journals of Mrs. Papendiek, Assistant Keeper of the Wardrobe and Reader to Her Majesty* (London: Richard Bentley & Son, 1887), vol. 2, 216.
7 Hadlow, *A Royal Experiment*, 473.
8 Papendiek, *Court and Private Life in the Time of Queen Charlotte*, 216.
9 Fraser, *Princesses*, 145.
10 Dorothy Margaret Stuart, *The Daughters of George III* (London: Fonthill, 1939), 179.
11 Stuart, *The Daughters of George III*, 182.
12 Hadlow, *A Royal Experiment*, 481.
13 Ibid.
14 Stuart, *The Daughters of George III*, 179.
15 Hadlow, *A Royal Experiment*, 481–82.
16 Fraser, *Princesses*, 90 & 122.
17 Ibid., 147.
18 "Queen Charlotte to George, Prince of Wales, 15 April 1793," GEO/MAIN/36406; "Queen Charlotte to George, Prince of Wales, 16 April 1793," GEO/MAIN/36407 & "Princess Sophia to the Prince of Wales, 18 April 1793," GEO/ADD/13/7, The Royal Archives, UK.
19 Although Sophia did develop a problem she labelled her swallow, the Queen doesn't mention it by name while discussing her illness with her brother. "Queen Charlotte to her brother Charles II, Grand Duke of Mecklenburg-Strelitz, 28 May 1793," MS. 12058/8/28–29, University of Virginia Special Collections, USA.
20 *The Diary of Lucy Kennedy (1790–1816)*, edited by Lorna J. Clark, *The Memoirs of the Court of George III*, ed. Michael Kassler (London: Routledge Taylor & Francis Group, 2016), vol. 3, 2.

21 "Embarkation of the Guards," *Times*, February 26, 1793, 2. *The Times Digital Archive*, accessed March 13, 2022, https://link-gale-com.libproxy. furman.edu/apps/doc/CS34082906/TTDA?u=furmanuniv&sid=bookmark-TTDA&xid=789b8a75.

22 "News," *Morning Chronicle* [1770], May 6, 1793. *Seventeenth and Eighteenth Century Burney Newspapers Collection*, accessed March 2, 2022, https://link-gale-com.libproxy.furman.edu/apps/doc/Z2000795759/ BBCN?u=furmanuniv&sid=bookmark-BBCN&xid=dc01fb77.

23 "Letter from Queen Charlotte to George, Prince of Wales 8 May 1793," GEO/ MAIN/36408, The Royal Archives, UK.

24 "News," *True Briton* [1793], June 14, 1793. *Seventeenth and Eighteenth Century Burney Newspapers Collection*, accessed March 2, 2022, https://link-gale-com.libproxy.furman.edu/apps/doc/Z2001552238/ BBCN?u=furmanuniv&sid=bookmark-BBCN&xid=a4d3af02.

25 "London," *Times*, July 25, 1793, 2. *The Times Digital Archive*, accessed March 3, 2022, https://link-gale-com.libproxy.furman.edu/apps/doc/CS33689849/ TTDA?u=furmanuniv&sid=bookmark-TTDA&xid=c02b0176.

26 *The Diary of Lucy Kennedy (1790–1816)*, edited by Lorna J. Clark, Vol 3 of *The Memoirs of the Court of George III*, ed. Michael Kassler (London: Routledge Taylor & Francis Group, 2016), 2.

27 "17 July 1793," Personal Accounts Robert Battiscombe (Royal Apothecary), 1780–1794, D239/F3, Dorset Record Office, UK.

28 Ibid.

29 "Windsor July 21 HER MAJESTY paid a visit to PRINCESS SOPHIA, at the Lower Lodge; she goes to Kew to-morrow for change of air." "News," *World*, July 22, 1793. *Seventeenth and Eighteenth Century Burney Newspapers Collection*, accessed March 2, 2022, https://link-gale-com.libproxy. furman.edu/apps/doc/Z2001540862/BBCN?u=furmanuniv&sid=bookmark-BBCN&xid=d3192fc3. Robert Battiscombe confirms this date stating "July 22 Prs Sophia went to Kew" "22 July 1793," Personal Accounts Robert Battiscombe (Royal Apothecary), 1780–1794, D239/F3, Dorset Record Office, UK.

30 *The Diary of Lucy Kennedy*, 2.

31 William Munk, *The Roll of the Royal College of Physicians of London*, 1701 to 1800 (London: Published by the College, Pall Mall East, 1878), vol. II, 306.

32 "Princess Mary to Lady Cathcart, 1793," Acc. 12686/40/1795/12, National Library of Scotland, UK & *The Diary of Lucy Kennedy*, 2. & Munk, *The Roll of the Royal College of Physicians of London*, 190.

33 Fraser, *Princesses*, 147.

34 "Yesterday the Prince of WALES dined with the Princesses MARY and SOPHIA, at Kew," *Times*, July 29, 1793, 2. *The Times Digital Archive*, accessed March 3, 2022, https://link-gale-com.libproxy.furman.edu/apps/doc/CS34083069/ TTDA?u=furmanuniv&sid=bookmark-TTDA&xid=afc91d88. & "Yesterday Evening THEIR MAJESTIES and Three Elder PRINCESSES Came from Windsor to," *Times*, July 31, 1793, 2. *The Times Digital Archive*, accessed March 3, 2022, https://link-gale-com.libproxy.furman.edu/apps/doc/CS3408 3071/TTDA?u=furmanuniv&sid=bookmark-TTDA&xid=2411c5f5.

35 Elizabeth (nee Elliot) Cathcart (d. 1847), daughter of the lieutenant-governor of New York. On April 10, 1779, she married William Schaw Cathcart (1755–1843), tenth Baron Cathcart, later Earl Cathcart (1814). She served as Lady of the Bedchamber to the junior princesses and was close to Queen Charlotte and all the daughters.

36 "Princess Mary to Lady Cathcart, 1793," Acc. 12686/40/1795/12, National Library of Scotland, UK

37 "Princess Sophia to George III, 19 August [1793]," GEO/ADD/13/9, The Royal Archives, UK.

38 "Advertisements and Notices," *World*, August 30, 1793. *Seventeenth and Eighteenth Century Burney Newspapers Collection*, accessed March 2, 2022, https://link-gale-com.libproxy.furman.edu/apps/doc/Z2001541630/BBCN?u=furmanuniv&sid=bookmark-BBCN&xid=3e178330.

39 *The Diary of Lucy Kennedy*, 2.

40 "Sophia to the Prince of Wales, Windsor 18 Sept. [1793]," GEO/ADD/13/10, The Royal Archives, UK.

41 Munk, *The Roll of the Royal College of Physicians of London*, 305.

42 "17 July 1793."

43 John Ball, *A New Compendious Dispensatory* (London: T. Cadell, 1769), 302.

44 "Sophia to the Prince of Wales, Windsor 18 Sept. [1793]," GEO/ADD/13/10, The Royal Archives, UK.

45 Stephen Hales, *Philosophical Experiments* (London: W. Innys and R. Manby, 1739), 99.

46 "Sophia to the Prince of Wales, Windsor 18 September [1793]," GEO/ADD/13/10, The Royal Archives, UK.

47 R. Brookes, *The Natural History of Waters, Earths, Stones, Fossils, and Minerals with their Virtues, Properties and Medicinal Uses* (London: J. Newberry, 1763), vol. V.

48 Jasper Sprange, *The Tunbridge Wells Guide* (Printed & Sold by J. Sprange at his Circulating Library, 1786), 52.

49 Ibid., 56.

50 *The Diary of Lucy Kennedy*, 2.

51 "Queen Charlotte to Lady Cathcart, 1793," Acc. 12686/40/1793/5, National Library of Scotland, UK.

52 *The Diary of Lucy Kennedy*, 2.

53 "17 July 1793."

54 "Lady Cathcart to Lord Cathcart, 7 October 1793," Letters to Lady Cathcart from Queen Charlotte, etc. 1791–1795, National Library of Scotland, UK.

55 "Queen Charlotte to Lady Cathcart, 11 October 1793," Letters to Lady Cathcart from Queen Charlotte, etc. 1791–1795, National Library of Scotland, UK. The Prince of Wales did visit on Thursday 17 October 1793. "October 18 [Friday]. On Thursday the Prince of Wales paid a visit to Princess Sophia, at Tunbridge, and afterwards returned to Brighton." "News," *World*, October 19, 1793. *Seventeenth and Eighteenth Century Burney Newspapers Collection*, accessed March 2, 2022, https://link-gale-com.libproxy.furman.edu/apps/doc/Z2001543209/BBCN?u=furmanuniv&sid=bookmark-BBCN&xid=810fd115.

56 "Much Especially P: Mary, Who Had Never Been Separated One Day in Her Life," *The Diary of Lucy Kennedy*, 2.

57 "Queen Charlotte to Lady Cathcart, 8 October 1793," Letters to Lady Cathcart from Queen Charlotte, etc. 1791–1795, National Library of Scotland, UK.

58 "Queen Charlotte to Lady Cathcart, 11 October 1793."

59 "Lady Cathcart to Lord Cathcart, 13 October 1793," Letters to Lady Cathcart from Queen Charlotte, etc. 1791–1795, National Library of Scotland, UK.

60 Ibid.

61 Letters from Princess Elizabeth and also Prince Augustus were disturbing to Sophia. "Lady Cathcart to Lord Cathcart, 13 October 1793."

62 "Lady Cathcart to Lord Cathcart, Tunbridge, Friday Eveng October 1793," Letters to Lady Cathcart from Queen Charlotte, etc. 1791–1795, National Library of Scotland, UK.

63 "Lady Cathcart to Lord Cathcart, Tunbridge, Friday Eveng October 1793," Letters to Lady Cathcart from Queen Charlotte etc. 1791–1795, National Library of Scotland, UK.

64 "Lady Cathcart to Lord Cathcart, 15 October 1793," Letters to Lady Cathcart from Queen Charlotte, etc. 1791–1795, National Library of Scotland, UK.

65 Paul Amsinck, *Tunbridge Wells, and Its Neighbourhood* (London: William Miller, 1810), 2.

66 These walks had once been tiled, but by the Princess's visit were paved with stone. Amsinck, *Tunbridge Wells, and Its Neighbourhood*, 2, 9–10 & 14. & Princess Sophia's accounts bills related to her stay in Tunbridge Wells GEO/MAIN/16849–16849A (Bill and receipt issued by the Sussex Tavern to princess Sophia to 'stable people's lodging', 27 October 1793), The Royal Archives, UK.

67 "Sr Lucas Has Wrote to Miss Goldsworthy to Say She Had Begun the Waters." "Queen Charlotte to Lady Cathcart 11 October 1793."

68 Princess Sophia's accounts bills related to her stay in Tunbridge Wells GEO/MAIN/16846A (Bill issued by Thos. Thomas for PS's apothecary treatment 23 Oct. 1793), The Royal Archives, UK.

69 Ball, *A New Compendious Dispensatory*, 302.

70 W. Lewis, *The New Dispensatory: Containing the Elements of Pharmacy* (London: C. Nourse, 1781), 307; Ball, *A New Compendious Dispensatory*, 302 & 307.

71 Ball, *A New Compendious Dispensatory*, 33.

72 "Lady Cathcart to Lord Cathcart, 19 October 1793," Letters to Lady Cathcart from Queen Charlotte, etc. 1791–1795, National Library of Scotland, UK.

73 Ibid.

74 Ibid.

75 Ibid.

76 "Queen Charlotte to Lady Cathcart, 19 October 1793," Acc. 12686/40/1793/3, National Library of Scotland, UK.

77 Princess Sophia's accounts and bills related to her stay in Tunbridge Wells GEO/MAIN/16848 (Bill and receipt issued by Adam Webb to Princess Sophia for acting as a guide [riding before her at Tunbridge Wells 20 Oct 1793]. For more on Princess Sophia's expenses while at Tunbridge, see GEO/MAIN/16848A, GEO/MAIN/16850–16850A, GEO/MAIN/16851, GEO/MAIN/16852–16852A, GEO/MAIN/16853.

78 "Lady Cathcart to Lord Cathcart, 22 October 1793," Letters to Lady Cathcart from Queen Charlotte, etc. 1791–1795, National Library of Scotland, UK. & "Lady Cathcart to Lord Cathcart, 22 October 1793," Letters to Lady Cathcart from Queen Charlotte, etc. 1791–1795, National Library of Scotland, UK.

79 "Charlotte to Lady Cathcart, 19 October 1793," Letters to Lady Cathcart from Queen Charlotte, etc. 1791–1795, National Library of Scotland, UK.

80 Ibid.

81 "Queen Charlotte to Lady Cathcart 11 October 1793."

82 "Charlotte to Lady Cathcart, 19 October 1793."

83 "Lady Cathcart to Lord Cathcart, 19 October 1793."

84 Ibid.

85 "Lady Cathcart to Lord Cathcart, 21 October 1793," Letters to Lady Cathcart from Queen Charlotte, etc. 1791–1795, National Library of Scotland, UK.

86 Ibid.

87 Ibid.

88 "Lady Cathcart to Lord Cathcart, 23 October 1793," Letters to Lady Cathcart from Queen Charlotte, etc. 1791–1795, National Library of Scotland, UK.

89 Ibid.

90 "Lady Cathcart to Lord Cathcart, 24 October 1793," Letters to Lady Cathcart from Queen Charlotte, etc. 1791–1795, National Library of Scotland, UK.

91 Fraser, Princesses, 144.

92 Ibid., 90.

93 "Queen Charlotte to Lady Cathcart, 1793," Acc. 12686/40/1793/5, National Library of Scotland, UK.

94 "Queen Charlotte to Lady Cathcart, 8 October 1793."

95 "Queen Charlotte to Lady Cathcart, 11 October 1793."

96 "Lady Cathcart to Lord Cathcart, 15 October 1793."

97 Ibid.

98 Letters from Princess Elizabeth and also Prince Augustus were disturbing to Sophia. "Lady Cathcart to Lord Cathcart, 13 October 1793."

99 "Lady Cathcart to Lord Cathcart, 24 October 1793."

100 Ibid.

101 "Lady Cathcart to Lord Cathcart, 25 October 1793," Letters to Lady Cathcart from Queen Charlotte, etc. 1791–1795, National Library of Scotland, UK.

102 "Lady Cathcart to Lord Cathcart, 26 October 1793," Letters to Lady Cathcart from Queen Charlotte, etc. 1791–1795, National Library of Scotland, UK.

103 "Lady Cathcart to Lord Cathcart, 27 October 1793."

104 "Business," *World*, October 30, 1793. *Seventeenth and Eighteenth Century Burney Newspapers Collection*, accessed March 2, 2022, https://link-gale-com.libproxy.furman.edu/apps/doc/Z2001543507/BBCN?u=furmanuniv&sid=bookmark-BBCN&xid=88434483.

105 "Princess S. talks of getting Home by the twenty fifth and I own to you fairly if she does not, nothing but my admiration and respect for the King & Qn shall prevent my quitting them intierly [sic] from disgust at their conduct." "Lady Cathcart to Lord Cathcart, 13 October 1793."

106 "London," *Times*, October 26, 1793, 2. *The Times Digital Archive*, accessed March 22, 2022, https://link-gale-com.libproxy.furman.edu/apps/doc/CS33689946/TTDA?u=furmanuniv&sid=bookmark-TTDA&xid=2e061276.

107 "Thursday ye 24 [October 1793]," *The Diary of Lucy Kennedy*, 9.

108 "Princess Sophia to Lady Harcourt, Weymouth, 24 August 1794," *The Harcourt Papers*, ed. Edward William Harcourt (Printed for Private Circulation by James Parker and Co. Oxford, 1880), vol. VI, 282.

109 A. Aspinall, "Letter 872 Prince Adolphus to The Prince of Wales, Head Quarters at Nimwegen, 15 October 1794," in *The Correspondence of George, Princes of Wales*, 1789–1794 (New York: Oxford University Press, 1963), vol. II, 467.

110 Fraser, *Princesses*, 149.

111 Aspinall, "Letter 872 Prince Adolphus to the Prince of Wales, Head Quarters at Nimwegen, 15 October 1794," 467.

112 "Letter from Lady Cathcart to Lord Cathcart, Tunbridge, 24 Oct. 1793," Acc. 12686, National Library of Scotland, UK.

Reference List

Primary—Archival

Dorset Record Office, UK

"17 July 1793," Personal Accounts Robert Battiscombe (Royal Apothecary), 1780–1794, D239/F3.
"22 July 1793," Personal Accounts Robert Battiscombe (Royal Apothecary), 1780–1794, D239/F3.

National Library of Scotland, UK

"Lady Cathcart to Lord Cathcart, 7 October 1793," Letters to Lady Cathcart from Queen Charlotte, etc. 1791–1795.
"Lady Cathcart to Lord Cathcart, 13 October 1793," Letters to Lady Cathcart from Queen Charlotte, etc. 1791–1795.
"Lady Cathcart to Lord Cathcart, 15 October 1793," Letters to Lady Cathcart from Queen Charlotte, etc. 1791–1795.
"Lady Cathcart to Lord Cathcart, 19 October 1793," Letters to Lady Cathcart from Queen Charlotte, etc. 1791–1795.
"Lady Cathcart to Lord Cathcart, 21 October 1793," Letters to Lady Cathcart from Queen Charlotte, etc. 1791–1795.
"Lady Cathcart to Lord Cathcart, 22 October 1793," Letters to Lady Cathcart from Queen Charlotte, etc. 1791–1795.
"Lady Cathcart to Lord Cathcart, 23 October 1793," Letters to Lady Cathcart from Queen Charlotte, etc. 1791–1795.
"Lady Cathcart to Lord Cathcart, 24 October 1793," Letters to Lady Cathcart from Queen Charlotte, etc. 1791–1795.
"Lady Cathcart to Lord Cathcart, 25 October 1793," Letters to Lady Cathcart from Queen Charlotte, etc. 1791–1795.
"Lady Cathcart to Lord Cathcart, 26 October 1793," Letters to Lady Cathcart from Queen Charlotte, etc. 1791–1795.
"Lady Cathcart to Lord Cathcart, 27 October 1793," Letters to Lady Cathcart from Queen Charlotte, etc. 1791–1795.
"Lady Cathcart to Lord Cathcart, Tunbridge, Friday Eveng Oct.1793," Letters to Lady Cathcart from Queen Charlotte, etc. 1791–1795.
"Letter from Lady Cathcart to Lord Cathcart, Tunbridge, 24 Oct. 1793." Acc. 12686.
"Princess Mary to Lady Cathcart, 1793," Acc. 12686/40/1795/12.
"Queen Charlotte to Lady Cathcart, 1793," Acc. 12686/40/1793/5.
"Queen Charlotte to Lady Cathcart, 8 October 1793," Letters to Lady Cathcart from Queen Charlotte, etc. 1791–1795.
"Queen Charlotte to Lady Cathcart, 11 October 1793," Letters to Lady Cathcart from Queen Charlotte, etc. 1791–1795.
"Queen Charlotte to Lady Cathcart, 19 October 1793," Acc. 12686/40/1793/3.
"Queen Charlotte to Lady Cathcart, 1793," Acc. 12686/40/1793/5.

The Royal Archives, UK

"Letter from Queen Charlotte to George, Prince of Wales 8 May 1793," GEO/MAIN/36408.

Princess Sophia's accounts bills related to her stay in Tunbridge Wells GEO/MAIN/16846A, 16848, GEO/MAIN/16848A, GEO/MAIN/16849–16849A, GEO/MAIN/16850–16850A, GEO/MAIN/16851, GEO/MAIN/16852–16852A, GEO/MAIN/16853.

"Princess Sophia to George III, 19 August [1793]," GEO/ADD/13/9, The Royal Archives, UK.

"Princess Sophia to the Prince of Wales, 18 April 1793," GEO/ADD/13/7.

"Queen Charlotte to George, Prince of Wales, 15 April 1793." GEO/MAIN/36406.

"Queen Charlotte to George, Prince of Wales, 16 April 1793," GEO/MAIN/36407.

"Sophia to the Prince of Wales, Windsor 18 Sept. [1793]," GEO/ADD/13/10, The Royal Archives, UK.

University of Virginia Special Collections, USA

"Queen Charlotte to Her Brother Charles II, Grand Duke of Mecklenburg-Strelitz, 28 May 1793." MS. 12058/8/28–29.

Primary—Newspaper Collections

"Advertisements and Notices." *World*, August 30, 1793. *Seventeenth and Eighteenth Century Burney Newspapers Collection.* Accessed March 2, 2022. https://link-gale-com.libproxy.furman.edu/apps/doc/Z2001541630/BBCN?u=furmanuniv&sid=bookmark-BBCN&xid=3e178330.

"Business." *World*, October 30, 1793. *Seventeenth and Eighteenth Century Burney Newspapers Collection.* Accessed March 2, 2022. https://link-gale-com.libproxy.furman.edu/apps/doc/Z2001543507/BBCN?u=furmanuniv&sid=bookmark-BBCN&xid=88434483.

"Embarkation of The Guards." *Times*, February 26, 1793, 2. *The Times Digital Archive.* Accessed March 13, 2022. https://link-gale-com.libproxy.furman.edu/apps/doc/CS34082906/TTDA?u=furmanuniv&sid=bookmark-TTDA&xid=789b8a75.

"London." *Times*, July 25, 1793, 2. *The Times Digital Archive.* Accessed March 3, 2022. https://link-gale-com.libproxy.furman.edu/apps/doc/CS33689849/TTDA?u=furmanuniv&sid=bookmark-TTDA&xid=c02b0176.

"London." *Times*, October 26, 1793, 2. *The Times Digital Archive.* Accessed March 22, 2022. https://link-gale-com.libproxy.furman.edu/apps/doc/CS33689946/TTDA?u=furmanuniv&sid=bookmark-TTDA&xid=2e061276.

"News." *Morning Chronicle* [1770], May 6, 1793. *Seventeenth and Eighteenth Century Burney Newspapers Collection.* Accessed March 2, 2022. https://link-gale-com.libproxy.furman.edu/apps/doc/Z2000795759/BBCN?u=furmanuniv&sid=bookmark-BBCN&xid=dc01fb77.

"News." *True Briton* [1793], June 14, 1793. *Seventeenth and Eighteenth Century Burney Newspapers Collection.* Accessed March 2, 2022. https://link-gale-com.libproxy.furman.edu/apps/doc/Z2001552238/BBCN?u=furmanuniv&sid=bookmark-BBCN&xid=a4d3af02.

"News." *World,* July 22, 1793. *Seventeenth and Eighteenth Century Burney Newspapers Collection.* Accessed March 2, 2022. https://link-gale-com.libproxy.furman.edu/apps/doc/Z2001540862/BBCN?u=furmanuniv&sid=bookmark-BBCN&xid=d3192fc3.

"News." *World,* October 19, 1793. *Seventeenth and Eighteenth Century Burney Newspapers Collection.* Accessed March 2, 2022. https://link-gale-com.libproxy.furman.edu/apps/doc/Z2001543209/BBCN?u=furmanuniv&sid=bookmark-BBCN&xid=810fd115.

"Yesterday Evening THEIR MAJESTIES and Three Elder PRINCESSES Came from Windsor to." *Times,* July 31, 1793, 2. *The Times Digital Archive.* Accessed March 3, 2022. https://link-gale-com.libproxy.furman.edu/apps/doc/CS34083071/TTDA?u=furmanuniv&sid=bookmark-TTDA&xid=2411c5f5.

"Yesterday the Prince of WALES Dined With the Princesses MARY and SOPHIA, at Kew." *Times,* July 29, 1793, 2. *The Times Digital Archive.* Accessed March 3, 2022. https://link-gale-com.libproxy.furman.edu/apps/doc/CS34083069/TTDA?u=furmanuniv&sid=bookmark-TTDA&xid=afc91d88.

Printed Primary

"25 March 1801," in *The Diaries of Sylvester Douglas, Lord Glenbervie,* edited by Francis Bickley, vol. I. London: Constable & Co., Ltd, 1928.

Amsinck, Paul. *Tunbridge Wells, and Its Neighbourhood.* London: William Miller, 1810.

Ball, John. *A New Compendious Dispensatory.* London: T. Cadell, 1769.

Brookes, R. *The Natural History of Waters, Earths, Stones, Fossils, and Minerals with their Virtues, Properties and Medicinal Uses.* Vol. V. London: J. Newbery, 1763.

The Diary of Lucy Kennedy (1790–1816). Edited by Lorna J. Clark. *The Memoirs of the Court of George III.* Vol. 3, edited by Michael Kassler. London: Routledge Taylor & Francis Group, 2016.

Hales, Stephen. *Philosophical Experiments.* London: W. Innys and R. Manby, 1739.

"Letter 872 Prince Adolphus to The Prince of Wales, Head Quarters at Nimwegen, 15 October 1794." In *The Correspondence of George, Princes of Wales,* edited by A. Aspinall, vol. II 1789–1794. New York: Oxford University Press, 1963.

"Letter Princess Elizabeth to Elizabeth, Lady Harcourt, 8 July 1793." Harcourt MSS. In *Princesses: The Six Daughters of George III,* edited by Flora Fraser. London: Bloomsbury, 2004.

Lewis, W. *The New Dispensatory: Containing the Elements of Pharmacy.* London: C. Nourse, 1781.

Munk, William. *The Roll of the Royal College of Physicians of London,* vol. II, 1701 to 1800. London: Published by the College, Pall Mall East, 1878.

Papendiek, Charlotte Louise Henrietta. *Court and Private Life in the Time of Queen Charlotte: Being the Journals of Mrs. Papendiek, Assistant Keeper of the Wardrobe and Reader to Her Majesty.* Vol. 2. London: Richard Bentley & Son, 1887.

"Princess Sophia to Lady Harcourt, Weymouth, 24 August 1794." In *The Harcourt Papers,* edited by Edward William Harcourt, vol. VI. Printed for Private Circulation by James Parker and Co. Oxford, 1880.

Sprange, Jasper. *The Tunbridge Wells Guide*. Printed & Sold by J. Sprange at his Circulating Library, 1786.

Secondary

Bickley, Francis, ed. *The Diaries of Sylvester Douglas, Lord Glenbervie*, vol. I. London: Constable & Co., Ltd, 1928.

Fraser, Flora. *Princesses: The Six Daughters of George III*. London: Bloomsbury, 2004.

Hadlow, Janice. *A Royal Experiment: The Private Life of King George III*. New York: Henry Holt and Company, 2014.

Stuart, Dorothy Margaret. *The Daughters of George III*. London: Fonthill, 1939.

Wardrober, John. *Wicked Ernest*. London: Shelfmark Books, 2002.

Part III

Regulations and Laws Against Malingering

8 Faking It
Thirteenth-Century Bolognese Responses to Feigning Leprosy

Courtney A. Krolikoski

In the Commune of Bologna between 1259 and 1276, there was a distinct concern over people who faked diseases, disabilities, and social status while begging to gain sympathy and, in turn, money. Referred to as the *falsarii* (counterfeiters) in the Bolognese *Statuti*, the Statutes of the commune contain increasingly strict regulations concerning individuals who sought to deceive the public for their own financial gain. Put simply, the Bolognese government was attempting to weed out charity scammers.[1] The *falsarii* who faked leprosy were specifically targeted for regulation and expulsion—a concern echoed in writings of contemporary Bolognese jurists and physicians—suggesting that the practice of feigning leprosy was likely a somewhat common occurrence in Bologna. This further confirms what has been suggested in the historiography of medieval leprosy in the last few decades that persons with leprosy were sought out, or at least recognized, by medieval citizens as valuable recipients of their alms.[2] What this also suggests, however, is that faking leprosy was also seen as a worthwhile and lucrative avenue for pre-modern charity scammers.

This chapter argues that during the High Middle Ages, a period wherein understandings of charity and salvation were in flux, urban centers like Bologna became more suspicious of false beggars and charity scammers. As the thirteenth century saw the development of new political institutions and systems, particularly at the local level, new relationships developed between urban governments and charitable institutions, like *leprosaria* and hospitals, that were mutually beneficial—so long as those institutions and the people they cared for remained worthy, the governments would continue to protect and support them.[3] In this environment, faking leprosy became one of the more problematic *falsarii* for the Bolognese government due to their unique place in medieval society. By analyzing two statutes found in the Bolognese *Statuti* of 1259 (and repeated in the Statuti of 1250–1261, 1264, and 1267–1276) that address how Bologna reacted to and attempted to regulate those who faked leprosy for personal gain, it is

DOI: 10.4324/9781003452324-12

possible to better understand how society understood and protected their neighbors who truly suffered from leprosy.[4]

Changes in Charity in the Later Middle Ages

From its foundations, Christianity has been intimately intertwined with the idea of poverty, with Christians being urged to care for their poor neighbors through charitable works and deeds. This command can be seen in the Second Epistle to the Corinthians where it is said that "for you know the grace of our Lord Jesus Christ, that though he was rich, yet for your sake he became poor, so that you through his poverty might become rich".[5] Poverty also held a privileged status within the Christian community, with Jesus proclaiming, "blessed are the poor: for yours is the kingdom of God".[6] Yet, not all of mankind was expected to experience poverty—voluntarily or otherwise—as the rich were meant to support the poor with their wealth in ways that were spiritually beneficial. Indeed, in the Gospel of Luke Jesus told a rich man that, instead of inviting friends, family, and his rich neighbors to his banquets, that he should "invite the poor, the crippled, the lame, the blind, and you will be blessed. Although they cannot repay you, you will be repaid at the resurrection of the righteous".[7] Those with material wealth were obligated to provide for the poor and the otherwise marginalized—as their spiritual health rested on following Jesus's example.[8] Moreover, as noted in the Rule of Saint Benedict, the poor themselves were Christ's representatives on Earth. "[G]reat care and concern" must be shown in "receiving poor people and pilgrims, because in them more particularly Christ is received".[9] In a society dominated by the ideology that good deeds and good works led to salvation, the rich and the poor were both necessary components. For people in medieval Europe, this meant that providing charity for those in need—physically or financially—was a celebrated virtue that was understood to be an act of mercy and love. Charity could take many forms and by providing hospitality, performing acts of service, or giving material bequests or gifts to those in need, Christians fulfilled their duty to God.[10]

In this system of charity and salvation, certain groups of the poor were understood to be more 'deserving' of the care of their neighbors and strangers than others. Distinctions thus formed between those who were deserving and those who were not. The 'deserving' poor were understood to be the 'poor of Christ', something that made them particularly worthy of alms. This group included those who were incapable of working, whose poverty was not considered a 'choice' but a result of an unfortunate circumstance; the orphaned, sick, disabled, elderly, and widowed. As the poor of Christ, the poor and the infirm were "a kind of natural-born intercessor, a guardian of heaven's gate".[11] Christians gave alms to disabled beggars because they were engaging in a system of exchange wherein the "generosity of the rich was transformed into the subsistence of the poor" but, even further, that generosity assured the donors of their own salvation.[12] The 'undeserving' poor, on the other hand, were seen as unruly, ungovernable, and a threat to society. These were the people who were capable of working and supporting themselves but did not seek out the employment necessary to do so. The worst of this group were those who chose to support their unemployed lifestyle by begging.

A significant shift occurred in the twelfth and thirteenth centuries, referred to as the 'Charitable Revolution', which changed the concept of poverty as well as its relationship to charity. While providing for the poor remained a key component of Christianity, this period (roughly 1130–1260) saw a notable increase in both pious works and donations by the lay population to charitable and assistive institutions.[13] Now, a cornerstone of the study of medieval charity and poor relief, the idea of the Charitable Revolution explains both the sudden uptick in the foundations of hospitals and *leprosaria* in this period as well as the increase in pious donations made to them. Moreover, this increase in donations has also been tied to the development of the idea of purgatory and its penitential value in the twelfth and thirteenth centuries.[14]

Purgatory, formally recognized by the Second Council of Lyons in 1274, was conceived of as a place where the souls of the dead went through a period of purification for their earthly sins while awaiting their admission into heaven. As the concept gained popularity, it became clarified that not only could the good works performed during one's lifetime alleviate their suffering and shorten their time in Purgatory after death, but so could the prayers and meritorious acts made in their name by the living.[15] Thus, the Charitable Revolution was further driven by the corporeal acts of mercy, which encouraged the laity feed the hungry, give drink to the thirsty, clothe the naked, shelter the homeless, visit the sick and imprisoned, and bury the dead.[16] Such acts and donations were therefore linked to the overwhelming growth of lay devotion. Through the desire to ensure their own salvation, medieval donors placed their faith in the intercessory powers of the sick and the poor as the recipients of their charity.[17] Serving *leprosaria* and other charitable institutions, through donations or acts—even by others after one's death—became a potent method for protecting one's soul from Purgatory.

The twelfth- and thirteenth-century growth of urban centers and the rise of the laity as a socioeconomic also led to the development of new forms of government and a boom in commercial activity across Europe. As urban centers grew in both size and wealth, migrants moved from the countryside to attempt to better their lives by engaging in the newly emerging monetary economy. However, the labor pools of a city often surpassed their needs, causing wages to fall and levels of indigence to rise.[18] As a result, poverty became more visible in the urban landscape, which led to new social and cultural understandings of poverty. By the late thirteenth century, Bologna reached its peak demographic numbers, with between 50,000 and 65,000 people calling the city home and another 50,000 people living in the surrounding *contado* (the countryside outside the district of Bologna, but still under the city's rule).[19] Like most (but not all) cities at this time, Bologna began to see a geographic segregation between the rich and the poor, with the rich living closer to the city center and the less rich to the poor living at increasing distances toward its edges.[20] With more and more people arriving in the city, it was impossible for individuals to intimately know the lives of all those they came into contact with, making it more difficult to know exactly to whom they were giving their charity. This made it imperative that the city establish a system for protecting donors by prohibiting individuals from faking a life that might be regarded as one worthy of receiving alms.

The emergence of new political systems within these urban centers likely also led to the development of new institutional systems of charity. As the motivations behind charitable giving reframed who could benefit from engaging in charitable works, broad popular support for these newly established institutions boomed.[21] Moreover, instead of solely being an individual or familial act, charity became something that could also be performed collectively by a community for the benefit of the whole. By the turn of the thirteenth century, this is exactly what occurred in Bologna—it pledged communal support to the city's religious and charitable institutions, including hospitals, monasteries, the houses of professed men or women, and, occasionally, private homes or small communities of pious men or women.[22] This was Bologna's *secolo d'oro,* their "Golden Age", wherein the city had become prosperous and well known within the region and beyond, thanks largely to the growth of the Studium.[23] Giving to charitable institutions that supported the commune's identity and culture reflects how important and beneficial the city fathers' considered them to be. Included on Bologna's annual list of charitable and assistive institutions that received support from the communal government was the *leprosarium* of San Lazzaro, Bologna's sole *leprosarium.* For a commune-like Bologna, donations to an institution like San Lazzaro could be used to express their own particular urban flair and political convictions.[24]

Non Alij Nisi Speciali Eorum Nuntio: Protecting Civic Charity

Bologna's government was no stranger to contemporary changes in conceptions of poverty and charity and their approach to both is reflected in their civic statutes, known as the *Statuti*. The first statute that hints at concern over the potential faking of leprosy is found in the *Statuti* of 1248–1260, 1250, 1259,[25] 1259–1265, 1264, 1267–1276, and 1288. In this statute, the commune of Bologna granted San Lazzaro 25 *corbe* of grain, a sum that remained constant throughout the period in question.[26] The *leprosarium* was not unique in receiving this support from the commune. Indeed, in each edition of the *Statuti* in question, the donation to San Lazzaro is nestled in the midst of a sizeable list of religious and charitable institutions that the commune promised to support. Between 1250 and 1267, these donations were placed toward the beginning of the statutes, in Book I, Rubric I, directly after the *sacramentum potestatis bononie*, the *podestà*'s oath. In the 1250 *Statuti*, for example, the *podestà* Rizzardo da Villa swears to oversee the maintenance and upkeep of a number of public works, including the gates of the city, the towers, the walls, and the waterways, to expel heretics from the city, and oversee a number of other related tasks.[27] After this, he promises to distribute the alms of certain quantities of grain or amounts of money to some of the city's pious houses.

The inclusion of these donations in the *podestà*'s oath is particularly interesting, when you consider what surrounds them. Beginning in 1259, there is an addition of a new Rubric II with the heading "On the due to sacred places for the honor and reverence of our lord Jesus Christ", which highlights the role that the institutions played within the commune as well as how it separates it directly from the oath.[28] This additional rubric heading would remain until 1267, with only some changes to the phrasing in each revision to the *Statuti*. While they may seem out of place, these donations were important for the upkeep of Bologna as a good and healthy city. By promising to do these things, the *podestà* ensures that the city remains pleasing to God, in terms of both appearance and morality; he promises to protect the health and bodies of citizens and commune, while simultaneously promising to care for those in need.

In the 1288 statutes, the donations to religious institutions, hospitals, or other groups are no longer included as part of the oath of the *podestà* or the oath of any other city official. Instead, the donations to pious institutions were relocated to Book XI, which deals primarily with the revenue and expenses of the commune. This change suggests that these donations were no longer seen as a prominent feature of city legislation nor understood to be a solemn commitment enshrined in the oath of a public official but were simply a routine civic expense. Though still described as a charity (*elimosine*), these donations became a matter of public accounting and accountability instead of part of a sworn oath to protect and provide for the Bolognese citizenry.[29]

Despite these changes, it is clear that Bologna, like its citizens, remained interested in ensuring that the commune's donations went to those who they were intended to support. In the earliest versions of this statute, the only mention of the residents of San Lazzaro is an allusion through the donations of grain made to the *leprosarium* from the city. However, beginning in 1259 it is stated that the 25 *corbe* of grain promised to San Lazzaro should be given directly "to the lepers or to a designated envoy".[30] Then, in 1288, the phrasing of the statute changes again, noting that the 25 *corbe* of grain are to go "to the lepers of San Lazzaro or to their legitimate master".[31] Interestingly, in no version of the Bolognese statutes are similar qualifications added to the donations for other hospitals or, for that matter, any other charitable or religious institution receiving aid from the commune. This measure was added, and increasingly tightened, to ensure that the donations actually went to those in San Lazzaro. And so, what is reflected in the progression of this statute is a continued effort to protect the good deeds of the commune toward its deserving residents so that it could receive the spiritual benefits of their actions.

There are a few possible reasons for these changes. It could potentially point to issues of corruption within the *leprosarium* or a desire to prevent any future corruption from occurring. As Anna M. Peterson has shown in the cases of Narbonne, France, and Siena, Italy, beginning in the mid-thirteenth century, there was a growing desire to "create accountable institutions and individuals" in order to "prevent corruption or, at the very least, uncover it before a house's integrity was compromised".[32] Though the church had attempted to regulate and eliminate corruption, scandal, and other forms of wrongdoing in hospitals since the early twelfth century, such intervention was often limited and sporadic.[33] The issue of corruption is interesting, as it points to a concern by the donors about the maintenance of the integrity of the institution. Indeed, historians have recently emphasized that civic and religious efforts in the thirteenth century to prevent corruption and fraud can be seen as responses to contemporary moral proscriptions.[34] Financial fraud was a particular concern for assistive institutions like *leprosaria* and hospitals. If Bologna's San Lazzaro was somehow tainted by corruption, either spiritually or morally, they risked their ability to holistically care for those who lived and served at the institution as well as their ability to offset the sins of their donors.

Indeed, issues of corruption within assistive institutions, particularly that related to charitable donations, were understood to be "tantamount to defrauding God and society".[35] One common fear was that of being deceived by those who served at a hospital who diverted the alms from the poor to their own pockets or tables either by outright fraud or by the misappropriation of the donations.[36] In the *Historia occidentalis* from around 1226, Jacques de Vitry makes it clear that while "[t]his pestilential corruption and hateful hypocrisy" did not affect all hospitals, it could.[37]

These corrupt hospitals, "under the pretext of hospitality and the guise of piety", become:

> alms-collectors, improperly extorting monies by lies and deception and by every means at their disposal, feasting on the poor, not caring for them except that they, by giving a little to the poor and infirm, are able to demand alms from the faithful.[38]

The addition of the clause to Bologna's donation to San Lazzaro regarding who could collect the commune's alms thus suggests that there might have indeed been some external scrutiny or trepidation about the house, particularly concerning civic charity.

The fear that the alms given to support an assistive institution would not actually benefit the sick poor was a pervasive and constant worry in this period. The inclusion of this designation might also be a response to people with no relationship to San Lazzaro collecting the grain, leaving the *leprosarium* without their expected and necessary support. In this case, it would not be a fear of corruption on the part of the *leprosarium*, but, instead, a fear that the city government and the commune would not gain the social and spiritual benefits of their charity.

Either way, the designation of "to the lepers themselves" or an envoy specifically determined by the *leprosarium* shows a concern on the part of the commune's government that, somehow, the lepers of San Lazzaro were not benefiting fully from their charity. The Bolognese government, by giving the grain "directly to the lepers or their special envoy", ensured that their donation facilitated the support and care of the sick poor at San Lazzaro. However, without a foundational charter or statutes of San Lazzaro, it is impossible to confirm whether there was a push for, or expectation of, the prevention of wrongdoing from within Bologna's *leprosarium*. As Peterson has shown with the Ospedale di Santa Maria della Scala, an institution's statutes can give us insight into their own concerns over fraud and corruption. In the Ospedale's 1305 and 1318 statutes, for example, the hospital promises to "love the Commune of Siena, and not to defraud it and to not let others defraud it in any way by any person of the aforesaid hospital".[39] This should be seen as a desire for the Ospedale's transparency, allowing them to remain uncorrupted in the eyes of the commune and continue to be a desirable outlet for charitable donations. However, the Bolognese inclusion of qualifications within the statute suggests that there likely had been a continuing issue of the donations being intercepted or gathered by persons not from the *leprosaria* and, moreover, that the city wanted to ensure that their charity ended up in the right hands.

Ad Hoc Ut Leprosi Videantur: Protecting Personal Charity

Over the course of the years covered by the *Statuti*, it is possible to trace the increasing protection (and potential legitimization) of San Lazzaro's begging rights and access to alms by following the communal policies which policed individuals who attempted to fake the disease within the city limits. The second statute that points to a fear of the potential faking of leprosy prohibits all those who "counterfeit" disabled or privileged statuses (*falsarii*) from entering Bologna or receiving hospitality within its walls.[40] This statute shows a pointed disdain for those who faked a protected status in order to beg in the city and gain money through the deception of Bolognese citizens. It presents an explicit list of the *falsarii* who were not allowed in the commune, including those who are made blind, those who "make themselves" blind, those who "stain themselves with herbs" in order to appear leprous, those who dress like monks and penitents, and any other *falsarii* who carry counterfeit begging licenses try and get rich "in a false way", so they can go into taverns, get drunk, and blaspheme God and the saints.[41] These were the people who city officials considered able to work for their wages and be productive member of the commune who, instead, faked a disability or privileged status in order to get rich (or, at least rich*er*) off the generosity of Bolognese citizens. This suggests that the Bolognese were already, in the mid-thirteenth century, wary of those who might be operating what might be considered a pre-modern 'charity scam' and thus forbidden from entering the commune or receiving hospitality from anyone within its walls.[42]

It is particularly interesting that Bologna's move to prohibit false beggars from entering the city to solicit alms begins with the 1259 *Statuti*. Elites, in particular, wanted to find a way to establish "distinguishing signs" that would demarcate a person's true status in the public sphere.[43] This was not initially intended to separate the true beggars from the false, but instead to visibly mark (through clothing, badges, and more) the different statuses and classes of individuals in society—from the royalty and elite rulers to the clergy to the Jews to the prostitutes and the beggars. As Sharon Farmer has noted, the idea that able-bodied beggars should be distinguishable from those who were truly disabled fits clearly into this broader worldview.[44] Bologna's attempt to do just this seems early when compared to other Western European institutionalized attempts to distinguish the deserving, true beggars from those faking a privileged status to collect alms. In France, for example, it was only in 1312 that Philip IV required blind beggars from the Hospice des Quinze-Vingts—the only group he granted the privilege to beg within Paris's city limits—to wear a yellow fleur-de-lys to identify their status and royal protection.[45]

This apprehension can be seen reflected in the policing false beggars by specifically highlighting those who distorted or changed their appearance in order to present as disabled. For example, the chapter *Contra dantes hastrionibus* (against giving charity to those who act like beggars) of Peter the Chanter's late twelfth-century *Verbum abbreviatum* condemns those beggars who "make themselves tremulous, and putting on the various forms of the sick, change their faces just like Proteus".[46] According to elite clerics like Peter, by tricking potential donors into believing they were doing a charitable deed by donating to the disabled put both the false beggars and their potential donors in great moral danger. In another example, Thomas of Chobham, a Parisian student of Peter the Chanter, wrote in a manual for confessors that beggars "frequently transfigure themselves into the appearance of the wretched, so that they seem more destitute than they really are, and thus they deceive others so that they will receive more".[47]

Encouraging, or even demanding, that those with leprosy seek membership in a *leprosarium* was likely paramount for a city. This is because leprosy sufferers, as far as both civic and ecclesiastic authorities were concerned, essentially fell into two distinct categories: the 'wild' and the 'tame'. Those leprosy sufferers labeled 'wild' were perceived as sexually voracious and sinful individuals who were often associated with prostitutes. The assumption was that, if left unattended and to their own devices, poor 'wild' leprosy sufferers would pose some sort of danger to the rest of society. 'Tame' leprosy sufferers, on the other hand, were safely housed in a *leprosarium* allowing them to satisfy their special purpose of being a religious intercessor for their community. By joining a *leprosarium*, 'tame' leprosy sufferers provided the local city and laity with a unique and potent devotional opportunity. This distinction between the 'wild' and the 'tame' is also echoed in literary and legislative texts that highlight *leprosaria* as the key feature that separated the two groups.[48] It conveniently allowed both civic and ecclesiastic powers to reconcile the "otherwise contradictory ideas about the disease".[49] As a social issue that was widely and uniformly condemned, vagrancy was seen as something that needed to be suppressed.[50] As a result, the idea of the 'wild' leprosy sufferer was closely aligned with the concept of the undeserving poor. This makes it even more clear as to how faking leprosy was seen as particularly problematic within this cultural and religious worldview.

As a whole, leprosy sufferers who were attached to a city or commune's *leprosaria* across Italy and throughout Europe enjoyed some freedom of movement or, at minimum, engagement with lay society, though the lengths of that freedom varied from place to place. While the founding charter, statutes, and records from San Lazzaro are either lost or no longer extant, the legislation and practices of other European *leprosaria* from this period can provide a sense of what may have been considered appropriate for its residents. In Siena, Italy, for example, a statute from the *Constituto* of 1262 stated that persons with leprosy who were associated with the city's *leprosaria* were allowed to enter the city during Holy Week.[51] At the Salle-aux-Puelles in Rouen, France, the leprous sisters were required to "first obtain the permission of the prioresses before speaking to lay people".[52] While this *leprosarium* was, in theory, enclosed, its boundaries were often crossed by lay persons who "enter[ed] the cloister and the kitchen and the workrooms" and "[went] among the sisters and speak with them".[53] In London, however, at the turn of the thirteenth century a civic regulation prohibited leprosy sufferers from "going about the city" or making "a sojourn in the city". They were instead permitted to select "a common attorney for themselves, to go each Sunday into the parish churches to collect alms for their sustenance".[54] Though this English example did prohibit leprosy sufferers from entering London, it did not cut the city's ties with the *leprosaria*. So, while there is no direct stipulation for when Bolognese leprosy sufferers were allowed to enter the city or engage with lay society, similar regulations from other *leprosaria* provide more evidence that it was unlikely that the rectors from San Lazzaro were meant to keep those who lived in the house locked away.

It is important to emphasize that those individuals who were actually diagnosed with leprosy are not addressed by this statute. Though Bolognese leprosy sufferers lived and received care at the *leprosarium* of San Lazzaro, it is likely that begging for alms in the city and the *contado* was a common practice for them to receive alimentary support for the house. Indeed, institutions that housed and cared for the poor, sick, or disabled often expected their residents to beg in the city streets to supplement the house's income.[55] While not explicitly stated in the *Statuti*, 'true' leprosy sufferers were likely permitted within Bologna's walls so long as they did not remain there as vagrants or loiterers. If this is the case for San Lazzaro, it would have been imperative that those who lived there had some sort of defining marker that indicated their privilege to do so—such as a designated article of clothing, badge, or license. As we see in the statute, a specific group of *falsarii* were listed as those who carried fake begging licenses in order to appear worthy of alms.[56] Though this may be tied in the statute specifically to penitents, as they would otherwise not look much different from regular citizens, this nevertheless suggests that the city may have indeed given begging licenses—a practice common in other urban centers in Western Europe—to known members of the deserving poor. As leprosy sufferers were seen as the ideal members of the deserving poor and therefore the ideal recipients of charity, particularly after the turn of the thirteenth century, a method of designating them as members of San Lazzaro is a likely possibility. This would make it easier for those moving through Bologna's city center or one of their busy markets to give alms to a leprosy sufferer without worry.

Bologna's statutes regulating the *falsarii* reflect a growing concern over the presence of beggars in the city who faked one of a number of disabilities and statuses in order to deceive others and collect false alms. This anxiety toward beggars who feigned protected and communally supported conditions to collect money instead of earning it through work is not unique to Bologna or even the Italian communes. While the stereotype of the lazy beggar has roots in Late Antiquity, it was in the thirteenth century when the suspicion toward this figure became particularly pronounced.[57] By projecting what was actually an "artificially disabled body", the charity-scammer thus pretended to be one thing while they were, in reality, something quite different.[58] In Touraine-Anjoy, for example, a chapter of the customs stated that if "there is a man who has nothing, and who lives in the town without earning anything, and he likes to go to the tavern", the town justices should "arrest him and ask what he lives on".[59] If the man is shown to be debauched (*de mauvaise vie*), then the justice should expel him from the town, according to the written law of the *Digest*, "*De officio praesidis*".[60] According to the learned elite, able-bodied men of lower statuses were part of society that was meant to work with their hands. To not do so and instead turn to the " 'soft' life of the beggar" meant that they had shunned their role in society and, in turn, their society as a whole.[61]

The inclusion of individuals *faking* leprosy by rubbing their bodies with herbs in the Bolognese statutes thus highlights the anxieties of the elite. Indeed, it was common in discussions of false beggars for members of the elite to accuse those of a lower status of altering or distorting their appearance in order to extort money from the rich. For example, between 1208 and 1210, the Bolognese jurist Azo wrote in his *Summa* on the *Corpus juris civilis* that some people "make themselves seem sick" by "applying herbs or ointments to their body in order to cause swollen wounds".[62] Azo also notes that such false beggars may also attempt to make their limbs look bent and shriveled, even when they were otherwise healthy and able to work. Though it is impossible to know whether Azo would have included the feigning of leprosy in this category, the descriptions of what he describes people doing to their bodies to appear sick and disabled are nearly identical to the symptoms of the advanced stages of leprosy. Yet, when we couple Azo's writing with the language of the statute prohibiting those who "stain themselves with herbs" to appear leprous, it suggests that the practice of feigning leprosy in this way may have been a somewhat common occurrence in Bologna. This is particularly interesting as it suggests that faking leprosy was a worthwhile and lucrative avenue for collecting alms from those passing by in the city streets. For this specific *falsarii* to be explicitly prohibited and policed, meant that those with leprosy were sought out or, at least, recognized as valuable recipients of alms by Bolognese residents.

The altering of appearance in the marketplace, via disguises or some form of cosmetics, in order to deceive was a fear that was felt more prominently in urban centers. Perhaps most concerning was the use of makeup by sex workers who were able to "transform undesirable bodies and faces into desirable ones".[63] In this way, by displaying their bodies as "products of charitable consumption" beggars were akin to sex workers, but false beggars had an affinity with the sex workers who transformed their appearances and bodies cosmetically to make them more appealing for consumption.[64] Thomas of Chobham, in the *Summa de arte praedicandi*, writes that the devil deceives a man much like a sex worker who "ornaments herself (*per ornamenta*)" in order to deceive potential customers.[65] Though sinful, a sex worker earned her wages licitly through the work of her body. However, if she altered her appearance with makeup, the money she earned became illicit, as she was luring men in under false pretenses. These women, according to Thomas, should not be allowed to keep their wages as "the one who hires [such a woman] believes that he has bought an appearance that is not there".[66] Sharon Farmer points out that, like the man who paid a sex worker, those who gave alms to beggars also expected an "intimate favor" in return for their actions: prayers for their souls.[67] However, as with the made-up sex worker, those who gave alms to beggars who feigned disabilities were "also, in a sense, buying an appearance that was not really there".[68] A false beggar who had altered their appearance in order to deceive was unable and, indeed, unworthy of keeping up their end of the bargain. For those who faked leprosy—a uniquely privileged status—the unequal nature of the bargain was even more dramatic.

This concern over counterfeit appearances also extended to those who altered their wares in the marketplace to fetch better prices for subpar products. For example, bakers were accused of selling smaller loaves of bread than the market weight or of producing adulterated bread that substituted other, often severely unwanted, materials for flour in order to make a greater profit. One example of the latter can be found in the case of Parisian bakers who, according to the chronicler Jean de Saint-Victor, were discovered to have "put many disgusting ingredients (*immunditias*)—the dregs of wine, pig droppings, and several other things" into the bread in order to cheat the "poor folk out of their money".[69] Craftsmen were similarly accused of using cheaper and lower quality materials for their wares, while selling them for the price of higher quality materials.[70] However, just as with the prohibition to keep the *falsarii* from the city, protections were enacted by governments and guilds statutes to similarly regulate goods. The Bolognese druggists, for example, stated at the beginning of their statutes that members were to operate "legitimately and legally" so as to not to commit fraud since they dealt with the "health of the human body" and needed to retain the trust of the commune.[71] Laws were enacted largely due to the same intimate relationship between contemporary moral assumptions and the idea of protecting the investments of individuals and the community.[72] In this way, we can see that the fear of being swindled in any manner—out of quality physical goods or quality spiritual benefits—was commonplace. This meant that it was necessary to combat fraud, in all its forms, at any cost.

Beginning in 1259, this statute aimed to keep those faking leprosy and all other *falsarii* from being accepted into the commune by fining anyone living in the city walls who provided them with shelter or any other form of hospitality. The fine for providing hospitality to a *falsarii* was steep: Every time a person was found to have done so they were fined 10 *lire*.[73] For comparison, being caught throwing "any stinking or dead animals or rotten fish or shellfish or any filthy or stinking thing" into the main piazzas of the city came with a 40 *soldi* fine, or 2 *lire*.[74] Moreover, if a person was discovered to *not* have denounced someone who they knew was breaking this law, they were similarly fined 10 *lire*. Finally, once collected, half of this fine was awarded to the person who made the accusation.[75] Fines, particularly steep fines, coupled with the naming of specific locations, are evidence that these practices both had previously occurred and, indeed, continued to occur in the city. These sorts of fines, wherein a portion was awarded to the person who denounced their neighbor for breaking the law, were common in medieval Europe. Such fines emphasize (and, indeed, incentivize) the role of the common citizens of the commune in protecting and safeguarding the health of the space they occupy. This use of the half of a fine going to the accuser is not unique to this case or Bologna in general. For example, in Bologna wherein accusers were granted half of the 40 *soldi* fine levied against butchers and fishmongers who butchered or slaughtered their animals within four houses of the piazza near the Ravenna gate so that there would be no "fetid animal parts or offal" at the market held there.[76] This sort of system of fines for a range of violations can also be seen in Lucca. In one instance, if a person was found to have used a public well for "washing, cleaning, or watering animals" a fine of 20 *lire* was mandated, with half going to the accuser.[77] The promise of a reward for denouncing neighbors who broke the law helped to ensure that the residents of the city were active in the policing of unwanted behaviors and persons.

Despite such a steep penalty, it seems that the *falsarii* continued to find their way into the commune. This can be seen, for example, in the 1259 statute which contains an explicit list of specific places and individuals, like the "house of *Jacobini in melle*", who were specifically targets as being prohibited from housing the *falsarii*.[78] Such a pointed declaration suggests that these were places and individuals who were specifically infamous for providing hospitality in some form to the *falsarii*—despite the commune's stance on their presence. This begs the question, then: Is it possible that these individuals were known crime bosses (much like *Oliver Twist*'s Fagin) who kept a portion of the loot brought back by the *falsarii* who lived on their property? If not, why would these people and institutions continue to provide shelter—at a steep cost—to those the commune actively sought to exclude?

The enforcement of some of these issues in Bologna fell under the mandate of the office of the *fango*. Established in the middle of the thirteenth century, the *fango* was mandated with monitoring and protecting many aspects of the city's health and safety.[79] The purview of the *fango* extended from issues, such as rogue pigs, clogged canals, and the improper butchering of animals, to monitoring market stalls, bridges, and stores of firewood within the city. At times, this meant that they were responsible for investigating the "presence of social undesirables such as false beggars, gamblers, vagabonds, and prostitutes" within the commune's walls.[80] The *fango* officials heard complaints about particular violations from residents, interviewed witnesses, and assigned fines or other penalties to offending parties for their violations.[81] It is therefore likely that they were the ones who would respond to accusations of criminal activity concerning the housing of *falsarii*. Though their mandate does not specifically include those who faked leprosy, it is likely that they were considered to fall under the heading of "false beggars". Thus, the *fango* served as an important piece in maintaining Bologna's social and civic order. It is interesting to note that true leprosy sufferers were not included in the *fango*'s mandate, as once might have been assumed. Indeed, leprosy sufferers have often been lumped together in the historiography with unwanted groups like prostitutes and vagabonds, thus supporting the narrative that medieval society was a so-called persecuting society.[82] However, as has been discussed, the commune was interested in protecting the credibility and support of those houses in *San Lazzaro,* and not removing those with the disease from their borders.

The faking of leprosy, or leprosy-like symptoms, becomes particularly interesting considering that in the thirteenth century the *judicium leprosorum* (the judgment of leprosy) became a medicalized legal procedure in Italy. This meant that university-trained physicians became the preferred figures to examine individuals who were suspected of having leprosy in order to determine whether they had the disease. Before this, juries of nonmedical laypersons or, in some cases, members of a local *leprosarium* came together at the behest of a court or town council in order to perform this examination. The first known recorded leprosy judgment by a medical practitioner in Europe comes from Siena in 1250, wherein four examining physicians "judged and sentenced" a man, Pierzivallus, to be leprous.[83] Similarly, in Pistoia in 1288 the *medicus* Master Laurentius, under oath "formally pronounced a sentence" of leprosy in the presence of three witnesses in the chapel of a priest.[84] While the practice of this more medicalized examination began in Italy, records of such cases become increasingly more prominent north of the Alps from the end of the thirteenth century. Though I have yet to come across an extant *judicium leprosorum* from Bologna, I believe it is likely that this procedure was similarly performed in the commune and, further, had similarly evolved to be conducted by medical doctors. With a prominent university and medical faculty, as well as a clear desire to root out those *falsarii* who faked leprosy, it is unlikely that such a practice would have been absent from the city.

Conclusion

What was the benefit, then, of faking leprosy in a city like Bologna in the Middle Ages? Bologna's prohibition against beggars who faked disability or a privileged status to gain alms and charity suggests that these conditions, when real, were seen by the commune and its citizens as legitimate reasons for a person to beg. Conditions like leprosy, blindness, and being an orphan were regarded as both chronic and permanent, rendering a person unable to work and earn a living (or, in the case of orphaned girls a dowry and orphaned boys an apprenticeship), granting them status as deserving of the charity of others. In a circular way, the prohibition against false beggars gave legitimacy to the rights of the truly disabled and others of a privileged status—theirs was a true and deserving condition that necessitated the charity of others. Moreover, by declaring these groups worthy of alms and other forms of charity meant that they were "prone to simulation" as, when true, they were marked as officially worthy by the commune.[85]

The concerns addressed in the *Statuti* are of attempts by people faking leprosy to usurp the alms meant for the leprosarium while also depriving the healthy of the benefits of their good works. Fears of fraudulent disability, that is of people faking the state of being disabled, were widespread in pre-modern Europe. Much like today, individuals, groups, and governments throughout the Middle Ages wanted to ensure that any donation of their hard-earned money was going to the people and institutions who were truly deserving. However, as long as people have been providing charity to the poor and the sick, there have also been people who were interested in taking advantage of them. While these concerns from the thirteenth and fourteenth centuries were rooted in different beliefs and traditions than our own, the concern for being swindled has remained a constant sore spot throughout the ages.

By clearly pointing out those who faked leprosy by "staining themselves with herbs" in the *Statuti* as a group who was not welcomed within the city limits suggests that this was a common, well-known practice for appearing leprous. Moreover, this suggests that the potential alms collected by leprosy sufferers made the facade a worthwhile charity scam and, further, that it was a well-known ruse. By drawing attention to this group, as well as those who faked other disabilities and privileged statuses, the efforts and concerns of the Bolognese government are accentuated. The more restrictive statutes illuminate a clear attempt made by the city to protect and support those in the city's *leprosarium*. While these may, on the surface, echo the exclusion narrative of leprosy sufferers, they actually highlight the city's desire to ensure that any donations and alms given to the leprous residents of Bologna and the *leprosarium* were actually reaching them so both parties could hold up their end of the salvation bargain.

Notes

1 This chapter was drawn from some of the work done for my dissertation "Neither Sinner nor Outcast: Communal Responses to Leprosy in Bologna, 1116–1347" (Ph.D. diss., McGill University, 2022). I owe my thanks to the support of so many in guiding me through the dissertation process and in discussing the topics addressed in this paper on so many occasions, most especially Travis Bruce and Faith Wallis.

2 For more on this topic, see Elma Brenner and François-Olivier Touati, eds., *Leprosy and Identity in the Middle Ages: From England to the Mediterranean* (Manchester: Manchester University Press, 2021); Elma Brenner, *Leprosy and Charity in Medieval Rouen* (Suffolk: Boydell & Brewer, 2015); Elma Brenner, "Outside the City Walls: Leprosy, Exclusion, and Social Identity in Twelfth- and Thirteenth-Century Rouen," in *Difference and Identity in Francia and Medieval France*, eds. Meredith Cohen and Justine Firnhaber-Baker (Farnham: Ashgate, 2010), 139–56; Luke Demaitre, *Leprosy in Premodern Medicine: A Malady of the Whole Body* (Baltimore: The Johns Hopkins University Press, 2007); Carole Rawcliffe, *Leprosy in Medieval England* (Woodbridge: Boydell Press, 2006); François Olivier-Touati, *Maladie et sociéte au Moyen Âge: la lèpre, les lépreux et les léproseries dans la province ecclésiastique de Sens jusqu'au milieu du XIVe siècle* (Bruxelles: De Boeck Université, 1998), 417–20; Nicole Bériou and François-Olivier Touati, eds., *Voluntate Dei Leprosus: Les lépreux entre conversion et exclusion aux XIIème et XIIIème siècles* (Spoleto: Centro Italiano di Studi Sull'Alto Medioevo, 1991).

3 For more on this topic, see Anna M. Peterson, "A Comparative Study of the Hospitals and Leprosaria in Narbonne, France and Siena, Italy (1080–1348)" (Ph.D. diss., University of St Andrews, 2017); Sharon Farmer, ed., *Approaches to Poverty in Medieval Europe: Complexities, Contradictions, Transformations, c. 1100–1500* (Turnhout: Brepolis, 2016); Sharon Farmer, *Surviving Poverty in Medieval Paris: Gender, Ideology, and the Daily Lives of the Poor* (Ithaca: Cornell University Press, 2002); James Brodman, *Charity and Religion in Medieval Europe* (Washington, DC: Catholic University of America Press, 2009); Miri Rubin, *Charity and Community in Medieval Cambridge* (Cambridge: Cambridge University Press, 1987); Richard C. Trexler, "Charity and the Defense of Urban Elites in the Italian Communes," in *The Rich, the*

Well Born, and the Powerful: Elites and Upper Classes in History, ed. Frederic Cople Jaher (Urbana: University of Illinois Press, 1973).

4 Archivio di Stato di Bologna (hereafter: ASB), *Governo, Statuti*, reg 37, fol. 41v. Transcriptions and translations are my own unless otherwise indicated.

5 2 Corinthians 8:9. Tell us what version you are using (or what you are translating from). This does not need to appear on your references cited page.

6 Luke 6:20.

7 Luke 14:13–4.

8 Miri Rubin, *Charity and Community in Medieval Cambridge*, Cambridge Studies in Medieval Life and thought, 4th Series, 4 (Cambridge: Cambridge University Press, 1987), 59.

9 Saint Benedict, "The Rule of Saint Benedict as Translated by Saint Æthelwold of Winchester," in *The Old English Rule of Saint Benedict: With Related Old English Texts*, ed. Jacob Riyeff (Collegeville, MN: Liturgical Press, 2017).

10 Adam J. Davis, "The Social and Religious Meanings of Charity in Medieval Europe," *History Compass* 12, no. 12 (2014): 936.

11 Michael Mollat, *The Poor in the Middle Ages: An Essay in Social History* (New London: Yale University Press, 1986), 112.

12 Henri-Jacques Stiker, *A History of Disability* (Ann Arbor: University of Michigan Press, 1999), 73–74.

13 André Vauchez, "Assistance et Charité en Occident, XIIIe-XVe Siècles," in *Domanda e Consumi Livelli e Strutture (Nei Secoli XIII-XVIII)*, ed. Vera Barbagli Bagnoli (Firenze: L. S. Olschki, 1978), 152–53.

14 Jacques Le Goff, *The Birth of Purgatory*, trans. Arthur Goldhammer (Chicago: University of Chicago, 1984), esp 130–53 and 284–88.

15 Miri Rubin, *Charity and Community in Medieval Cambridge* (Cambridge: Cambridge University Press, 1987), 65.

16 Matthew 25: 31–46; Tobit 12:12; Frederico Botana, *The Works of Mercy in Italian Medieval Art (c. 1050–1400)* (Turnhout: Brepolis, 2011), 15–48; Vauchez, "Assistance et Charité," 152–53.

17 Adam J. Davis, "Hospitals, Charity, and the Culture of Compassion in the Twelfth and Thirteenth Centuries," in *Approaches to Poverty in Medieval Europe: Complexities, Contradictions, Transformations, c. 1100–1500*, ed. Sharon Farmer (Turnhout: Brepolis: 2016), 23.

18 Rubin, *Charity and Community*, 8.

19 Sarah Rubin Blanshei, "Introduction," in *Violence and Justice in Bologna, 1250–1700*, ed. Sarah Rubin Blanshei (Lanham: Lexington Books, 2018), xii; Antonio Ivan Pini, "Problemi demografici di Bologna nel Duecento," *Atti e Memorie della Deptazione di Storia Patria per le Province di Romagna* 16–17 (1969): 180–22; Rosa Smurra, "Progetto Fonti medievali in rete," *Centro Gina Fasoli:* www.centrofasoli.unibo.it, accessed 5 March 2020; Rosa Smurra, "Fiscal Sources: The Estimi," in *A Companion to Medieval and Renaissance Bologna*, ed. Sarah Rubin Blanshei (Leiden: Brill, 2018), 42–55; Shona Kelly Wray also estimates that, prior to the Black Death in 1348, the city proper of Bologna had between 45,000 and 50,000 people. Shona Kelly Wray, *Communities and Crisis: Bologna During the Black Death* (Leiden: Brill, 2009), 2.

20 David Nichols, *Urban Europe, 1100–1700* (New York: Palgrave Macmillan, 2003), 152–53.

21 Sethina Watson, "City as Charter: Charity and the Lordship of English Towns, 1170–1250," in *Cities, Texts and Social Networks 400–1500: Experiences ad*

Perceptions of Medieval Urban Space, eds. Caroline Goodson, Anne E. Lester, and Carol Symes (Farnham: Ashgate, 2010), 235–62.

22 Sherri Franks Johnson, *Monastic Women and Religious Orders in Late Medieval Bologna* (Cambridge: Cambridge University Press, 2014), 135.

23 For more on civic life in Bologna at this time, see Wray, *Communities in Crisis*, esp. 57–98; Johnson, *Monastic Women*, esp. 129–36.

24 Watson, "City as Charter," 235.

25 Note that it is not that the *Statuti* of 1250–1261 did not include charitable donations to the leprosaria, but instead that the book wherein charitable donations would have been listed is not extant within the volume.

26 *Item hospitali misellorum XXV corb. frumenti et predictus numerus corbium detur ipsis miselli et non alii nisi eorum speciali nuntio.* ASB, Governo, Statuti, reg. 37, fol. 3v.

27 ASB, Governo, Statuti, reg. 35, fol. 1r–5r.

28 *de elimosinis ad pia loca faciendis a honorem et reverentiam domini nostri ihesu christi.* ASB, Governo, Statuti, reg. 37, fol. 3r.

29 *De ellimoxinis ad pia loca concessis.* ASB, Governo, Statuti, reg. 42, fol. 110v.

30 *et predictus numerus corbium detur ipsis misellis et non alij nisi speciali eorum nuntio.* ASB, Governo, Statuti, reg. 37, fol. 3v.

31 *Leprosis de Sancto Lazzaro seu eorum legittimo sindico.* ASB, Governo, Statuti, reg. 42, fol. 110v.

32 Anna M. Peterson, "A Comparative Study of the Hospitals and Leprosaria in Narbonne, France and Siena, Italy (1080–1348)" (Ph.D. diss., University of St Andrews, 2017), 106.

33 We see instances of a broad approach to ecclesiastic oversight of hospitals at this time with a number of scattered instances that fluctuated with respect to their location. Brodman, *Charity and Religion in Medieval Europe*, 77–85.

34 William Chester Jordan, "Anti-Corruption Campaigns in Thirteenth-Century Europe," *Journal of Medieval History* 35 (2009): 205–7; Marie Dejoux, *Les enquêtes de Saint Louis: Gouverner et sauver son âme* (Paris: PUF, 2014), 9; Odd Langholm, *Economics in the Medieval Schools. Wealth, Exchange, Value, Money and Usury According to the Paris Theological Tradition, 1200–1350* (Leiden: Brill, 1992), 533–35.

35 Brodman, *Charity and Religion in Medieval Europe*, 87.

36 Ibid., 79.

37 Jacques de Vitry, *The History occidentalis of Jacques de Vitry*, ed. J. F. Hinnebusch (Freibourg: The University Press, 1972), 148–49.

38 Ibid.

39 Translation from Peterson, "A Comparative Study," 124.

40 *Quod orbi <u>auocoli</u> asidrati ostendentes se leprosi et fratres penitentales et aliqui <u>infrascripti</u> falsarii non hospitentur in hiis locis.* Though there are some minor differences in the lexicon used and the division of this statute between the years that it appears in the Statuti, there are none that significantly alter its meaning or intent. ASB, Governo, Statuti, reg 37, fol. 41v.

41 *orbos et asidratos et avoculos et qui faciunt se avoculos et tingunt se de herbis ad hoc ut leprosi videantur et qui faciunt se fratres et penitentiales qui deferunt stamignas dicontes cum tabulis bulatis et etiam si velle penitentiam exercere et aliis diversis vii et modis falso nituntur lucrari et sunt falsatores dei et homnium et propter eorum ebrietates constent cotidie in tabernis blasfemando deum et sanctos.* ASB, Governo, Statuti, reg 37, fol. 41v.

42 *et aliis diversis vii et modis falso nituntur lucrari et sunt falsatores dei et hom-nium.* ASB, *Governo, Statuti,* reg. 37, fol 41v.

43 Diane Owen Hughes, "Distinguishing Signs: Ear-Rings, Jews and Franciscan Rhetoric in the Italian Renaissance City," *Past and Present* 112 (1986): 3–59; Sharon Farmer, "The Beggar's Body: Intersections of Gender and Social Status in High Medieval Paris," in *Monks and Nuns, Saints and Outcasts: Religion in Medieval Society,* eds. Sharon Farmer and Barbara H. Rosenwein (Ithaca: Cornell University Press, 2018), 161.

44 Farmer, "The Beggar's Body," 161.

45 Edward Wheatley, *Stumbling Blocks Before the Blind: Medieval Constructions of a Disability* (Ann Arbor: The University of Michigan Press, 2010), 74.

46 *Sunt alii omni tempore calamitosi et inimici trivialiter se inflantes, tremulosi, et varias figuras aegrotantium induentes, vultum sicut Protea mutantes.* Peter the Chanter, *Verbum abbreviatum,* c. 48, PL 205, col. 152, as quoted in Farmer, "The Beggar's Body," 160, n. 24.

47 *Sepe transfigueant se in habitu miserabili, ut videantur magis egeni quam sunt, et ita decipiunt alios ut plus accipiant.* Thomas de Chobham, *Summa confessorum,* Art. 5, dist. 4m quaest. 6, ed. F Broomfield (Louvain, 1968), 297, as quoted in Farmer, "The Beggar's Body," 161 n. 26.

48 Bruno Tabuteau, *Lépreux et sociabilité du Moyen Age aux temps modernes* (Rouen: Publications de l'Université du Rouen, 2000), 11.

49 Carole Rawcliffe, *Leprosy in Medieval England* (Woodbridge: The Boydell Press, 2006), 284.

50 Damien Jeanne, "Lepers and Leper-Houses: Between Human Law and God's Law (6th-15th Centuries)," in *Social Dimensions of Medieval Disease and Disability,* eds. Sally Crawford and Christina Lee (Oxford: BAR Publications, 2014), 70.

51 *si alii malagdi foretanei intraverint civitatem, per bampnum missum faciam eos de civitate eici, et stare non permittam, excepta de edomada sancta.* Lodovico Zdekauer, ed., *Il Constituto del Comune di Siena dell'anno 1262* (Bologna: A. Forni, 1983), 51.

52 Brenner, *Leprosy and Charity,* 74.

53 Ibid.

54 Rawcliffe, *Leprosy in Medieval England,* 288.

55 Sharon Farmer, "From Personal Charity to Centralized Poor Relief: The Evolution of Responses to the Poor in Paris, *c.* 1250—1600," in *Experiences of Charity, 1250–1650,* ed. Anne M. Scott (Farnham: Ashgate, 2015).

56 *qui deferunt stamignas dicontes cum tabulis bulatis*—literally: "with tablets bearing seals." ASB, *Governo, Statuti,* reg. 37, fol 41v.

57 Farmer, "The Beggar's Body," 159.

58 Irena Metzler, *A Social History of Disability in the Middle Ages* (London: Routledge, 2013), 169.

59 F. R. P. Akehurst, *The Etablissements de Saint Louis: Thirteenth-Century Law Texts from Tours, Orleans, and Paris* (Philadelphia: University of Pennsylvania Press, 2015), 27.

60 Ibid.

61 Farmer, "The Beggar's Body," 159.

62 *Vel loquitur auth. specialiter in his, qui in sacra urbe reperiuntur: quasi cum eis mitius sit agendum: vel loquitur de his qui per Quaestorem fuerint reperti, vel de his qui non simulant corporis debilitatem, quasi quod hic dicitur, speciale*

sit in his, qui cum sint validi et robusti, corporis simulant infirmitatem, aliquas herbas, sive appositoria corpori apponentes: propter quae tumidi, vel vulnerati [alias curuati videntur: sicut plures, gallioti. Nam et quidam contracti, alias curuati] pedibus et manibus videntur cum non sint. Azo, *Azonis Summa avrea recens, pristinae suae fideri restituta, ac archetypo collata* (Lvgdvni: Excudebat Petrus Fradin, 1557), 252r.

63   Sharon Farmer, *Surviving Poverty in Medieval Paris: Gender, Ideology, and the Daily Lives of the Poor* (Ithaca: Cornell University Press, 2005), 68.

64   Ibid.

65   *Unde, meretrici purpurate conparatur que per ornamenta sua homines decipit.* Cambridge, Corpus Christi College, MS 455, fol. 58v.

66   *Item, si meretrix inungit se et ornat se ut decipiat lascivos et mentiatur pulcritudinem suam et speciem qual non habet, quia tunc locator credit emere speciem que ibi non est, peccar meretrix nec licite potest retinere quod si accipit.* Thomas of Chobham, *Summa confessorum,* ed. F. Broomfield (Louvain: Éditions Nauwelaerts, 1968), 296.

67   Farmer, "The Beggar's Body," 163.

68   Ibid.

69   *Cum autem illo anno esset maxima caristia, inventum est quod pistores panis in pane multas immunditias posuerunt, fæces vini, stercora porcorum: quae et alia plura famelici homines comedebant; et sic panifici pauperum pecunias emungebant. Cognita ergo veritate, positæ sunt rotæ in campellis Parisius sexdecim super palos, et super eas singuli tales panifici constituti, tenentes manibus elevatis panum frusta taliter corrupotrum. Potea sunt de Francia banniti.* Jean of St. Victor, "Excerpta e Memoriali Historiarum, auctore Johanne Parisiensi, Sancti Victoris Parisiensis canonico regulari," *Recueil des Historiens des Gaules et de la France,* ed. Martin Bouquet et al. (Paris: Imprimerie royale, 1738–1904), 21:663; trans. in William Chester Jordan, *The Great Famine: Northern Europe in the Early Fourteenth Century* (Princeton: Princeton University Press, 1997), 162.

70   Dennis Romano, *Markets and Marketplaces in Medieval Italy, c.1100–c.1400* (New Haven: Yale University Press, 2015), 153–90; Brigit van den Hoven, *Work in Ancient and Medieval Thought: Ancient Philosophers, Medieval Monks and Theologians and Their Concept of Work, Occupation, and Technology* (Amsterdam: J. C. Gieben, 1996), 240.

71   ASB, *Capitano del Popolo, Società d'arti e d'armi, Società d'arte,* b.9, *Statutes of the Speziali* 1303, n.p.

72   James Davis, *Medieval Market Morality: Life, Law and Ethics in the English Marketplace, 1200–1500* (Cambridge: Cambridge University Press, 2012), 137.

73   *Et qui tenuerit aliquem de predictis personis sive hospitatus fuerit et qui sterint solvat nomine banni X lib. bon.* ASB, *Governo, Statuti,* reg. 37, fol 41v.

74   *Ordinamus quod nemo prohiciat vel prohici faciat in plateam comunis Bononie vel in trivium porte Ravennatis aliqua animalia fetida vel morticina, nec pisces vel gambaros mortuos seumarcidos nec aliquam turpem vel fetidam . . . Et qui contra predicta vel aliquod predictorum fecerit vel ea . . . pro qualibet vice in quadraginta solidis bononinorum.* ASB, *Governo, Statuti,* reg. 42, fol 104v.

75   *qualibet vice qua contrafecerit medietas sit comunis et alia accusantis.* ASB, *Governo, Statuti,* reg. 37, fol 41v.

76   Gina Fasoli and Pietro Sella, eds., *Statuti di Bologna dall'anno 1288* (Città del Vaticano: Biblioteca Apostolica Vaticana, 1937), vol. 2, 135.

77 State Archive of Lucca, ASLu, CVP 1, fols. 1r—8v, as presented in Guy Geltner, *Roads to Health: Infrastructure and Urban Wellbeing in Later Medieval Italy* (Philadelphia: University of Pennsylvania Press, 2019), 173.

78 *in domo rose et guilielmi orbi et iacobini de sancto severio et iacobini in melle et iacobini de triario et per petri bergogononi et aliorum que continent et contrata podiali et poncte morandi et ospitantur.* ASB, Governo, Statuti, reg. 37, fol 41v.

79 Guy Geltner, "Finding Matter Out of Place: Bolognas *fango* ("dirt") Notary in the History of Premodern Public Health," in *Lo sguardo lungimirante delle capitali: saggi in onore di Francesca Bocchi*, eds. Rosa Smurra, Hubert Houben, and Manuela Ghizzoni (Rome: Viella, 2014), 308.

80 Guy Geltner, "Finding Matter Out of Place: Bologna's Dirt (*Fango*) Officials in the History of Premodern Public Health," in *The Far-Sighted Gaze of Capital Cities: Essays in Honor of Francesca Bocchi*, eds. Rosa Smurra, Houbert Houben, and Manuela Ghizzoni (Rome: Viella, 2014), 311.

81 Geltner also notes that the records of such officials also "reveal that complaints could be made publicly, for instance by neighbors and at court, and that the officials entertained secret accusations as well as made their own *in situ* inquiries." Guy Geltner, "Public Health and the Pre-Modern City: A Research Agenda," *History Compass* 10, no. 3 (2012): 236.

82 R. I. Moore, *The Formation of a Persecuting Society: Power and Deviance in Western Europe, 950–1250* (Oxford: Basil Blackwell, 1987), esp. 45–65, 73–80; Wheatley, *Stumbling Blocks Before the Blind*, 3.

83 Though, as Demaitre notes, this document was particularly focused on the "remuneration for the service" that the physicians "performed at the command of the podesta and the court." Demaitre, *Leprosy in Premodern Medicine*, 37.

84 Demaitre, *Leprosy in Premodern Medicine*, 37.

85 Metzler, *A Social History of Disability in the Middle Ages*, 172.

Reference List

Archival Sources

Archivio di Stato di Bologna: The State Archive of Bologna

ASB, *Capitano del Popolo, Società d'arti e d'armi, Società d'arte*, b.9, Statutes of the Speziali 1303, n.p.

ASB, *Governo, Statuti*, reg. 35, fol. 1r-5r.

ASB, *Governo, Statuti*, reg. 37, fol. 3r.

ASB, *Governo, Statuti*, reg. 37, fol. 3v.

ASB, *Governo, Statuti*, reg 37, fol. 41v.

ASB, *Governo, Statuti*, reg. 42, fol 104v.

ASB, *Governo, Statuti*, reg. 42, fol. 110v.

Cambridge, Corpus Christi College

MS 455, fol. 58v.

Archivio di Stato di Lucca: State Archive of Lucca

ASLu, CVP 1, fols. 1r-8v. Found in Guy Geltner. *Roads to Health: Infrastructure and Urban Wellbeing in Later Medieval Italy*. See reference below.

Printed Primary

Azo. *Azonis Summa avrea recens, pristinae suae fideri restituta, ac archetypo collate*. Lvgdvni: Excudebat Petrus Fradin, 1557.

Benedict, Saint. "The Rule of Saint Benedict as Translated by Saint Æthelwold of Winchester." In *The Old English Rule of Saint Benedict: With Related Old English Texts*, edited by Jacob Riyeff. Collegeville, MN: Liturgical Press, 2017.

Chanter, Peter. *Verbum abbreviatum*. As found in Farmer, "The Beggar's Body." Reference below.

Chobham, Thomas de. *Summa confessorum*. Edited by F Broomfield (Louvain, 1968). As found in Farmer, "The Beggar's Body." Reference below.

Jean of St. Victor. "Excerpta e Memoriali Historiarum, auctore Johanne Parisiensi, Sancti Victoris Parisiensis canonico regulari." In *Recueil des Historiens des Gaules et de la France*, edited by Martin Bouquet, et al. Paris: Imprimerie Royale, 1738–1904.

Secondary Materials

Akehurst, F. R. P. *The Etablissements de Saint Louis: Thirteenth-Century Law Texts from Tours, Orleans, and Paris*. Philadelphia: University of Pennsylvania Press, 2015.

Bériou, Nicole, and François-Olivier Touati, eds. *Voluntate Dei Leprosus: Les lépreux entre conversion et exclusion aux XIIème et XIIIème siècles*. Spoleto: Centro Italiano di Studi Sull'Alto Medioevo, 1991.

Blanshei, Sarah Rubin. "Introduction." In *Violence and Justice in Bologna, 1250–1700*, edited by Sarah Rubin Blanshei. Lanham: Lexington Books, 2018.

Botana, Frederico. *The Works of Mercy in Italian Medieval Art (c. 1050–1400)*. Turnhout: Brepols, 2011.

Brenner, Elma. "Outside the City Walls: Leprosy, Exclusion, and Social Identity in Twelfth- and Thirteenth-Century Rouen." In *Difference and Identity in Francia and Medieval France*, edited by Meredith Cohen and Justine Firnhaber-Baker. Farnham: Ashgate, 2010.

———. *Leprosy and Charity in Medieval Rouen*. Suffolk: Boydell & Brewer, 2015.

Brenner, Elma, and François-Olivier Touati, eds. *Leprosy and Identity in the Middle Ages: From England to the Mediterranean*. Manchester: Manchester University Press, 2021.

Brodman, James William. *Charity and Religion in Medieval Europe*. Washington, DC: The Catholic University of America Press, 2009.

Davis, Adam J. "Hospitals, Charity, and the Culture of Compassion in the Twelfth and Thirteenth Centuries." In *Approaches to Poverty in Medieval Europe: Complexities, Contradictions, Transformations, c. 1100–1500*, edited by Sharon Farmer. Turnhout: Brepols, 2016.

———. *Medieval Market Morality: Life, Law and Ethics in the English Marketplace, 1200–1500*. Cambridge: Cambridge University Press, 2012.

———. "The Social and Religious Meanings of Charity in Medieval Europe." *History Compass* 12, no. 12 (2014): 936.

Dejoux, Marie. *Les enquêtes de Saint Louis: Gouverner et sauver son âme*. Paris: PUF, 2014.

Demaitre, Luke. *Leprosy in Premodern Medicine: A Malady of the Whole Body.* Baltimore: The Johns Hopkins University Press, 2007.

Farmer, Sharon, ed. *Approaches to Poverty in Medieval Europe: Complexities, Contradictions, Transformations, c. 1100–1500.* Turnhout: Brepols, 2016.

———. "The Beggar's Body: Intersections of Gender and Social Status in High Medieval Paris." In *Monks and Nuns, Saints and Outcasts: Religion in Medieval Society*, edited by Sharon Farmer and Barbara H. Rosenwein. Ithaca: Cornell University Press, 2018.

———. "From Personal Charity to Centralised Poor Relief: The Evolution of Responses to the Poor in Paris, c. 1250—1600." In *Experiences of Charity, 1250–1650*, edited by Anne M. Scott. Farnham: Ashgate, 2015.

———. *Surviving Poverty in Medieval Paris: Gender, Ideology, and the Daily Lives of the Poor.* Ithaca: Cornell University Press, 2002.

Fasoli, Gina, and Pietro Sella, eds. *Statuti di Bologna dall'anno 1288.* Vol. 2. Città del Vaticano: Biblioteca Apostolica Vaticana, 1937.

Geltner, Guy. "Finding Matter Out of Place: Bologna's Dirt (*Fango*) Officials in the History of Premodern Public Health." In *The Far-Sighted Gaze of Capital Cities: Essays in Honor of Francesca Bocchi*, edited by Rosa Smurra, Houbert Houben, and Manuela Ghizzoni. Rome: Viella, 2014. Also published as: "Finding Matter Out of Place: Bolognas *fango* ("dirt") Notary in the History of Premodern Public Health." In *Lo sguardo lungimirante delle capitali: saggi in onore di Francesca Bocchi*, edited by Rosa Smurra, Hubert Houben, and Manuela Ghizzoni. Rome: Viella, 2014.

———. "Public Health and the Pre-Modern City: A Research Agenda." *History Compass* 10, no. 3 (2012): 236.

———. *Roads to Health: Infrastructure and Urban Wellbeing in Later Medieval Italy.* Philadelphia: University of Pennsylvania Press, 2019.

Hughes, Diane Owen. "Distinguishing Signs: Ear-Rings, Jews and Franciscan Rhetoric in the Italian Renaissance City." *Past and Present* 112 (1986): 3–59.

Jeanne, Damien. "Lepers and Leper-Houses: Between Human Law and God's Law (6th-15th Centuries)." In *Social Dimensions of Medieval Disease and Disability*, edited by Sally Crawford and Christina Lee. Oxford: BAR Publications, 2014.

Johnson, Sherri Franks. *Monastic Women and Religious Orders in Late Medieval Bologna.* Cambridge: Cambridge University Press, 2014.

Jordan, William Chester. "Anti-Corruption Campaigns in Thirteenth-Century Europe." *Journal of Medieval History* 35 (2009): 205–7.

———. *The Great Famine: Northern Europe in the Early Fourteenth Century.* Princeton: Princeton University Press, 1997.

Langholm, Odd. *Economics in the Medieval Schools. Wealth, Exchange, Value, Money and Usury According to the Paris Theological Tradition, 1200–1350.* Leiden: Brill, 1992.

Le Goff, Jacques. *The Birth of Purgatory.* Translated by Arthur Goldhammer. Chicago: University of Chicago, 1984.

Metzler, Irina. *A Social History of Disability in the Middle Ages: Cultural Considerations of Physical Impairment.* London: Routledge, 2013.

Mollat, Michael. *The Poor in the Middle Ages: An Essay in Social History.* New London: Yale University Press, 1986.

Moore, R. I. *The Formation of a Persecuting Society: Power and Deviance in Western Europe, 950–1250.* Oxford: Basil Blackwell, 1987.

Nichols, David. *Urban Europe, 1100–1700.* New York: Palgrave Macmillan, 2003.

Olivier-Touati, François. *Maladie et sociéte au Moyen Âge: la lèpre, les lépreux et les léproseries dans la province ecclésiastique de Sens jusqu'au milieu du XIVe siècle.* Bruxelles: De Boeck Université, 1998.

Peterson, Anna M. "A Comparative Study of the Hospitals and Leprosaria in Narbonne, France and Siena, Italy (1080–1348)." Ph.D. diss., University of St Andrews, 2017.

Pini, Antonio Ivan. "Problemi demografici di Bologna nel Duecento." *Atti e Memorie della Deptazione di Storia Patria per le Province di Romagna (AMR)* 17–19 (1966–68): 147–222.

Rawcliffe, Carole. *Leprosy in Medieval England.* Woodbridge: Boydell, 2006.

Romano, Dennis. *Markets and Marketplaces in Medieval Italy, c.1100–c.1400.* New Haven: Yale University Press, 2015.

Rubin, Miri. *Charity and Community in Medieval Cambridge.* Cambridge Studies in Medieval Life and thought, 4th Series, 4. Cambridge: Cambridge University Press, 1987.

Smurra, Rosa. "Fiscal Sources: The Estimi." In *A Companion to Medieval and Renaissance Bologna,* edited by Sarah Rubin Blanshei. Leiden: Brill, 2018.

———. "Progetto Fonti medievali in rete." Software, 2007. *Centro Gina Fasoli.* Accessed March 5, 2020. www.centrofasoli.unibo.it.

Stiker, Henri-Jacques. *A History of Disability.* Ann Arbor: University of Michigan Press, 1999.

Tabuteau, Bruno. *Lépreux et sociabilité du Moyen Age aux temps modernes.* Rouen: Publications de l'Université du Rouen, 2000.

Trexler, Richard C. "Charity and the Defense of Urban Elites in the Italian Communes." In *The Rich, the Well Born, and the Powerful: Elites and Upper Classes in History,* edited by Frederic Cople Jaher. Urbana: University of Illinois Press, 1973.

van den Hoven, Brigit. *Work in Ancient and Medieval Thought: Ancient Philosophers, Medieval Monks and Theologians and Their Concept of Work, Occupation, and Technology.* Amsterdam: J.C. Gieben, 1996.

Vauchez, André. "Assistance et Charité en Occident, XIIIe-XVe Siècles." In *Domanda e Consumi Livelli e Strutture (Nei Secoli XIII-XVIII),* edited by Vera Barbagli Bagnoli. Firenze: L.S. Olschki, 1978.

Vitry, Jacques de. *The History Occidentalis of Jacques de Vitry.* Edited by J. F. Hinnebusch. Freibourg: The University Press, 1972.

Watson, Sethina. "City as Charter: Charity and the Lordship of English Towns, 1170–1250." In *Cities, Texts and Social Networks 400–1500: Experiences and Perceptions of Medieval Urban Space,* edited by Caroline Goodson, Anne E. Lester, and Carol Symes. Farnham: Ashgate, 2010.

Wheatley, Edward. *Stumbling Blocks Before the Blind: Medieval Constructions of a Disability.* Ann Arbor: The University of Michigan Press, 2010.

Wray, Shona Kelly. *Communities and Crisis: Bologna During the Black Death.* Leiden: Brill, 2009.

Zdekauer, Lodovico, ed. *Il Constituto del Comune di Siena dell'anno 1262.* Bologna: A. Forni, 1983.

9 Expertis Medicis Videatur

Legal Medical Expertise in the Apostolic Chancery's Assessment of Personal Injury Damages During the Avignon Period (1309–1378)

Ninon Dubourg

Assessing personal injury is a central concern of modern insurance companies tasked with determining the eligibility of claimants to often substantial damages. Documents from the fourteenth century demonstrate the long history of such investigations and offer vital context to some of the issues that preoccupy our contemporary legal systems and insurance sector. The necessity to determine the extent of personal injury has been long established, and protocols to do so have existed for centuries. For example, we find processes to undertake such investigations in Egypt at the time of Ptolemy and the Romans, in Germanic laws of the fifth to eighth centuries, and eighteenth-century judicial investigations and forensic examinations.[1] The pontifical institution was one of the first, and certainly most influential, organizations to devote significant resources to such concerns, although its activities have remained largely unexplored. In this chapter, I address this gap by examining the role of forensic medicine in the institution's adjudication procedures between 1309 and 1378, while the papacy was resident in Avignon.

The modern public policy typically foregrounds a personalized conception of disability in assessing personal injury and any associated damages, taking into account the interaction between an individual and his or her environment alongside doctors' expertise and any valid insurance policies.[2] In other words, public policy determines the extent of an individual's disability in terms of a relative inability to undertake routine tasks and any decrease in functionality that could, for example, limit one's ability to work.[3] Crucially, calculations of what is known as an individual's "personal disability rate" are not based solely on the nature of the medical condition, but rather on the effect of that condition on everyday functioning; to put it in another way, it is the degree of incapacity caused by the disability that matters. It appears that this personalized vision of disability is very close to the model used by the Apostolic Chancery at the end of

DOI: 10.4324/9781003452324-13

the medieval period. The ecclesiastical institution thus functioned in much the same way as a modern state or supranational bloc in dictating public policy. An analysis of the petitions received by the Chancery and the letters sent in return during the Avignon period demonstrates that the Curia recognized the condition of disabled individuals who, within the limits of the law, wished to adapt their duties, as clerics and as Christians, according to their physical limitations. Disabled petitioners, men and women alike, wrote to the Chancery in order to secure a dispensation that would allow them either to continue working as secular or regular clerics or to contravene religious prohibitions regarding worship.

Similar to modern insurance companies, the pontifical institution sometimes called upon medical experts to determine the validity of petitioners' appeals and to oversee grants of privilege, indulgence, dispensation, exemption, or grace. Broadly speaking, these experts were responsible for determining the extent of an individual's incapacity resulting from physical, mental and sensory disabilities, illnesses, and/or incapacitating old age. In reality, physicians adopted a variety of roles. For instance, the petitioners themselves could call upon medical experts whom they identified as authorities of their condition and thus able to offer vital testimony to support the submitted requests for accommodations. At the same time, these medical personnel served the papal institution directly by evaluating petitioners' bodily or mental functionality in an advisory role and acted as decision makers with the power to authorize or reject an application, depending on the patient's condition. In the Middle Ages as today, claims could be assessed using medical evidence provided by the petitioner's doctor, conditioned by a positive assessment from a physician retrospectively or, in some cases, using reports provided by an independent doctor commissioned by the Apostolic Chancery. Physicians served as gatekeepers, and as conduits for the dispensation of pontifical grace, demonstrating the trust that the popes placed in them. Such procedures reinforced both *medicus'* own authority and that of the institution.

The epistolary sources discussed here are necessarily concise. Despite their brevity, however, these texts reveal physicians' essential role in granting pardons.[4] As such, this chapter's operating hypothesis is that physicians were acknowledged as experts in determining disability for the Apostolic Chancery in the fourteenth century. They were accorded a share of the popes' institutional authority, in the same way that a modern insurance company or a state defers to medical experts to judge an individual's relative disability and thus define the exact nature of his or her limitations and any necessary accommodations. The Church's reliance on physicians' specialist judgments reveals above all the institution's concern about fraudulent petitions: The risk of fraud was high and the Chancery sought to dispense grace and dispensations only in cases of real and verified disability. To do so, it turned to medical experts to provide vital information.

The theoretical framework for this study is supported by disability history. Before the 1980s, researchers approached disability history through the lens of a social history of marginality, poverty, and impairment as a physical anomaly. In this approach, they followed in particular public assistance policies that conceived of disabled people as indigents, patients, or objects of charity (the medical model).[5] In the 1980s, however, the question of accessibility became crucial: society itself became the vector of disability, highlighting a distinction between impairment (as a biomedical phenomenon) and disability (as a restriction on activity caused by society) (the social model).[6] In the 2000s, the notion that disability is not limited to material conditions and does not have a fixed existence gained currency, whether studied with or without the help of a model.[7] Indeed, the nature and experience of disability change according to the period and culture under consideration.[8] Therefore, studying disability in history requires us to modify our understanding of society as a whole, as demonstrated in the past decade by seminal research on physical and mental disability.[9]

The topic of forensic medical expertise has long been discussed in scholarship in the history of medicine and health.[10] Researchers have paid particular interest to the commissions that were established to determine whether a diagnosed leper should join a *leprosarium*, or in cases of suspected poisoning.[11] Historians have also focused on specific geographic areas, such as medieval Provence, the kingdom of Valencia, and Italian courts in the late Middle Ages.[12] The role of physicians in determining a criminal petitioner's mental state, and thus eligibility for pardon, has also been studied in the context of the procedures conducted in the Parliament of Paris and in early modern Florence.[13] While forensic medicine remains a strong historiographical trend in scholarship on the history of medicine; however, it thus far has been neglected—and certainly underexplored—in the discipline of disability history, especially when it comes to considering the role of medical authorities in classifying individuals' relative disability.[14]

Petitions sent to the popes and response letters prepared by the Apostolic Chancery offer insight into the role of the physician in medieval society and about the Chancery's participation in medical forensic investigations. The Apostolic Chancery, which managed the petitions received and the letters sent, was created in the late twelfth century during the papacy of Innocent III (1198–1213); these petition-response documents purportedly contain the first mention of legal medical expertise.[15] The establishment of the pontifical theocracy (i.e., a political system wherein the pope is considered superior to secular powers such as counts, dukes, kings, emperors) then led to an increase in the number of petitions made during the thirteenth and fourteenth centuries.[16] This growth was particularly evident when the Papacy moved to Avignon in order to occupy the "center of gravity of Christendom—a rational center, that is to say, a geographic center", as Jacques Le Goff writes in 1977.[17] The Papal Curia remained there from 1309 to 1378, consolidating the papal position over France and southwestern Europe in general, notably thanks to the French monarchy immense influence over the papacy. The year 1378 marked the return of the papacy to the Eternal City and the beginning of the Western Schism (1378–1417), which divided Christians into multiple factions, each supporting a different pontifical candidate, for some 40 years. Such discord generated a colossal diplomatic output of documents. As a consequence, Chancery staff progressively gained quality control over the content and form of their correspondence, ultimately establishing a formulaic tradition of petition- and letter-writing.

The petitions, copied in registers from the reign of Clement VI (in 1342) onward, contain the cases made by petitioners, composed mostly of medieval elites who had the financial means and necessary contacts to write to the popes themselves, to obtain grace. Notaries or procurators subsequently transposed these requests into Curia's style, rigorously reformulating the disabled petitioners' experiences. Then, in a specific and strictly adhered-to format called a 'minute', these requests were presented to the pope in the hope that the pontifical institution would recognize the petitioner's disability.[18] These stylistic formatting rules allow the papal institution to adapt to the increasing number of documents that it received and produced.[19] However, the Apostolic Chancery's rewriting of the petitioner's request during the composition of the response letter largely removed the supplicants' original words. A close study of these documents nevertheless reveals that, despite the institutional context in which they were written by pontifical scribes, the voices and experiences of disabled people are still present. Thus, it is not so much the words of the popes, scribes, notaries, or chancellor that can be discovered in these papal letters, but rather the weight of the institution and tradition that guided the petitioners' discourses as they transmitted their experiences.[20]

The Apostolic Chancery typically dealt with issues such as restrictions on becoming a priest (age, legitimate birth, and disability), but some also concerned people with disabilities whose condition prevented them from physically going to the mass (they could then benefit from portable altars, private priests or personal confessors), fulfilling their pilgrimage vows (which could be commuted), or respecting dietary restrictions (Lent or fasting, for example). In these documents, the physicians appeared as medical authorities, advisors, or decision makers, entrusted to justify, evaluate, or verify the personal injury damages report.

Secundum Assertionem Et Consilium Medicorum: Physicians and Medical Authority

Among other medical practitioners, the physician is a key figure in medieval culture. For example, in his *Quodlibetic Questions*, Thomas Aquinas, a famous thirteenth-century theologian, states that:

> Someone subjected to bodily sickness (*morbo corporali*), would commit himself to danger unless he would seek the remedy of medicine as quickly as he could, and he would sin out of negligence. . . . It must be said that bodily sickness, unless it is extinguished through the remedy of medicine, always grows unto the worse, unless perhaps it should be extinguished even by the power of nature.[21]

In the documents explored for this chapter, physicians positioned themselves as mediators between the petitioner (as a patient) and the Apostolic Chancery (as an institution). In that dialogue, physicians appeared as crucial characters who helped the petitioners not only to understand their limitations but also to present them in words that would be understood by other medieval elites. They can be found as consultants in numerous supplications, highlighting their growing influence on medieval elites and their families. However, their absence in other supplications also reflects the growing medicalization of medieval elites, revealing the extent to which they have integrated medical discourse into their requests.

A Crucial Actor in Medieval Society

Physicians played a role in the prevention of disease and disability through their recommendations and the expertise they brought to bear in granting pardons through pontifical letters. In the first instance, they acted as advisors to their patients, recommending ways for them to maintain their good health. They could act also by restoring humoral balances, that is, by treating their clients. For Cornelius Celsus, an encyclopaedist of the first century, the art of medicine was comprised of three parts: the first healed through diet (*victus*), the second, with the help of medicines (*medicamentum*), and the last, by the hand of the surgeon (*manus*). According to the Hippocratic and Galenic traditions, the human body is composed of four elements (fire, air, water, and earth) representing four qualities (hot, cold, wet, and dry) and forming four humors (yellow bile, blood, phlegm, and black bile). These criteria together constitute the temperaments (humours) that characterize the patient's complexion (qualities). Those constitutive principles of the physiology of the human body are called "natural things". This theory does not reflect a binary opposition between good health and bad health, however. On the contrary, it allows for a multitude of personal situations of health or ill health that fall between these two poles.[22] Each human being is indeed made up of a personal complexion that changes over the course of life.

Petitioners seeking papal dispensation increasingly made reference to doctors in their supplication. A request presented by Manfred, count of Clermont, to Clement VI and addressed by the Apostolic Chancery on April 2, 1347, testifies to this:

> Our dearest brother Manfred, Count of Clermont, has notified us that his only son, named Simon, aged 12, has such a weak complexion and delicate health that he must, according to the advice of the doctors, eat meat, as fish is not recommended during Lent, because his complexion does not allow him to eat fish due to his cold nature so that he will often be sick. Therefore, the count humbly begs us that the said Simon may eat meat and other foods during Lent until he is 25 years old in order to maintain his health, by special grace of apostolic authority—This is possible at certain times according to the advice of doctors, we place the responsibility of this authorization on their consciences.[23]

The missive relates the situation of Simon, aged 12 and only son of Manfred, who suffered from a weak complexion. On the advice of doctors, Pope Clement VI authorized the child to eat meat during Lent, a practice that was otherwise forbidden during the many lean days of the Christian calendar (at least one hundred each year: the 40 days of Lent, Friday of each week, and several days or eves of feasts). Simon's condition was clearly linked in some way to his age, as the letter later explains that this authorization would be valid until Simon reached the age of 25 years. Indeed, one's complexion evolves several times, according to the moments of life, "like the seasons".[24] It passes from a childhood with a wet complexion, too fluid to function satisfactorily, to a hot and wet adolescence, thence a hot and dry youth and a cold and wet old age, culminating in a cold and dry senility. A person could influence the "natural things" to recover his or her complexion by addressing the six "non-natural things".[25] These involved the food and drinks one consumed, repletion and secretion, the alternation between exercise and rest and between sleep and wakefulness, as well as the ambient air and passion and emotions.[26] Literature on the regulation of the six "non-natural things", which gained popularity in the years 1300–1348, had a considerable influence on the requests of supplicants and pontifical decisions during the Avignon period.[27]

To eat meat during Lent for Simon meant avoiding fish, the food normally used as a meat substitute. Although fish was frequently consumed by medieval people, and otherwise valued in the Christian context, texts that address dietary concerns often criticized it as a food source.[28] These texts highlight the cold and wet nature of fish caused by their environment of origin (rivers or seas). Accordingly, it is a food that is not well adapted to the human complexion, even dangerous in certain cases, as here for young Simon. Indeed, the letter states that cold and wet fish did not go well with Simon's weak complexion and cold nature. On the contrary, he needed food that was dry and warm to counterbalance his natural inclinations. The therapeutic theory was well known in the Papal Curia's circle, as well as among the lay and ecclesiastical elites who called upon it. Understanding the good and bad mixing of humors was a must for doctors, who had to know the cause of illness (i.e., imbalanced humors) in order to make a diagnosis. Indeed, health could be completely lost from a humoral imbalance. Practitioners therefore had to consider the individuality of the patient in order to produce a specific and adapted medical therapy.[29]

According to Hippocratic–Galenic theories, each person is formed by his or her "natural" environment, and understanding that environment allows one to gain a deeper conception of the sick person's body. Thus, good health is subject to the optimal adjustment of several parameters. It is not only a question of considering a disturbance to the qualities of health but also of comprehending the role played by the environment and "non-natural things" in causing that disturbance. Duraguerre, the aged and very ill abbot of the Cistercian monastery of San Sebastiano fuori le mura in Rome, claimed that he suffered from bad weather because of his old age. He therefore wished to be transferred elsewhere to regain his good health. Duraguerre thus sought not only to benefit from medical treatment but also perhaps to change the nature of the environment in which he lived:

> Your petition presents to us that, in a decrepit age and frequently suffering from serious illness in your body because of the bad weather, well known in your Cistercian monastery of San Sebastiano fuori le mura, you cannot conveniently and without personal danger reside in your monastery. Therefore, you ask us to transfer you to one of the hospitals of a monastery within the city walls in order to survive with the care of the doctors that our authority can grant. We authorize you to transfer to the city and join the hospice that belongs to your monastery and to live and reside there on an interim basis in order to receive the care of the doctors.[30]

This missive highlights the belief in the Hippocratic–Galenic tradition that climate and diet influenced the body. It likewise reflects the essential role of "non-natural things" in human health. According to Duraguerre, he could no longer reside in his monastery, where he faced bad weather, not without danger. The pope then authorized him to go to the monastic hospital that belonged to his order in the city of Rome, although he could return occasionally to his community "on an interim" basis. The transfer can be explained by the danger to health posed by certain places, according to the petitioner's own considerations. Thus, the Chancery believed that Duraguerre's transfer from one place to another would be very beneficial from a medical point of view. The pontifical institution did not hesitate, under this pretext, to authorize numerous infringements of monastic and canonical laws to allow clerics to regain their good health when they were suffering from the climate or the environment.[31]

Another letter, sent on the same day by the Chancery of Urban V to Duraguerre, uses the same wording to relate the illness, almost word for word. However, this letter was written in response to a separate supplication by which Duraguerre sought an indulgence concerning food prohibitions. Here, the pope authorized him to eat meat and dairy products, following the advice of doctors:

> You are writing to us because, at a decrepit age and suffering continuously from serious illnesses in your body, according to the advice and counsel of doctors, you are in danger of death if you do not eat meat and milk. In this regard, we wish to authorize you to eat meat and milk freely during Lent and Advent, provided that necessity demands it and that you see knowledgeable physicians.[32]

According to the letter, the indulgence received by Duraguerre was to avoid the "dangers of death", to which he seemed especially exposed during Lent and Advent Sunday. Just as in the case of the child Simon, Duraguerre's age—in this case being quite advanced—called for a particular diet. Since old age embodied a cold, wet state, eating hot, dry meat was considered to be a good way to influence "non-natural things". Health regimens recommended a drastic moderation of diet for the elderly, but the deprivations of Lent and fasting times were more harmful than beneficial for Duraguerre, according to the doctors' expertise. Respect for a good measure of food was propagated by ecclesiastical elites who had access to medical manuscripts, and especially to health regimens. This respect was then imported into the cloisters through monastic reforms led by these same elites. Finally, the therapeutic conception shared by the monks was relayed to the secular population during the twelfth century thanks to the increasing access to numerous learned medical works, which became popular before the end of the medieval period.[33] Key to these sources was a moderate lifestyle for all members of Christian society based on the conventual model, in which a diet without excess was deemed essential.

In the first letter, Duraguerre also received authorization to receive care from doctors who worked at the monastic hospital.[34] The traditional monastic orders, and later the mendicant orders, employed physicians as society became more medicalized, although a certain freedom was already permitted by the monastic rules. The Augustinian rule, for example, allowed the religious to break their vow of poverty and hire a doctor when the situation required it.[35] Doctors gradually acquired a privileged place in monasteries as supplicants hired trained practitioners for their medical advice and counsel: Papal letters thus authorized certain convents to recruit several doctors and surgeons.[36] However, medicine never was limited to conventual spaces: People had access to all kinds of medical care provided by a wide range of providers.[37] It varies greatly throughout Europe, but there was overall a growing distinction between university-trained physicians and all other kinds of medical providers. During the thirteenth century, lay and ecclesiastical elites progressively hired the services of university-educated doctors, who became increasingly professionalized which in turn enabled the social ascension of the physicians themselves. The new professionalism of the practitioners was asserted in particular thanks to a wealthy clientele that grew as the number of doctors increased. They certainly participated actively in the health of elite medieval society and were consulted in other cases as well. Their participation is particularly emphasized when the supplication offers a detailed diagnosis that could only have been made by a qualified expert.

The Medicalization of Medieval Elites

Recurrent appeals to the physician in petitions to the papacy appeared in the general context of the medicalization of medieval elites. The "democratization" of medical knowledge was made possible by numerous contemporary translation works that rendered Latin texts into the vernacular, such as that carried out by the physician Gilbertus Anglicus in the first half of the thirteenth century.[38] In his work, which represents one of the essential sources of therapeutic vocabulary, Gilbert anglicized Latin terms by producing numerous neologisms to transpose medical knowledge into the vernacular. During the thirteenth and fourteenth centuries, the representation of diseases as they were conveyed in our documentation evolved thanks to the establishment of medical discourse among the lay and ecclesiastical elites. A "medicalization of theological discourse" likewise influenced diagnoses and understanding of physical and mental disabilities, which can also be found in other documents.[39]

The staff in the Papal Curia who "revised" what was submitted by the petitioner into a standard format began to offer more detailed diagnoses, including naming the condition from which the supplicants suffered. This is illustrated by a petition written to Innocent VI by Simon, a deacon in the diocese of Artois, who was suffering from a serious fever: "At the time the synod [to which he was to go] was celebrated, [Simon] was suffering from a serious illness called tertian fever, so much so that he was unable to go even if he wished".[40] One can assume that Simon commissioned a physician at some point during his illness because he used the Latin term for tertian fever. Indeed, the ailment from which he suffered, constituted a chronic incapacitating condition, since it caused high fevers every other day. The fever prevented Simon from attending the synod, as he could not move around. The recurrent nature of this illness, in modern parlance malarial fever, ensured that symptoms recurred for months or even years. In fact, in this example, and in an increasingly systematic way in the fourteenth century, the words used in supplications or by the Apostolic Chancery may enable us to identify the affliction related to the missive. Yet, there is no question of making a retrospective diagnosis, for the illness presented by the suppliant may in fact have represented a variety of complaints with similar symptoms, even if a physician gave a diagnosis. It does not matter what the diagnosis was, as long as the author of the document considered himself to be suffering from this condition.[41]

Details about the disability or illness conveyed by the suppliants using a doctor's diagnosis, as well as knowledge of the illness and its consequences among members of the Curia, influenced the papal decision. Simon depicted a condition that was in principle incurable, and in this sense deployed a detailed presentation for the reader or reviewer using precise and culturally understood medical terms. This reflects the medicalization of medieval society more broadly, as therapeutic concepts became increasingly accessible to laymen and clerics alike. Many words were used by suppliants, procurators, scribes and members of the Chancery to relate physical and/or mental disabilities. But this, in turn, causes a challenge with these sources: a difficulty with translation, which is further reinforced by the double recording of these texts and the use in them of different terminology. A supplication and letter, exchanged by Aubertus Martini, cantor of the church of Saint Médéric de Linays, in Paris, and Urban V on May 6 1364, qualify his disability with several synonyms:

> [petition] Aubertus Martini because of the fragility of his head and also of the diseases (*egritudino*) and affections (*epidemie*) like the gout from which he had suffered and from which he suffers in an almost incessant way, cannot and does not risk to go to the church or in other public places to celebrate the masses. You humbly and devoutly ask us to have an altar in your house, located in a suitable and honest place— Authorized for four years.[42]

> [letter] According to your petition, you cannot and do not dare to go to church or other public places to celebrate mass, both because of your weakness (*debilis*) in the head and because of the various illnesses

(*egritudo*) from which you have suffered and suffer almost incessantly. We therefore authorize you to have a portable altar for a minimum of four years.[43]

Both the supplication and the letter tell us that Aubertus, because of a "weakness of his head", is incessantly afflicted with multiple diseases, both "epidemics" and gout. Some of these words seem clearly interchangeable, such as *fragilitas*, used in the supplication, or *debilitas*, used in the letter, to describe the condition from which the supplicant suffers. Hagiographic and theological texts use the word *debilitas* as a generic of *infirmitas* to mean illness or debility (sometimes old age), but also the state caused by these conditions.[44] The word *fragilitas* depicts Aubertus's vulnerability to illness, just as *debilitas* relates to his weakness. One can then think that Aubertus is not affected by a traumatic physical impairment, but because of the fragility of his head which can mean headaches, or dizziness, or some kind of mental incapacity, rather by a disturbance of the humours that causes all his illnesses. This situation leads to almost incessant suffering, according to the petition and the letter: Aubertus cannot go to church to hear mass. He is allowed by the Chancery to use a portable altar for four years. The context of the events recounted by the missive shows that *debilitas* is a generic term like *fragilitas* and does not correspond to illnesses, rather referred to by the word *egritudines*. Thus, bodily weakness seems to be included in the idea of disease and impairment, since it is associated with these words. However, in order to specify the illnesses with which the suppliant is still affected, the supplication goes into more detail than the letter. According to this first missive, Aubertus could be a victim of general diseases (*epidemiae*) as well as very specific ones (*gutta*), causing him incessant suffering, putting in opposition generic diseases and a well-defined disease. On the contrary, the letter does not take up this information and only relates that he always endures various diseases.

The development of medical knowledge and its transmission to the popes and then to the lay and ecclesiastical elites explain the medicalization of the terminology used. The choice of these words allowed the pontifical institution to recognize the disabled condition. It was important both for the petitioner, whose condition needed to be understood, and for the institution that granted or denied the petition based on its own assessment of the physical or mental consequences faced by the petitioners. In this way, the words constituted criteria that legitimized the relative inclusion or exclusion of clerics and laymen in the ecclesial body and the Christian community. Physicians helped the suppliants in that wording, then highlighting the cultural significance of their condition, understood by other medieval elites. But the doctors also served as experts for the pontifical institution to assess the petitioners' physical and/or mental limitations.

Medicorum, Super Hoc Conscientias Oneramus: Physicians and Evaluation of the Damages

Physicians had an important advisory role in diagnosing the condition from which the supplicants suffered. Another of their objectives was to assess the exact nature of the limitations experienced by the petitioners in order to delimit pontifical grace. The Apostolic Chancery was eager to have an evaluation of personal abilities according to assigned roles. While clerics had to meet certain standards of physical perfection (in order to be able to serve in worship, for example), the laity had to be in good enough health to fulfil their Christian duties, which often required a good physical condition (pilgrimage to the Holy Land or Santiago de Compostela, vows of fasting, etc.). In that event, doctors' advice was used to both legitimize the request from the petitioners' point of view and justify the Chancery's response.

The Physical or Mental Capacity

Physical or mental inability to perform clerical functions appears to be paramount in the definition of disability contained in the petitions and letters.[45] One of the most important decisions made by the Apostolic Chancery in this situation was whether the persons could accomplish what was expected of them in case of ill health. Indeed, Galenic medicine mobilized by these documents established a functional approach to disability in which, according to Thomas Aquinas, "A member is said to be weak (*infirmus*), when it cannot do the work of a healthy (*sanus*) member, the eye, for instance, when it cannot see clearly, as the Philosopher [Aristotle] states (De Hist. Animal. x, 1)".[46] The author then used a practical meaning of physical ability in which there is a difference between a limb or organ unable to function properly and a healthy one. Aquinas is here making a distinction between health, strength and ability on one side, and weakness, nonfunctional and, then, disability on another side. This definition of functionality was clearly linked to an individual's ability to perform various social and occupational functions. In this case, nonfunctionality, as a disability, was seen as a deviation from the norm, the latter being defined both by the efforts that healthy members of society could make and by the expectations of the pontifical institution. Disability was defined as an obstacle to the accomplishment of certain activities. With that in mind, the authors of the letters examined here considered the effects of their disabilities rather than their medical causes. The diagnosis was thus important, but what mattered most was the description of the effects on the petitioners, insofar as the consequences of the same illness could vary from one person to another.

The challenges posed by physical or mental disabilities on the management of ecclesiastical benefits are often clearly identifiable through the content of the requested grace. Well aware of this, the pontifical institution had to judge the health of petitioners on a case-by-case basis. A letter addressed by Alexander IV on August 9, 1257, to the Bishop of Sparta illustrates the extent to which the criterion of capacity was essential for the pontifical institution to be able to define the petitioner's integrity:

> We accept that, since your body is seriously impotent due to illness, you should withdraw from the execution of the pastoral office. We concede with our authority that, consequently, you may, with God's help and in order to fulfil your wish to recover your health, go to Salerno or Montpellier or to a different place and that you be able to stay there for the time you deem necessary.[47]

In this letter, the pope authorizes the bishop to remain in the region of Salerno or Montpellier, for example, far from his Spartan benefice, because the petitioner is unable to carry out his pastoral functions due to a serious illness. The Chancery does not linger on the causes of this "serious bodily infirmity", since it is not clearly identified. The classic formulation used by Alexander IV, insisting on the petitioner's impotence to exercise his pastoral office, provides a crucial clue that the problem does not lie in impotence as a type of defilement, for example, but rather as the consequence of his physical disability on his abilities.

Indeed, canon law was more concerned with the cleric's functionality.[48] The canonist Henry of Segusio (1200–71) indicated in his work that there are three criteria of irregularity *ex defectu corporis* (defect of the body) that would make one unfit for divine service: mutilation, weakness, and deformity.[49] One also finds in medieval canon law, notably in the Decree of Gratian written in the middle of the twelfth century, that a man who, weighed down by old age or illness and prevented from performing his office, was authorized to substitute a person in his place.[50] In the letter noted earlier, the bishop, for his part, sought to recover his health, and the pontifical institution did not seek to prevent him from doing so. It even allowed him to go to Salerno or Montpellier—the two greatest medical centres in medieval Europe.

The fact that the Curia emphasized the concrete consequences of ill health is explained pragmatically. The letters issued by the Apostolic See are first and foremost sources of practice written to address a specific problem. Their purpose was to find a solution to the disabling effects rather than to seek a way to deal with the physical impairment (although this was often a desired corollary effect): A supplicant asked for grace because he or she foresaw that the situation would last until it constituted a disability, completely preventing him or her from performing a specific task for a given moment. Then, the Chancery had to adapt to the physical incapacity of the cleric requesting the pardon according to what he could or could not carry out. This flexibility implies granting different dispensations not only according to the type of disability and its perceived duration, but also according to the status of the applicant and the functions he or she was supposed to perform. This link is very clearly found in canon 47 of the *Apostolic Constitutions*, written in the fourth century and then repeated in the canon law of the twelfth and thirteenth centuries, because it allowed for limitations to be set on physical incapacity caused by certain impairments. "The deaf (*surdus*) or the blind (*caecus*) will not become a bishop; not because he is defiled (*pollutus*), but so that the affairs of the Church do not suffer".[51] It appears, then, that the pontifical institution was particularly interested in the management of goods and ecclesiastical affairs, one of its principal missions. It was willing to offer pardons according to the ability or inability of the supplicant to fulfil his prescribed duties. This provision makes sense in letters written "*in casu*" (in case of). These applied only when the condition for which the dispensation was granted was fulfilled; in the context of this study, in the event that the illness occurred. Louis I of Blois-Châtillon (died in 1346), Count of Blois, and his wife, Jeanne de Hainaut (died in 1374), were authorized by Clement VI on August 4, 1343, to eat meat on fast days and lean days "in case of infirmitas":

> That on the days of fasting that are instituted by the Church and on the other days on which it is forbidden to eat meat, you may, in case of illness, eat meat following the advice of the Doctors in case the confessor and the aforementioned doctor think that it would be useful for you, we place the responsibility of this authorization on their consciences.[52]

According to the letter, the couple was to follow the advice of their doctor and confessor. A large majority of the cases handled by the Apostolic Chancery invoking a grace "in case" concerned lay elites. Indeed, one must have had the financial means to initiate a petition in order to receive a letter that applied only in cases of illness. In this way, the noble laity forged a special bond with the pope and affirmed their faith. They participated in 'dialogue' with the Chancery, under the influence of their priests and confessors representing the ecclesiastical authority, but also following a phenomenon of class mimicry by wanting to have their own pontifical grace and personal devotional space.[53] These speeches testify to what Jacques Chiffoleau calls the "flamboyant piety".[54] They also reveal an elite adherence to the pontifical conception of salvation. The supplications and letters likewise attest to the fact that both laymen and clerics asked for future accommodations in the event that their health deteriorated, without waiting until they were dying or otherwise incapacitated.

In cases of irregularities or temporary impediments, the Chancery had to rule on the actual capacity of the cleric to hold his benefice at the time the request was made. Although the Chancery could not know in advance how long the physical disability would last, its mission was to adapt the clerk's duties according to the effects of the disability or illness, so that the applicant was able to perform his duties.

The Submission of Grace to the Advice of Experts

Doctors played an active role in defining the abilities of a supplicant and helping him or her choose the optimal diet. In fact, they determined the patient's complexion and made a diagnosis that allowed the supplicant to clearly present his or her ill health to the pope. In the papal letters written in response to the petitions, the scribes emphasized whether or not the petitioner had sought medical advice. They did not hesitate to repeat this information during the *narratio*—the presentation of the applicant's motivations—attesting to the influence of the medical guarantee on the verdict of the patient's condition. During the petition process, the Apostolic Chancery relied on the statements of the supplicants who related medical diagnoses in order to gain a pardon in accordance with the medical recommendations. The exchange of letters also allows us to follow the evolution of the health of the people who wrote the petitions, thanks to a strong archival memory.

According to the obligation contained in the tenth rule of Chancery, written under Pope Benedict XII, a newly elected pope had to validate the graces granted by his predecessors that could not be executed because of their deaths.[55] Benedict's successor, Pope Clement VI, thus invited clerics to present their exceptional requests to the court of Avignon.[56] In this context, he was asked to renew an indulgence for illness less than a year after his coronation, on April 28, 1343. Bernardus de Taxio, a monk from the Cistercian monastery of Fontfroide, had written to the pope because he was afraid that the previously requested pardon (given at an unknown date) would not be valid.

> You obtained [this grace] from our predecessor of blessed memory, Pope Benedict XII, when he was elected Supreme Pontiff, because, for twelve years and more, you have been continually harassed by the disease of gout and burdened by arthritis, we agree to allow you, since this is in accordance with the advice of doctors, to place on yours and their consciences the responsibility of the authorisation to eat meat in the

Cistercian Order on the days and times when it is forbidden in a general way by law or custom.[57]

Bernardus, sick with gout and suffering from arthritis for more than 12 years, said that he had been authorized by Benedict XII to eat meat on medical advice. Pope Clement VI again allowed Bernardus to not respect the rigour of the order to which he belonged, provided that the grace requested was the result of medical advice. In fact, despite the resolution of the supplicants to abide by monastic rules, the rigorous way of life of the religious orders or the chronic nature of certain illnesses led to their inability to remain in these communities.[58] Concerns about the care of sick monks and nuns forced the popes to clarify their reading of the institution's rule and to clearly define the rights of the disabled in the statutes and customs of religious orders.[59] The papal letters also added certain relaxations to several monastic statutes, as Gregory IX did for the Cistercian statutes enacted in 1235, in order to facilitate the following of Benedictine rules.[60]

The letter cited earlier also demonstrates that the granting of grace was subject to the act of consulting a doctor in order to ensure the validity of this breach of the law. Indeed, as illustrated earlier, physicians were supposed to help the staff of the Curia to know the exact nature of the supplicants' limitations. In some cases, petitioners invoked ill health as a cleverly formulated excuse to obtain a pardon, which in fact hides an inability to live daily under a rule that the petitioner considered too harsh. This is a technique still used today, as demonstrated by currently published books that help people increase their chances of success during personal injury cases.[61] The use of well-oiled rhetoric that appealed to the reader's mercy while also calling on the expertise of doctors seems to have always existed.

In order to make that rhetoric easier to use, notaries and scribes gathered letters in "chancery forms", collecting various models of awarded graces since the eleventh century.[62] Those documents were stylistic and legal tools that allowed the staff of the Curia to prepare missives more quickly and uniformly. The scribes only had to follow the pre-established formulas repeated in the different models of letters, like a checklist to complete their theoretical knowledge.[63] They also serve the notaries, who were agents of the Curia in charge of standardizing the speeches of the petitioners to the applicable forms, and thus rewriting the petitions before they were presented to the popes.[64] It is their version that is finally recorded. An example from a thirteenth-century form edited by Henry Charles Lea shows that supplicants' notaries may have used such standard letters. This letter, initially written to an unnamed abbey, was supposed to provide a template for relating a case of disability in order to receive grace:

A monk of your order has presented to your representative a request containing the fact that, while he was once suffering from the disease of epilepsy which he contracted in the order, he approached the physician of your order, then finally refused to follow his advice, and left your monastery; the application of this medical advice then permitted the softening of the disease and the hope of a cure. So, he asks that the Apostolic See authorize him to return to your order, on condition that the Doctors persuade him to be vigilant about a remedy for intemperance and the other asperities of the order which can lead to the extreme fatigue of his head. Thus, we authorize that if this is so, it is possible to moderate the rigor of your order as satisfying the authorization of relaxation and the necessary temperance of the rule on which his salvation depends.[65]

This epileptic monk asked his order to do something to make his illness easier to live with, after having followed the advice of doctors. While he seemed reluctant to follow the advice at first, perhaps because it did not fit with how he lived his life, its effectiveness seems to have changed his mind. Thus, the unnamed monk wished to return to the order while continuing to follow the medical recommendations. The letter's call to temperance in order to make the asperities of order life more agreeable constitutes one aspect of a model letter, testifying to the standardization of invocations of doctors. For some historians, a certain lack of originality results from the writing of these documents to the point that they become "suspect".[66] On the contrary, this standardization can help historians to highlight the specificities of each supplicant's request: Since it offers a framework through which all the deviations become visible, it reveals the originality of the supplicant's words. For the pontifical institution, though, there was no question of granting a pardon under false pretences.

By mobilizing medical discourse, the Chancery strengthened the basis of the pardon and the authority of the Church. Indeed, by basing itself on the opinion of recognized experts, the decisions it rendered or the advice it sent through letters gained both accuracy and authority. The doctors thus served as safeguards and medical guarantees to determine the limitations of each supplicant and to legitimize the requests. They also appeared as allies during the control procedure that the Chancery put in place to verify and confirm the physical condition of the supplicant before the pardon was considered to be valid.

Medicorum Expertorum: Physicians and Graces' Implementation

Doctors were not limited to an advisory role but also actively participated in the granting of grace. The letters reveal the growing influence of physicians who worked to heal bodies rather than souls, when the saints and their miracles were absent. The pontifical institution used its skills and placed its trust in doctors to recognize disabled people's condition, and physicians were then used to confirm the petitioners' diagnosis at the express request of the pope. They were also sometimes called in as a second expert to validate a colleague's diagnosis.

The Confirmation of the Diagnosis

Petitioners did not always appeal to a physician before sending their petitions to the Chancery, or at least did not always mention doing so. Therefore, popes sometimes needed to request that petitioners seek an expert medical opinion about their health. This directive indicates that the institution had confidence in physicians render a valid verdict,[67] and, in fact, that the pontiffs sometimes submitted the granting of a pardon to the opinions and advice of doctors. Through this tradition of correspondence, which kept the supplicant's hierarchy informed, the pope or his staff utilized the specialist's verdict to strengthen the decision and controlled the favours granted.

The validity of the letter may be conditioned by the expert's confirmation of the diagnosis presented in the petition, which appears just after the papal *fiat* ("done"). For example, through Nicolus de Alifia, chancellor of the kingdom of Sicily, Fulconus Ruffus de Calabria, count of Synopolis in Calabria, asked to be able to eat meat during Lent in a supplication addressed to Urban V:

> Idem Fulconus Ruffus, count of Synopolis, a man of delicate health, who, because of the Lenten food, easily gets several invalidities threatening him with serious illnesses and endangering his person, ask to be considered worthy to eat meat and other foods of animal origin during Lent—I put the conscience in the hands of God-fearing medical experts.[68]

At the end of the supplication, the pope allowed Fulconus Ruffus to consume meat and other foods of animal origin during this period on the express condition that he requested the advice of medical experts. This stipulation meant that, since the petitioner had not mentioned a doctor in his original supplication, he must consult one before the pardon could become valid. The letter sent to him in response, dated August 27, 1363, repeated the speech of Fulconus contained earlier, in which he explains that he suffers from various threatening illnesses due to deficiencies caused by Lent:

> You have devoutly asked the Apostolic See to give you a grace to be able, because of your weak complexion, . . . to eat meat, milk and eggs during Lent, following the advice of your confessor and medical experts.[69]

The wording of the letter of reply contains the final papal decision, indicating that Fulconus must follow the advice of his confessor and doctors in order to have the right to eat meat and dairy products. This appeal to experts (*expertae*) is already found in the requests for autopsies contained in the decretals of Innocent III (1198–1216).[70] The term "expert", however, does not clearly refer to a doctor, surgeon, barber, or other representative of the therapeutic professions. It is possible to assume that the missive requests the appointment of a qualified physician to ratify the papal verdict. The petitioners' hierarchical superiors or colleagues, who had to verify the conduct of the examination, undoubtedly took the petitioners to health professionals they approved. At this time, doctors began to control the practice of their profession, notably through the creation of professional titles. Medical expertise was also exported to civil law: Doctors took on a new social role, as they were in the best position to judge impairment or illness. This role is transposed into forensic medicine, insofar as their diagnosis could be used as evidence in legal proceedings, in the same way that papal letters mobilize their expertise to render a pardon effective or not. Second, the pope adds that the doctor must fear God: Even if this might only be a standard expression, it might also reveal that the pope worried that the petitioner did not take Lent seriously. Thus, he could have wished to have a God-fearer expert to check on Fulconus physical condition before granting the grace, in order to make a valid decision. This letter makes it clear that, for the pontifical institution, a good doctor was respectful of divine judgment.

The vow concerning food constitutes a question that particularly mobilized medical experts, since they were the only ones capable of judging the poor health of the supplicants and of skilfully describing their complexions. This is, in any case, the opinion of the Chancery of Pope Innocent VI. A letter sent by Pierre de Lusignan, Count of Tripoli and first son of the King of Cyprus who was treated on August 3, 1354, asked that he to be released from his vow to fast on bread and water. "If the advice of the doctors attests that it is not possible for you to fulfil your vow without significant damage to your body, the bishop of Paphos will be able to commute and dispense your vow".[71] The pope's verdict, which is included in that one sentence at the end of the letter, puts forward the role of the doctor as a witness. Indeed, the count wished to benefit from a confessor who could enable him to commute his vow into a pious work. The pope authorized it, provided that Pierre met a doctor and that the latter estimated that he could carry out his oath without causing serious damage to his body. If the result of this examination was positive, the bishop of Paphos was to authorize Peter to elect a confessor and to commute his vow.

As experts, physicians were supposed to verify a patient's symptoms. This verification was meant to minimize the fraudulent granting of graces, following the same type of investigation conducted for the miracle trials. Indeed, during those, physicians were commissioned to certify miraculous cures and to testify to their own inability to treat the person seeking the miracle.[72] In those documents, we can also see the medicalization of elitist discourse from the twelfth century onwards. It is evidenced in the use of medical terms by people who related their experiences and through the frequent invocation of doctors in their speeches.[73] These actors were more and more frequently consulted, especially about the potential curability of a disease from which the ill person suffered since a curable condition could not appear as one miraculously cured.[74] For example, a quarter of the children presented in the canonization process of Nicholas of Tolentino written in 1325 benefitted from the visit of a helpless doctor during their illness.

As for miracles, medical expertise helped the pontifical institution to control the presence of fraud and lies.[75] In the same way that it was absolutely necessary to control the incurability of a person who experienced a miraculous cure in order to prove the miracle, it was absolutely necessary to control the veracity of the incapacities of clerics and laymen who asked for a letter of grace. This legal expertise allowed the Church to distribute its favours without ambiguity, since the medical verdict guaranteed the authenticity of the missives.[76]

The Need for a Second Opinion

Doctors were, therefore, considered experts in diagnosis, able to say whether or not the pontifical pardon should be validated. They were sometimes charged with determining whether the petitioners' impairments were real and consistent with those described in their petitions. The Chancery staff sometimes requested a second opinion or asked the recipients of their letters to set up a council to determine the state of health of a supplicant. This happened, for example, in a purported leprosy case brought to the attention of Pope Honorius III on May 16, 1222.[77] The pope ordered the examination of Theobaldus, treasurer of Rouen, to silence people who were spreading rumours that Theobaldus was leprous. He commissioned a medical test administered by both lawyers and doctors, comparable to what would have happened in a lay trial. He asked for judges who were the most learned scholars in the field of medical investigation and who worked the most meticulously.[78] There are no other letters in the records regarding this investigation, except for one requesting that another suitable person be elected to celebrate mass in his place during the investigation. The original letter speaks to the need for a thorough investigation to determine the truth about a clergyman's physical condition that may taint the sacredness of the church.

Another petition, this time addressed to Urban V on August 30, 1363, by Joan of Kent, Princess of Aquitaine and Wales in a *rotulus* (grouped registration of several requests by a prestigious supplicant for several of his or her people), related Margerie de Mere's request to be allowed to eat something other than fish during Lent, in particular milk and eggs. The pope's *fiat* (done) conditioned the attribution by stating that:

> In the rotulus of Joan of Kent, Princess of Aquitaine and Wales, it is requested that the noblewoman Margerie de Mere, lord of that principality, who cannot eat fish during Lent, may eat milk and eggs—Done, according to the advice of the doctors and in case, in any other way, a second judgment of these doctors can fill this weakness by vegetables rather than by milk and eggs.[79]

Here, the Chancery required that the granting of the grace be conditioned by the advice of doctors, in case Margerie's health could be restored by eating vegetables rather than milk and eggs. This time, Urban V was not quick to grant the pardon to the petitioner and asked that the medical judgment be made in two stages: the first to determine her dietary deficiencies; the second to verify whether a diet of soup and vegetable-based dishes would be sufficient to restore her health. Then, if one reads the letter more closely, the Curia staff (and/or, possibly, the pope himself) proposed a dietary alternative to the nonobservance of Lent. Vegetables and their nutritional qualities, the basis of the medieval diet, could indeed compensate for the energy losses caused by a purely vegan diet over short periods. This reveals that Popes and their entourage knew medicine and had some therapeutic opinions about human health. Indeed, doctors were present in Curia as early as the thirteenth century, which could explain how Urban V's Chancery could offer such medical advice. The link between medicine, doctors, popes, and the papal entourage was not new. Innocent III founded a hospital in 1201 where the members of the Curia could be treated and was the first pontiff for whom the existence of a pontifical doctor is attested.[80] Thus, from the beginning of the thirteenth century, papal physicians remained in the vicinity of St Peter's Basilica: there were more than 70 during this century.

During the fourteenth century, when the Curia moved to Avignon, many medical books could be seen on the shelves of the papal libraries.[81] The presence of these writings proves the interest of the pontiffs and their entourage in the care of the body, especially through medical works of practice. Some popes commissioned the writing of medical works on their own behalf, testifying to their involvement in the study of medicine. For example, the *Opus Majus*, the *Opus minus*, and the *Opus tertium* were composed by Roger Bacon on the subject of old age and rejuvenation of the body at the request of Clement VI, himself sick of gout and treated on this occasion by the famous doctor Guy de Chauliac. We learn more about Clement VI's disease in a letter dated December 18, 1351, written to Peter, king of Aragon, to warn him of the recent consequences of his illness the day after his encounter with Guy de Chauliac, who had diagnosed his kidney stones. In his letter, the pope declared that he would put his recovery in the hands of God, although he admitted to suffering greatly.[82]

Even better than asking for a second opinion to validate a request, in at least one case Pope John XXII sent one of his personal physicians to a petitioner. Informed of his illness, this pope notified Robert Albaron, lord of Monfrin, that he had sent the doctor Bernard de Cannassio on April 6, 1334:

> Because we desire that you, our son, be freed from a serious illness of the body by the grace of God, here is the dear son master Bernard de Cannassio, archdeacon of Lombés in the church of Albi, our physician, so that he can comfort you and relieve you in your function, for he is endowed by God with experience, we attach him to your service, urging divine attention to you, in the hope that you will be comforted by God, as you are worthy of receiving this merciful visit and this favour thank to your humble spirit; May you welcome with placid zeal the said physician for your salvation, and may he offer you his salubrious advice for the salvation of your body by the grace of God and be at the service of your tranquillity.[83]

At that time, John XXII was 90 years old and died a few months later, on December 4, 1334. Even still, he did not hesitate to send one of his own doctors to the lord of Montfort (living about 20 kilometres from Avignon). Moreover, this was not an ordinary doctor, but a member of his *familia* (close circle), which we know thanks to a letter giving an indulgence *"in articulo mortis"* (on the verge of death) to Bernard where he is presented in this way.[84] Some of the high officials of the Roman Curia were themselves doctors or had members of their *familia* who were doctors to the popes. Popes and members of the Apostolic Chancery were frequently in contact with doctors and their medical works. The growing authority of the university-trained physician ensured that he appeared in various aspects of medieval life, not the least of which was the role he played in the papal entourage.[85] Certainly, as Agostino Paravicini Bagliani writes, "medical knowledge was not incompatible with high functions in the Roman Curia".[86] For example, learned physicians held crucial positions in the Avignon Papal Curia, even as scribes (as Gasbert de Septemfontanis for Benedict XII), and thus might have had a fundamental influence on the writing of the documents consulted here.[87] Moreover, the private doctors of the popes did not put aside their personal careers and were, on the contrary, among the most prolific in their profession. The pontiffs, armed with this medical knowledge just like ecclesiastical and lay elites, dealt with the Galenic theory of complexion and proposed alternatives to religious dietary obligations. Consequently, they adopted and used the same functional definition of disease and impairment as the therapeutic practice.

Conclusions

The role of professional medical practitioners gradually grew in medieval society, and supplicants increasingly called on them to support their petitions. In this instance, supplicants were considered patients whose incapacity had been validated by a medical authority. The study of supplications and papal letters reveals that the petitioners mobilized medical and theological knowledge to present themselves as good candidates for grace. Then, the papacy based its decisions on the advice of its doctors, on whom it relied to grant pardons. It used the speeches of the supplicants to categorize them according to physical or mental abilities. Finally, popes sometimes also requested that the granting of grace be subject to the verification of one or more doctors who were charged with confirming the diagnosis or giving a second opinion. By requesting doctors or surgeons, the Chancery posed as a connoisseur of the human race; not as a healer, but as a supporter. The documentation underlines the growing interest of the papacy in the suffering and care of the body in the fourteenth century and reveals how the expected functions was the main criterion for determining the granting of the requested favour. Moreover, by often making the application of grace conditional on the opinion of these experts, the pontifical institution found in them a new means of controlling the granting of grace and a way to mutually reinforce their influence on the Christian bodies.

The power and function of the doctors were also strengthened by the pontifical institution, which one might say participated in the general movement of the professionalization of these actors. Through their dialogue, the supplications and papal letters reinforced the authority and role of physicians, just as the ecclesiastical institution consolidated its own power by conditioning its decisions on their expertise. The physicians could serve as a relay for pontifical grace, demonstrating the trust that the popes place in them. This process reinforced their authority as well as that of the institution. Thus, the physician was a delegate of the popes' power in the fourteenth century in the same way that an insurance company or a state today commissions a physician to judge the percentage of incapacity of a person in order to know the exact nature of their limitations.

A trace of this medical culture deeply embedded in everyday life can be found in the supplications recorded by the Apostolic Penitentiary in the fifteenth century. Arnold Esch's work shows that supplicants demonstrated a solid medical knowledge and dispensed with doctors most of the time.[88] However, the doctor's authority over bodies continued to be summoned in very specific circumstances. As in the Avignon period, the role of the doctors was to provide preventive care and advice on diet and general hygiene (food, baths, contagion risks), but they were mainly summoned by the popes to produce death or illness certificates that corroborated petition requests. Thus, they seem to have retained and even strengthened their function as experts in cases of disability and ill health.

Notes

1 Darrel W. Amundsen and Gary B. Ferngren, "The Forensic Role of Physicians in Ptolemaic and Roman Egypt," *Bulletin of the History of Medicine* 52–53 (Fall 1978): 336–53; Oliver Lisi, *The Body Legal in Barbarian Law* (Toronto: University of Toronto Press, 2011); Fabrice Brandli et al., *Les corps meurtris. Investigations judiciaires et expertises médico-légales au xviiiᵉ siècle* (Rennes: Presses Universitaires de Rennes, 2014).

2 Anne-Marie Naveau, "Quelques réflexions concernant le nouveau rôle du médecin-expert en droit commun," in *Justice et dommage corporel: Panorama du handicap au travers des divers systèmes d'aide et de réparation,* ed. Jean-Pol Beauthier (Bruxelles: Larcier, 2011).

3 Christopher J. Bruce, Kelly A. Rathje, and Laura J. Weir, *Assessment of Personal Injury Damages,* 6th ed. (Toronto: LexisNexis Canada, 2019).

4 Marilyn Nicoud, *Le prince et le médecin. Pensée et pratiques médicales à Milan (1402–1476)* (Rome: École française de Rome, 2014).

5 Colin Barnes, "A Legacy of Oppression: A History of Disability in Western Culture," in *Disability Studies: Past, Present and Future,* eds. Len Barton et Michael Oliver (Leeds: Disability Press, 1997), 3-24.

6 Michael Oliver, "A New Model of the Social Work Role in Relation to Disability," *The Handicapped Person: A New Perspective for Social Workers?* ed. Jo Campling (London: RADAR, 1981), 19–32; Henri Jacques Stiker, *Corps infirmes et sociétés: Essais d'anthropologie historique,* 3rd ed. (Paris: Aubier, 1982).

7 On those models, see Wendy J. Turner, "Models of Disability: Connecting the Past to the Present," *Zeitschrift für Disability Studies* 1 (2022), https://diglib. uibk.ac.at/zds/content/titleinfo/7323860/full.pdf.

8 Ian Hacking, *The Social Construction of What?* (Cambridge: Harvard University Press, 1999); Sharon L. Snyder and David T. Mitchell, *Cultural Locations of Disability* (Chicago: University of Chicago Press, 2006).

9 On physical disability, see Irina Metzler, *Disability in Medieval Europe: Thinking About Physical Impairment During the High Middle Ages, c. 1100–1400* (London: Routledge, 2006); Cordula Nolte et al., eds., *Homo debilis: Behinderte, Kranke, Versehrte in der Gesellschaft des Mittelalters* (Korb: Didymos-Verlag, 2009); Valérie Delattre, ed., *Décrypter la différence* (Paris: CQFD, 2009); Joshua Eyler, ed., *Disability in the Middle Ages: Reconsiderations and Reverberations* (Farnham: Ashgate, 2010); Wendy J. Turner and Tory V. Pearman, eds., *The Treatment of Disabled Persons in Medieval Europe: Examining Disability in the Historical, Legal, Literary, Medical, and Religious Discourses of the Middle Ages* (Lewiston: Edwin Mellen Press, 2010); Franck Collard and Evelyne Samama, eds., *Handicaps et sociétés dans l'histoire* (Condé sur Noireau: L'Harmattan, 2010); Irina Metzler, *A Social History of Disability in the Middle Ages: Cultural Considerations of Physical Impairment* (London:

Routledge, 2013). On mental disability, see Wendy J. Turner, *Care and Custody of the Mentally Ill, Incompetent, and Disabled in Medieval England* (Turnhout: Brepols, 2013); Wendy J. Turner, ed., *Madness in Medieval Law and Custom* (Leiden: Brill, 2010); Irina Metzler, *Fools and Idiots? Intellectual Disability in the Middle Ages* (Manchester: Manchester University Press, 2016).

10 See, for example, Sarah M. Butler, *Forensic Medicine and Death Investigation in Medieval England* (New York: Routledge, 2016).

11 On leprosarium, see François-Olivier Touati, *Maladie et société au Moyen Âge: la lèpre, les lépreux et les léproseries dans la province ecclésiastique de Sens jusqu'au milieu du xive siècle* (Bruxelles: De Boeck, 1998); Johan Picot, " 'La Purge': une expertise juridicomédicale de la lèpre en Auvergne au Moyen Âge," *Revue historique* 66–22 (2012): 292–321; on poison, see Franck Collard, "*Secundum artem et peritiam medicine*. Les expertises dans les affaires d'empoisonnement à la fin du Moyen Âge," in *Expertises et conseils au Moyen Âge* (Paris: Pub. de la Sorbonne, 2012), 161–73. Note also an important chapter on forensic medicine in Italy written by Ann G. Carmichael, "The Legal Foundations of Post-Mortem Diagnosis in Later Medieval Milan," in *Death and Disease in the Medieval and Early Modern World: Perspectives from Across the Mediterranean and Beyond*, eds. Lori Jones and Nükhet Varlık (York: York Medieval Press, 2022).

12 On medieval Provence, see Joseph Shatzmiller, *Médecine et justice en Provence médiévale, Documents de Manosque, 1262–1348* (Aix-en-Provence: Publications de l'Université de Provence, 1989). On Valencia, see Carmel Farragud, "Expert Examination of Wounds in the Criminal Court of Justice in Cocentaina (Kingdom of Valencia) During the Late Middle Ages," in *Medicine and the Law in the Middle Ages*, eds. Wendy J. Turner and Sarah M. Butler (Leiden: Brill, 2014), 109–32. On Italian courts, see Joanna Carraway Vitiello, "Forensic Evidence, Lay Witnesses and Medical Expertise in the Criminal Courts of Late Medieval Italy," in *Medicine and the Law in the Middle Ages*, eds. Wendy J. Turner and Sarah M. Butler (Leiden: Brill, 2014), 133–56.

13 On the Parliament of Paris, see Maud Ternon, *Juger les fous au Moyen Âge: dans les tribunaux royaux en France xive–xve siècles* (Paris: Presses universitaires de France, 2018); Sasha Pfau, *Medieval Communities and the Mad: Narratives of Crime and Mental Illness in Late Medieval France* (Amsterdam: Amsterdam University Press, 2020). On Early Modern Florence, see Elizabeth W. Mellyn, *Mad Tuscans and Their Families: A History of Mental Disorder in Early Modern Italy* (Philadelphia: University of Pennsylvania Press, 2014).

14 Giovanni Ceccarelli, *Il gioco e il peccato. Economia e rischio nel tardo Medioevo* (Bologna: Il Mulino, 2003).

15 Ynez V. O'Neill, "Innocent III and the Evolution of Anatomy," *Medical History* 20, no. 4 (1976): 429–33.

16 Brett E. Whalen, *Dominion of God* (Cambridge, MA: Harvard University Press, 2010), 3.

17 Jacques Le Goff, "1274, année charnière: mutations et continuités," in *Actes du colloque international du Centre national de la recherche scientifique* (Paris: Édition du CNRS, 1977), 481–89, reedited in Jacques Le Goff, *Pour un autre Moyen Âge: temps, travail et culture en Occident: 18 essais* (Paris: Gallimard, 2013), 516 (my translation).

18 Patrick Zutshi, "The Political and Administrative Correspondence of the Avignon Popes, 1305-1378: A Contribution to Papal Diplomatic," in *Aux origines*

de l'État moderne. Le fonctionnement administratif de la papauté d'Avignon (Rome: École française de Rome, 1991), 371–84.

19 Armand Jamme, "Écrire pour le pape du xie au xive siècle. Formes et problems," *Mélanges de l'École française de Rome—Moyen Âge* (2016): 128–31, https://journals.openedition.org/mefrm/3121.

20 On the supplicants "subjectivity" in French remission letters, see Pfau, *Medieval Communities*, 42 and following. It is interesting to note that she did not find more than one mention of physician's aid in her letters on madness, but mentioned that physicians "were called as witnesses for other physical illnesses" and "were brought into the court to provide testimony in the form of prognosis for the injured party, determining whether or not the wounds were likely to prove fatal" (p. 141).

21 Thomas Aquinas, *Disputed Questions*, transl. Urban Hannon for The Aquinas Institute, URL consulted on January 10, 2022, https://aquinas.cc/. Quodlibet 1, "On Man", article 2.

22 Ortrun Riha, "Chronisch Kranke in der medizinischen Fachliteratur des Mittelalters. Eine Suche nach der Patientenperspektive," in *Homo debilis: Behinderte, Kranke, Versehrte in der Gesellschaft des Mittelalters*, ed. C. Nolte (Korb: Didymos-Verlag, 2009), 99–120.

23 RS13, f. 198V—Manfredus, to Clément VI, 2 May 1347. Inedited text:

> *Significat s. v. devotus filius vester Manfredus, comes Claromonte quod ipsem unicum filium habet nomine Simonetum in XII anno constitutum complexionis debilis et nimium dellicate cuius sanitati pisces non congruunt iuxta consilium medicorum cum eumdem symonetum quadragesimali tempore propter frigiditatem piscium dicte sue complexioni contraxeram contingat sepius infirmari. Quare idem come humiliter supplicatur quatenus prefato symoneco que carnes et alia cibaria dicto quadragesima tempore comedere usque ad XXV anni pro sanitate sua conservanda valeat dignemini de speciali graciam auctoritate apostolica indulgere. Possit predicte de consilio medicorum dispensari ad tempus super quibus eius conscientias oneramus.*

24 Metzler, *Fools and Idiots?* 69.

25 Neville Morley, *Theories, Models, and Concepts in Ancient History* (London: Routledge, 2004), 57.

26 Pedro Gil-Sostres, "Les régimes de santé," in *Histoire de la pensée médicale en occident. 1, Antiquité et Moyen Âge*, ed. Mirko D. Grmek (Paris: Édition du Seuil, 1995), 257–82.

27 Marilyn Nicoud, *Les régimes de santé au Moyen Âge: naissance et diffusion d'une écriture médicale, xiiie-xve siècle* (Rome: École française de Rome, 2007), introduction.

28 Paul Freedman, "Food Histories of the Middle Ages," in *Writing Food History: A Global Perspective*, eds. Kyri W. Claflin and Peter Scholliers (London: Berg, 2012), 24–37.

29 Danielle Jacquart, "The Introduction of Arabic Medicine Into the West. The Question of Etiology," in *Health, Disease and Healing in Medieval Culture*, ed. Sheila D. Campbell (Basingstoke: Macmillan, 1997), vol. III, 186–95.

30 RV 260, f. 5 V—Urban V to Duraguerre, Cistercian abbot of San Sebastiano fuori le mura (Roma), 13 December 1369. Text analyzed by François Avril et al., eds., *Urbain V (1362–1370): lettres communes analysées d'après les*

registres dits d'Avignon et du Vatican, series: Bibliothèque des écoles françaises d'Athènes et de Rome (Paris: École française de Rome, 1954), n° 26 392:

> *Sane petitio pro parte tua nobis nuper exhibita continebat quod tu qui in decrepita etate ut asseris constitutus existis et assidue graves infirmitates in tuo corpore pateris propter aeris intemperiem qui in tuo monasterio sancti Sebastiani extra muros urbis, Cisterciensis ordinis, sepius vigere dinoscitur in eodem monasterio non potes commode et sine persone tue periculo residere. Quare pro parte tua nobis fuit humiliter supplicatum ut tibi morandi in aliquo hospitiorum que prefatum monasterium infra muros urbis predicte habere dinoscitur quamdiu sub medicorum cura extiteris licentiam concedere de benignitate apostolica dignaremur. Nos igitur huiusmodi supplicationibus inclinati tibi ut in prefata urbe in aliquo de huiusmodi hospitiis ad dictum tuum monasterium pertinentibus quamdiu sub cura medicorum ut prefertur te necesserio esse contigerit licite habitare valeas et ad residendum interim in eodem monasterio minime tenearis.*

31 Ninon Dubourg, "L'incapacité dans les lettres de dispenses pontificales: aller à l'encontre de la réglementation ecclésiastique médiévale pour franchir la clôture," in *L'exception et la Règle, les pratiques d'entrée et de sortie des couvents, de la fin du Moyen Âge au XIXe siècle,* eds. Albrecht Burkardt and Alexandra Roger (Rennes: Presse universitaire de Rennes, 2022), 41–54.

32 RV 260, f. 5 V (RA 172, f. 348)—Urban V to Duraguerre, abbot of the Cistercian monastery of Sebastian outside the walls of Rome on 13 December 1369. Text analysed by Avril et al., *Urbain V (1362–1370),* n° 26 391:

> *Cum itaque tu qui sicut accesseris in decrepita etate constitutus existis propter nonnullas graves infirmitates quas in tuo corpore assidue pateris nequeas secundum assertionem et consilium medicorum vitam tuam sine esu carnium et lacticinorum absque periculo mortis sustentare. Nos tuis in hac parte supplicationibus inclinati tibi ut etiam tempore quadragesimali et adventus Domini vesci carnibus et lacticiniis libere valeas, dummodo necessitas id exigat et expertis medicis videatur.*

33 Georges Vigarello, *Le sain et le malsain: santé et mieux-être depuis le Moyen Âge* (Paris: Éditions du Seuil, 1993), 46.

34 Andrew T. Crislip, *From Monastery to Hospital: Christian Monasticism and the Transformation of Health Care in Late Antiquity* (Ann Arbor: University of Michigan Press, 2008).

35 Luc Verheijen, eds., *La Règle de saint Augustin* (Paris: Études augustiniennes, 1967), 35, chapitre 5, article 35: "If a sister declares herself ill (*dolor in corpore*), she must be believed; but if there is any doubt as to the remedies to be taken (*sanando illi dolori*), a doctor (*medicus*) must be consulted" (my translation).

36 AN, L 248, n° 215 (olim n° 216)—Innocent IV to the Master and the Brothers of the Hospital of Jerusalem, October 21, 1252, text analyzed by Bernard Barbiche, ed., *Les actes pontificaux originaux des archives nationales de Paris 1, 1198–1261* (Vatican: Biblioteca Apostolica Vaticana, 1975), n° 704, 268.

37 Caroline Darricau-Lugat, "Regards sur la profession médicale en France médiévale (xiie-xve)," *Cahiers de recherches médiévales et humanistes,* Vulgariser la science: les encyclopédies médiévales 6 (1999), https://journals.openedition.org/crm/939.

38 Faye M. Getz, *Healing and Society in Medieval England a Middle English Translation of the Pharmaceutical Writings of Gilbertus Anglicus* (Madison: University of Wisconsin Press, 1991), xlix.

39 Aurélien Robert, "Contagion morale et transmission des maladies: histoire d'un chiasme (xiiie-xixe siècle)," *Tracés. Revue de Sciences humaines* 21 (2011): 41-60 (my translation).

40 RS 34, f. 11 R—Simon, deacon in the diocese of Artois to Innocent VI, February 14, 1351. Unedited text: ". . . *Esset tempore quo dicta synodus fuit celebrata, gravi infirmitate febrorum tertiane detentus, quod non potuisset etiam si valuisset in dicta synodo interesse.*"

41 On parallel diagnosis, see Wendy J. Turner, "Medieval English Understanding of Mental Illness and Parallel Diagnosis to Contemporary Neuroscience," in *Cognitive Sciences and Medieval Studies: An Introduction*, eds. Juliana Dresvina and Victoria Blud (Cardiff: University of Wales Press, 2020), 97–120.

42 RS 42 f. 149 V—Aubertus Martini, cantor of the church of Saint Médéric de Linays, in Paris to Urban V, May 6, 1364. Text analysed by Anne-Marie Hayez, Janine Mathieu and Marie-France Yvan, eds., *Urbain V: suppliques de 1362 à 1365 (années I à IV)* (Turnhout: Brepols, 1978), n° 1 187:

> *Pater beatissime devotus orator vester Aubertus Martini, . . . propter fragilitatem sui capitis ac etiam propter varias egritudines tam epidemie quam gute quas hactenus passus fuit et adhuc quasi incessanter patitur, non potest nec audet in ecclesia aut alio loco publico missarum solemnia celebrare . . .. Supplicat igitur s. v. humiliter et devote quatenus ut in oratoris domus habitationis sue loco idoneo et honesto . . ., fiat ad quadriennium.*

43 RV 251, f. 424 V—Urban V to Aubertus Martini, cantor of the church of Saint Médéric de Linays, in Paris, May 6, 1364. Text analyzed by Avril et al., *Urbain V (1362–1370)*, n° 8 877:

> *Cum itaque sicut exhibita nobis tua petitio continebat quod tu, tam propter debilitatem tui capitis quam etiam propter varias egritudines quas hactenus passus fuisti et adhuc quasi incessanter pateris non possis nec audeas in ecclesiam aut loco publico missarum solemnia celebrare . . . liceat tibi habere altare portatile . . . post quadriennium minime valituris.*

44 Hans-Werner Goetz, "'*Debilis*'. Vorstellungen von menschlicher Gebrechlichkeit im frühen Mittelalter," in *Homo debilis: Behinderte, Kranke, Versehrte in der Gesellschaft des Mittelalters*, eds. Cordula Nolte et al. (Korb: Didymos-Verlag, 2009), 21–56.

45 Paolo Ostinelli, "I chierici e il '*defectus corporis*': Definizioni canonistiche, suppliche, dispense," in *Deformità fisica e identità della persona tra medioevo ed età moderna*, ed. Gian Maria Varanini (Firenze: University of Firenze, 2015), 3–30.

46 Thomas Aquinas, *Summa Theologiae I-II*, q. 77, article 3, "Whether a sin committed through passion should be called a sin of weakness?" transl. by Laurence Shapcote for The Aquinas Institute, URL consulted on the December 31, 2021, https://aquinas.cc/.

47 RV 25, f. 74 V—Alexander IV to G., bishop of Sparta, August 9, 1257. Text edited by Joseph de Loye, Pierre de Cenival, Auguste Coulon and Charles de La

Roncière, ed., *Les registres d'Alexandre IV: recueil des bulles de ce pape* (Paris: Boccard, 1953), n° 2 180:

> *Multam ex eo, prout accepimus, cordis angustiam pateris, quod pro tui corporis infirmitate gravissima impotens ad pastoralis officii executionem debitam inveniris. Nos itaque paterno tibi super hoc condolentes affectu et benigne tuis precibus annuentes, fraternitati tue presentium auctoritate concedimus, ut pro consequenda, Deo propitio, sospitate votiva, Salerni vel apud Montempesulanum sive alibi, quandiu expedire videbitur, valeas commorari.*

48 Brandon Parlopiano, "*Propter deformitatem*: Towards a Concept of Disability in Medieval Canon Law," *Canadian Journal of Disability Studies* 4–3 (2015): 72–102.

49 Henry of Segusio, *Summa Aurea* (Venice: Bernardo Giunta, 1570) 1.20.

50 Gratiani, "Decretum Gratiani," in *Corpus Iuris Canonici I*, ed. Emil Friedberg (Liepzig, 1878; reprint Styria: Graz, 1956) second part, causa 7–11, online with Bayerische Staatsbibliothek, Munich, https://geschichte.digitale-sammlungen. de/decretum-gratiani/online/angebot.

51 Jean Hardouin, *Conciliorum collectio Regia Maxima: Act Conciliorum*, 12 vols. (Paris: Ex Typographia Regia, 1714–15), tome I, p. 27.

52 RV 159, f. 275 R—Clement VI to Louis I of Blois-Châtillon, Count of Blois, and his wife, Jeanne de Hainaut (diocese of Chartres), August 4, 1343. Unedited text:

> *ut diebus quibus ieiunia sunt per ecclesiam instituta et aliis in quibus est esus carnium interdictus possitis in casu infirmitatis vesci carnibus de consilio medicorum quotiens confessor et medici predicti hoc vobis viderint expedire, quorum quidem confessoris et medicorum super hoc conscientias oneramus.*

53 Florian Mazel, *La noblesse et l'Église en Provence, fin x^e-début xive siècle* (Paris: Comité des travaux historiques et scientifiques—CTHS, 2002), 516.

54 Jacques Chiffoleau, *La Comptabilité de l'au-delà: les hommes, la mort et la religion dans la région d'Avignon à la fin du Moyen Âge (~1320-~1480)* (Paris: Albin Michel, 2011).

55 Lucius Ferraris and Jacques-Paul Migne, *Prompta bibliotheca, canonica, juridica, moralis, theologica, nec non ascetica, polemica, rubricistica, historica* (Paris: J. P. Migne, 1861), 54. Edited in Emil Von Ottenthal, ed., *Regulae cancellariae apostolicae. Die päpstlichen Kanzleiregeln von Johannes XXII bis Nikolaus V* (Aalen: Scientia-Verlag, 1968).

56 The medieval chronicler of the popes Pierre d'Herenthals, prior of Floreffe, states that 100,000 impetrants (mostly poor clerics) went to Rome following the request of Clement VI. See Étienne Baluze and G Mollat, eds., *Vitae Paparum Avenionensium, hoc est, Historia Pontificium Romanorum qui in Gallia sederunt ab anno Christi 1305 usque ad annum 1394* (Paris: Letouzey, 1921), 298.

57 RV 155, f. 263 R—Clement VI to Bernardus de Taxio, monk of the Cistercian monastery of Fontfroide, 28 April 1343. Inedited text:

> *Cum itaque tu qui sicut asseris felicis recordationis Benedicti pape XII, predecessoris nostri serviciis priusque in summum pontificem promotus existeret duodecim annis et amplius institisti continue infirmitate podagrica et artetica te asseras laborare, nos tuis supplicationibus inclinati ut si de consilio id processerit medicorum super quo tuam et ipsorum conscientias oneramus diebus illis*

et temporibus quibus alter de iure vel consuetudine non est esus carnium secularibus communiter interdictus licite carnibus vesci possis ordinis Cisterciensis.

58 Angela Montford, "Fit to Preach and Pray: Considerations of Occupational Health in the Mendicant Orders," in *The Use and Abuse of Time in Christian History*, ed. R. N. Swanson (Woodbridge: Boydell & Brewer, 2002), 95–106.

59 M. K. K. Yearl, "Medieval Monastic Customaries on Minuti and Infirmi," in *The Medieval Hospital and Medical Practice*, ed. Barbara S. Bowers (Aldershot: Ashgate, 2007), 175–94.

60 RV 18, f. 21 V—Gregory IX, statutes for the monks and nuns of the black order (Cistercians), 1235. Text edited by Lucien Auvray et al., eds., *Les registres de Grégoire IX: recueil des bulles de ce pape* (Paris: Albert Fontemoing, 1896), n° 3 045 A. See statute 18 on food in the infirmary: "Regarding the infirmary, no one can eat meat, except monks or lay brothers who are sick (*infirmus*) and have been sent to the infirmary because of the weakness (*debilitas*) of their body". Statute 19 gives them the right to eat meat elsewhere if they are ill; Statute 21 returns to the care of the sick and the monks.

61 See, for example, Ellsworth T. Rundlett III, *Maximizing Damages in Small Personal Injury Cases*, 22nd ed. (Costa Mesa: James Publishing, 2021).

62 Geoffrey Barraclough, *Public Notaries and the Papal Curia; A Calendar and a Study of a Formularium Notariorum Curie From the Early Years of the Fourteenth Century* (London: Macmillan and Co., 1934), 9.

63 Benoît Grévin, *Rhétorique du pouvoir médiéval: les lettres de Pierre de la Vigne et la formation du langage politique européen (xiiie-xve siècles)* (Rome: École française de Rome, 2013), 21.

64 Patrick N. R. Zutshi, "The Office of Notary in the Papal Chancery in the Mid-fourteenth Century," in *Forschungen zur Reichs-, Papst- und Landesgeschichte*, eds. Enno Bünz, Karl Borchhardt and Peter Herd (Stuttgart: Hiersemann, 1998), vol. 2, 665–83.

65 Henry C. Lea, *A Formulary of the Papal Penitentiary in the Thirteenth Century* (Philadelphia: Lea, 1892), 147, n° 152:

> *Monachi vestri latoris presentium relatio continebat quod cum ipse olim epileptico morbo quem incurrit in ordine laboraret ac physicus vestri ordinis accessit [et] exhibere consilium denegaret, idem monachus monasterium vestrum egressus, et usus consilio medicorum sensit aliquid mitigationis in morbo et spem remedii ad medelam. Verum cum ad ordinem vestrum redire metuat ne sicut medici persuadent propter vigiliarum immoderantiam et aliorum asperitatum ordinis remedium [reincidentiam] et capitis exinanitionem incurrat, supplicavit super hoc sedis apostolice providentia subveniri. Nos igitur auctoritate etc. quatenus si est ita temperetis rigorem vestri [ordinis] circa ipsum vel indulgeatis licentiam laxioris prout eius saluti expedire videritis et temperantiam decuerit regularem.*

66 Jacques Verger, "Que peut-on attendre d'un traitement automatique des suppliques?" *Publications de l'École française de Rome* 31-1 (1977): 73–78.

67 Darricau-Lugat, "Regards sur la profession médicale."

68 RS40, f.53V—Fulconus Ruffus de Calabria to Urban V, 27 August 1363. Text analyzed by Hayez et al., *Urbain V: suppliques de 1362 à 1365*, n° 395:

> *Item quatenus Fulconi Ruffus de Calabria, militi comiti Synopolis genero suo, homino satis delicato, qui propter esum ciborum quadragesimalium de facili*

incurrit varias invalitudines minantes sibi graves infirmitates et periculum persone, concedere dignemini in quadragesima esus carnium et aliorum trahunt sementinam carnis originem, remitto conscientie expertorum medicorum Deum timentium.

69 RA155, f.463V—Urban V to Fulconus Ruffus, 27 August 1363. Text analyzed by Avril et al., *Urbain V (1362–1370)*, n° 6 482:

> . . . *Ut eo Sedi apostolice te devocionem exhibeas quo te noveris amplius illius gracie ubertate foveri tibi qui sicut asseris debilis complexionis existis,* . . . *carnibus et lactis vesci possis de consilio dicti confessoris et medicorum expertorum.*

70 J. Ziegler, "Practitioners and Saints: Medical Men in Canonization Processes in the Thirteenth to Fifteenth Centuries," *Social History of Medicine* 12–2 (1999): 191–225.

71 RS 27, f. 199 R—Peter of Lusignan, Count of Tripoli, first son of the king of Cyprus, to Innocent VI, August 3, 1354. Inedited text: ". . . *Si iudico medicorum videatur quod non possit adimplere votum sine notabiliter corporum laesionum commutetur et dispensetur per episcopum Paphensis.*"

72 Didier Lett, "*Judicium Medicine* and *Judicium Sanctitatis*. Medical Doctors in the Canonization Process of Nicholas of Tolentino (1325): Experts Subject to the Inquisitorial Logic," in *Church and Belief in the Middle Ages. Popes, Saints, and Crusaders*, eds. Kirsi Salonen and Sari Katajala-Peltomaa (Amsterdam: Amsterdam University Press, 2016), 153–70.

73 Sally Crumplin, "Modernizing St Cuthbert: Reginald of Durham's Miracles Collection," in *Signs, Wonders, Miracles. Representations of Divine Power in the Life of the Church* (Woodbridge: Boydell, 2005), 179–91.

74 Jenni Kuuliala, *Childhood Disability and Social Integration in the Middle Ages: Constructions of Impairments in Thirteenth and Fourteenth-Century Canonization Processes* (Turnhout: Brepols, 2016), 198.

75 Rachel Koopmans, *Wonderful to Relate: Miracle Stories and Miracle Collecting in High Medieval England* (Philadelphia: University of Pennsylvania Press, 2011), 183.

76 Joël Chandelier and Marilyn Nicoud, "Les médecins en justice (Bologne, xiiie-xive siècles)," in *Experts et expertise au Moyen Âge. « Consilium quaeritur a perito »* (Paris: Publications de la Sorbonne, 2012), 149–60.

77 Ninon Dubourg, "Clerical Leprosy and the Ecclesiastical Office: Dis/Ability and Canon Law," in *New Approaches to Disease, Disability, and Medicine in Medieval Europe*, eds. Erin Connelly and Stefanie Künzel (Oxford: Archaeopress, 2018), 62–77.

78 RV 11, f. 237 V—Honorius III to Gervasius, bishop of Séez, to the major archdeacon of Reims and to the deacon of Amiens, May 16, 1222. Text analysed by Pietro Pressutti, ed., *I regesti del pontefice Onorio III dall'anno 1216 all'anno 1227* (Rome: Tipogr. A. Befani, 1884), n° 3951.

79 RS40, f.95R—Joan of Kent, princess of Aquitaine—Wales, to Urban V, 30 August 1363. Text analysed by Hayez et al., *Urbain V: suppliques de 1362 à 1365*, n° 761:

> Item [rotulus domine johannie principisse aquitanie et wallie], quatenus nobilis mulier Margeria de mere, domicella dicte principisse, que nunquam pisces

commedere potuit, nec pro tempore quadragesimali lacticiniis et ovis uti pos-
sit ut in forma, fiat de consilio medicorum et ubi alter per potagia non possit
secundum eorum judicium satisfieri ejus debilitati.

80 Agostino Paravicini Bagliani, *Medicina e scienze della natura alla corte dei papi*
nel Duecento (Spoleto: Centro italiano di studi sull'alto Medioevo, 1991), 214.

81 Ninon Dubourg, "*Deo iudicio percusset* - l'idée de contamination d'après les
suppliques et les lettres pontificales," in *Alter-habilitas. Perception of Disability*
Among People, Towards the Creation of an International Network of Studies,
ed. Sylvia Cararo (Vérone: Alteritas, 2018), 89–114. A list of medical books
is given by the Clement V's chancery on the 8 September 1309 (see RV 57, f.
269, text edited by Benedictine Monks, *Registres de Clément V* (Paris: E. de
Boccard, 1948), n° 6 273.

82 RV 145, f. 143 V—Clement VI to Peter, king of Aragon, 18 December 1351.
Inedited text.

83 RV 117, f. 302 V—John XXII to Robert Albaron, lord of Monfrin, 6 April 1334,
text edited by de Loye et al., *Les registres d'Alexandre IV*, n° 5 458.

84 RV 116, f. 207—John XXII to Bernard de Cannassio, 30 August 1332. Text
analyzed by Auguste Coulon and Suzanne Clemencet, eds., *Lettres secrètes et*
curiales du pape Jean XXII (1316–1334) relatives à la France (Paris: Boccard,
1961), n° 3 939:

Quia te, fili, ab infirmitate corporali qua gravaris visitante Domino cupimus
liberari, ecce dilectum filium magistrum B[ernardum] de Cannassio, archidi-
aconum Lomberiensem in ecclesia Albiensi, phisicum nostrum qui tibi consolationis et adjutor ministerium juxta datam sibi a Deo experientiam exhibeat
tibi providimus destinandum, nobilitatem tuam in Domino attencius exhor-
tantes quatinus in Deo qui tocius consolationis est auctor spem figens et ei qui
te visitare misericorditer dignatus est gratiarum referens in humilitate spiritus
actiones, prefatum phisicum tue salutis specialem utique zelatorem placide sus-
cipias, ejusque salubribus consiliis que pro tui salute corporis suffragante sibi
divina gratia tibi dederit et ministraverit acquiescas.

85 Agostino Paravicini Bagliani, *Medicina e scienze della natura alla corte dei papi*
nel Duecento (Spoleto: Centro italiano di studi sull'alto Medioevo, 1991), 214.

86 Agostino Paravicini Bagliani, *La cour des papes au xiiie siècle* (Paris: Hachette,
1995), 204.

87 Danielle Jacquart, *Le milieu médical en France du xiie au xve siècle* (Genève:
Droz, 1981), 99.

88 Arnold Esch, "Medicina del tardo Medioevo. Testimonianze di pazienti e
medici nelle suppliche della Penitenzieria Apostolica," *Bullettino dell'Istituto*
storico italiano per il medio evo 119 (2017): 375–404.

Reference list

Edited Primary Sources

Aquinas, Thomas. *Disputed Questions.* Translated by Urban Hannon for The
Aquinas Institute. January 10, 2022. https://aquinas.cc/.

———. *Summa Theologiae I-II*, q. 77, article 3, "Whether a Sin Committed Through Passion Should Be Called a Sin of Weakness?" Translated by Laurence Shapcote for The Aquinas Institute. December 31, 2021. https://aquinas.cc/.

Auvray, Lucien, et al., eds. *Les registres de Grégoire IX: recueil des bulles de ce pape*. Paris: Albert Fontemoing, 1896.

Avril, François, et al., eds. *Urbain V (1362–1370): lettres communes analysées d'après les registres dits d'Avignon et du Vatican*. Paris: BEFRA, 1954.

Baluze, Étienne, and G. Mollat, eds. *Vitae Paparum Avenionensium, hoc est, Historia Pontificium Romanorum qui in Gallia sederunt ab anno Christi 1305 usque ad annum 1394*. Paris: Letouzey, 1921

Barbiche, Bernard, ed. *Les actes pontificaux originaux des archives nationales de Paris 1, 1198–1261*. Vatican: Biblioteca Apostolica Vaticana, 1975.

The Benedictine Monks. *Registres de Clément V*. Paris: E. de Boccard, 1948.

Coulon, Auguste, and Suzanne Clemencet, eds. *Lettres secrètes et curiales du pape Jean XXII (1316–1334) relatives à la France*. Paris: Boccard, 1961.

de Loye, Joseph, Pierre de Cenival, Auguste Coulon, and Charles de La Roncière, eds. *Les registres d'Alexandre IV: recueil des bulles de ce pape*. Paris: Boccard, 1953.

Ferraris, Lucius, and Jacques-Paul Migne. *Prompta bibliotheca, canonica, juridica, moralis, theologica, nec non ascetica, polemica, rubricistica, historica* (org. Paris: J.P. Migne, 1861). Edited by Emil Von Ottenthal, in *Regulae cancellariae apostolicae. Die päpstlichen Kanzleiregeln von Johannes XXII bis Nikolaus V.* Aalen: Scientia-Verlag, 1968.

Gratiani, *Decretum Gratiani*, in *Corpus Iuris Canonici I*. Edited by Emil Friedberg (Liepzig, 1878; reprint Styria: Graz, 1956). Online with Bayerische Staatsbibliothek, Munich. https://geschichte.digitale-sammlungen.de/decretum-gratiani/online/angebot.

Hardouin. *Conciliorum Collectio Regia Maxima: Act Conciliorum*, 12 vols. Paris: Ex Typographia Regia, 1714–15.

Hayez, Anne-Marie, Janine Mathieu, and Marie-France Yvan, eds. *Urbain V: suppliques de 1362 à 1365 (années I à IV)*. Turnhout: Brepols, 1978.

Henry of Segusio, *Summa Aurea*. Venice: Bernardo Giunta, 1570, 1.20.

Lea, Henry C. *A Formulary of the Papal Penitentiary in the Thirteenth Century*. Philadelphia: Lea, 1892.

Pressutti, Pietro, ed. *I regesti del pontefice Onorio III dall'anno 1216 all'anno 1227*. Rome: Tipogr. A. Befani, 1884.

Verheijen, Luc, ed. *La Règle de saint Augustin*. Paris: Études augustiniennes, 1967.

Secondary sources

Amundsen, Darrel W., and Gary B. Ferngren. "The Forensic Role of Physicians in Ptolemaic and Roman Egypt." *Bulletin of the History of Medicine* 52–53 (Fall 1978): 336–53.

Barnes, Colin. "A Legacy of Oppression: A History of Disability in Western Culture." In *Disability Studies: Past, Present and Future*, edited by Len Barton and Michael Oliver, 3–24. Leeds: Disability Press, 1997.

Barraclough, Geoffrey. *Public Notaries and the Papal Curia; A Calendar and a Study of a Formularium Notariorum Curie From the Early Years of the Fourteenth Century.* London: Macmillan and Co., 1934.

Brandli Fabrice, et al. *Les corps meurtris. Investigations judiciaires et expertises médico-légales au xviiie siècle.* Rennes: Presses Universitaires de Rennes, 2014.

Bruce, Christopher J., Kelly A. Rathje, and Laura J. Weir. *Assessment of Personal Injury Damages.* 6th ed. Toronto: LexisNexis Canada, 2019.

Butler, Sarah M. *Forensic Medicine and Death Investigation in Medieval England.* New York: Routledge, 2016.

Carmichael, Ann G. "The Legal Foundations of Post-Mortem Diagnosis in Later Medieval Milan." In *Death and Disease in the Medieval and Early Modern World: Perspectives From Across the Mediterranean and Beyond*, edited by Lori Jones and Nükhet Varlık. York: York Medieval Press, 2022.

Carraway-Vitiello, Joanna. "Forensic Evidence, Lay Witnesses and Medical Expertise in the Criminal Courts of Late Medieval Italy." In *Medicine and the Law in the Middle Ages*, edited by Wendy J. Turner and Sarah M. Butler, 133–56. Leiden: Brill, 2014.

Ceccarelli, Giovanni. *Il gioco e il peccato. Economia e rischio nel tardo Medioevo.* Bologna: Il Mulino, 2003.

Chandelier, Joël, and Marilyn Nicoud. "Les médecins en justice (Bologne, xiiie-xive siècles)." In *Experts et expertise au Moyen Âge. "Consilium quaeritur a perito"*, 149–60. Paris: Publications de la Sorbonne, 2012.

Chiffoleau, Jacques. *La Comptabilité de l'au-delà: les hommes, la mort et la religion dans la région d'Avignon à la fin du Moyen Âge (~1320-~1480).* Paris: Albin Michel, 2011.

Collard, Franck. "*Secundum artem et peritiam medicine*. Les expertises dans les affaires d'empoisonnement à la fin du Moyen Âge." In *Expertises et conseils au Moyen Âge*, 161–73. Paris: Pub. de la Sorbonne, 2012.

Collard, Franck, and Evelyne Samama, eds. *Handicaps et sociétés dans l'histoire.* Condé sur Noireau: L'Harmattan, 2010.

Crislip, Andrew T. *From Monastery to Hospital: Christian Monasticism and the Transformation of Health Care in Late Antiquity.* Ann Arbor: University of Michigan Press, 2008.

Crumplin, Sally. "Modernizing St Cuthbert: Reginald of Durham's Miracles Collection." In *Signs, Wonders, Miracles. Representations of Divine Power in the Life of the Church*, 179–91. Woodbridge: Boydell, 2005.

Darricau-Lugat, Caroline. "Regards sur la profession médicale en France médiévale (xiie-xve)." In *Cahiers de recherches médiévales et humanistes*, vol. 6. Vulgariser la science: les encyclopédies médiévales, 1999. https://journals.openedition.org/crm/939.

Delattre, Valérie, ed. *Décrypter la différence.* Paris: CQFD, 2009.

Dubourg, Ninon. "Clerical Leprosy and the Ecclesiastical Office: Dis/Ability and Canon Law." In *New Approaches to Disease, Disability, and Medicine in Medieval Europe*, edited by Erin Connelly and Stefanie Künzel, 62–77. Oxford: Archaeopress, 2018.

———. "*Deo iudicio percusset* - l'idée de contamination d'après les suppliques et les lettres pontificales." In *Alter-habilitas. Perception of Disability Among*

People, Towards the Creation of an International Network of Studies, edited by Sylvia Cararo, 89–114. Vérone: Alteritas, 2018.

———. "L'incapacité dans les lettres de dispenses pontificales: aller à l'encontre de la réglementation ecclésiastique médiévale pour franchir la clôture." In *L'exception et la Règle, les pratiques d'entrée et de sortie des couvents, de la fin du Moyen Âge au XIXᵉ siècle*, edited by Albrecht Burkardt and Alexandra Roger, 41–54. Rennes: Presse universitaire de Rennes, 2022.

Esch, Arnold. "Medicina del tardo Medioevo. Testimonianze di pazienti e medici nelle suppliche della Penitenzieria Apostolica." *Bullettino dell'Istituto storico italiano per il medio evo* 119 (2017): 375–404.

Eyler, Joshua, ed. *Disability in the Middle Ages: Reconsiderations and Reverberations*. Farnham: Ashgate, 2010.

Farragud, Carmel. "Expert Examination of Wounds in the Criminal Court of Justice in Cocentaina (Kingdom of Valencia) During the Late Middle Ages.". In *Medicine and the Law in the Middle Ages*, edited by Wendy J. Turner and Sarah M. Butler, 109–32. Leiden: Brill, 2014.

Freedman, Paul. "Food Histories of the Middle Ages.". In *Writing Food History: A Global Perspective*, edited by Kyri W. Claflin and Peter Scholliers, 24–37. London: Berg, 2012.

Getz, Faye M. *Healing and Society in Medieval England: A Middle English Translation of the Pharmaceutical Writings of Gilbertus Anglicus*. Madison: University of Wisconsin Press, 1991.

Gil-Sostres, Pedro. "Les régimes de santé." In *Histoire de la pensée médicale en occident. 1, Antiquité et Moyen Âge*, edited by Mirko D. Grmek, 257–82. Paris: Édition du Seuil, 1995.

Goetz, Hans-Werner. "'Debilis'. Vorstellungen von menschlicher Gebrechlichkeit im frühen Mittelalter." In *Homo debilis: Behinderte, Kranke, Versehrte in der Gesellschaft des Mittelalters*, edited by Cordula Nolte, 21–56. Korb: Didymos-Verlag, 2009.

Grévin, Benoît. *Rhétorique du pouvoir médiéval: les lettres de Pierre de la Vigne et la formation du langage politique européen (xiiiᵉ-xvᵉ siècles)*. Rome: École française de Rome, 2013.

Hacking, Ian. *The Social Construction of What?* Cambridge: Harvard University Press, 1999.

Jacquart, Danielle. "The Introduction of Arabic Medicine into the West. The Question of Etiology." In *Health, Disease and Healing in Medieval Culture*, edited by Sheila D. Campbell, 186–95, vol. III. Basingstoke: Macmillan, 1997.

———. *Le milieu médical en France du xiiᵉ au xvᵉ siècle*. Genève: Droz, 1981.

Jamme, Armand. "Écrire pour le pape du xiᵉ au xivᵉ siècle. Formes et problems." *Mélanges de l'École française de Rome—Moyen Âge* 128-1 (2016). https://journals.openedition.org/mefrm/3121.

Koopmans, Rachel. *Wonderful to Relate: Miracle Stories and Miracle Collecting in High Medieval England*. Philadelphia: University of Pennsylvania Press, 2011.

Kuuliala, Jenni. *Childhood Disability and Social Integration in the Middle Ages: Constructions of Impairments in Thirteenth and Fourteenth-Century Canonization Processes*. Turnhout: Brepols, 2016.

Le Goff, Jacques. "1274, année charnière: mutations et continuités." In *Actes du colloque international du Centre national de la recherche scientifique*, 481–89. Paris:

Édition du CNRS, 1977. Re-edited and published in Jacques Le Goff, *Pour un autre Moyen Âge: temps, travail et culture en Occident: 18 essais*. Paris: Gallimard, 2013.

Lett, Didier. *"Judicium Medicine and Judicium Sanctitatis*. Medical Doctors in the Canonization Process of Nicholas of Tolentino (1325): Experts Subject to the Inquisitorial Logic." In *Church and Belief in the Middle Ages. Popes, Saints, and Crusaders*, edited by Kirsi Salonen and Sari Katajala-Peltomaa, 153–70. Amsterdam: Amsterdam University Press, 2016.

Lisi, Oliver. *The Body Legal in Barbarian Law*. Toronto: University of Toronto Press, 2011.

Mazel, Florian. *La noblesse et l'Église en Provence, fin x^e-début xive siècle*. Paris: Comité des travaux historiques et scientifiques—CTHS, 2002.

Mellyn, Elizabeth W. *Mad Tuscans and Their Families: A History of Mental Disorder in Early Modern Italy*. Philadelphia: University of Pennsylvania Press, 2014.

Metzler, Irina. *Disability in Medieval Europe: Thinking About Physical Impairment During the High Middle Ages, c. 1100–1400*. London: Routledge, 2006.

———. *Fools and Idiots? Intellectual Disability in the Middle Ages*. Manchester: Manchester University Press, 2016.

———. *A Social History of Disability in the Middle Ages: Cultural Considerations of Physical Impairment*. London: Routledge, 2013.

Montford, Angela. "Fit to Preach and Pray: Considerations of Occupational Health in the Mendicant Orders." In *The Use and Abuse of Time in Christian History*, edited by R. N. Swanson, 95–106. Woodbridge: Boydell & Brewer, 2002.

Morley, Neville. *Theories, Models, and Concepts in Ancient History*. London: Routledge, 2004.

Naveau, Anne-Marie. "Quelques réflexions concernant le nouveau rôle du médecin-expert en droit commun." In *Justice et dommage corporel: Panorama du handicap au travers des divers systèmes d'aide et de reparation*, edited by Jean-Pol Beauthier. Bruxelles: Larcier, 2011.

Nicoud, Marilyn. *Le prince et le médecin. Pensée et pratiques médicales à Milan (1402–1476)*. Rome: École française de Rome, 2014.

———. *Les régimes de santé au Moyen Âge: naissance et diffusion d'une écriture médicale, xiiie-xve siècle*. Rome: École française de Rome, 2007.

Nolte, Cordula, ed. *Homo debilis: Behinderte, Kranke, Versehrte in der Gesellschaft des Mittelalters*. Korb: Didymos-Verlag, 2009.

Oliver, Michael. "A New Model of the Social Work Role in Relation to Disability.". In *The Handicapped Person: A New Perspective for Social Workers?* edited by Jo Campling, 19–32. London: RADAR, 1981.

O'Neill, Ynez V. "Innocent III and the Evolution of Anatomy." *Medical History* 20, no. 4 (1976): 429–33.

Ostinelli, Paolo. "I chierici e il *"defectus corporis"*: Definizioni canonistiche, suppliche, dispense." In *Deformità fisica e identità della persona tra medioevo ed età moderna*, edited by Gian Maria Varanini, 3–30. Firenze: University of Firenze, 2015.

Paravicini Bagliani, Agostino. *La cour des papes au xiiie siècle*. Paris: Hachette, 1995.

———. *Medicina e scienze della natura alla corte dei papi nel Duecento*. Spoleto: Centro italiano di studi sull'alto Medioevo, 1991.

Parlopiano, Brandon. "*Propter deformitatem*: Towards a Concept of Disability in Medieval Canon Law." *Canadian Journal of Disability Studies* 4, no. 3 (2015): 72-102.

Pfau, Sasha. *Medieval Communities and the Mad: Narratives of Crime and Mental Illness in Late Medieval France*. Amsterdam: Amsterdam University Press, 2020.

Picot, Johan. " 'La Purge': une expertise juridicomédicale de la lèpre en Auvergne au Moyen Âge." *Revue historique* 66, no. 22 (2012): 292–321.

Riha, Ortrun. "Chronisch Kranke in der medizinischen Fachliteratur des Mittelalters. Eine Suche nach der Patientenperspektive." In *Homo debilis: Behinderte, Kranke, Versehrte in der Gesellschaft des Mittelalters*, edited by Cordula Nolte, 99–120. Korb: Didymos-Verlag, 2009.

Robert, Aurélien. "Contagion morale et transmission des maladies: histoire d'un chiasme (xiiie-xixe siècle)." *Tracés. Revue de Sciences humaines* 21 (2011): 41–60.

Rundlett III, Ellsworth T. *Maximizing Damages in Small Personal Injury Cases*. 22nd ed. Costa Mesa: James Publications, 2021.

Shatzmiller, Joseph. *Médecine et justice en Provence médiévale, Documents de Manosque, 1262–1348*. Aix-en-Provence: Publications de l'Université de Provence, 1989.

Snyder, Sharon L., and David T. Mitchell. *Cultural Locations of Disability*. Chicago: University of Chicago Press, 2006.

Stiker, Henri Jacques. *Corps infirmes et sociétés: Essais d'anthropologie historique*. 3rd ed. Paris: Aubier, 1982.

Ternon, Maud. *Juger les fous au Moyen Âge: dans les tribunaux royaux en France xiv^{e}xve siècles*. Paris: Presses universitaires de France, 2018.

Touati, François-Olivier. *Maladie et société au Moyen Âge: la lèpre, les lépreux et les léproseries dans la province ecclésiastique de Sens jusqu'au milieu du xive siècle*. Bruxelles: De Boeck, 1998.

Turner, Wendy J. *Care and Custody of the Mentally Ill, Incompetent, and Disabled in Medieval England*. Turnhout: Brepols, 2013.

———, ed. *Madness in Medieval Law and Custom*. Leiden: Brill, 2010.

———. "Medieval English Understanding of Mental Illness and Parallel Diagnosis to Contemporary Neuroscience." In *Cognitive sciences and medieval studies: An introduction*, edited by Juliana Dresvina and Victoria Blud. Cardiff: University of Wales Press, 2020.

———. "Models of Disability: Connecting the Past to the Present." *Zeitschrift für Disability Studies* 1 (2022). https://diglib.uibk.ac.at/zds/content/titleinfo/7323860/full.pdf.

Turner, Wendy J., and Tory V. Pearman, eds. *The Treatment of Disabled Persons in Medieval Europe: Examining Disability in the Historical, Legal, Literary, Medical, and Religious Discourses of the Middle Ages*. Lewiston: Edwin Mellen Press, 2010.

Verger, Jacques. "Que peut-on attendre d'un traitement automatique des suppliques?" *Publications de l'École française de Rome* 31, no. 1 (1977): 73-78.

Vigarello, Georges. *Le sain et le malsain: santé et mieux-être depuis le Moyen Âge*. Paris: Éditions du Seuil, 1993.

Whalen, Brett E. *Dominion of God*. Cambridge, MA: Harvard University Press, 2010.

Yearl, M. K. K. "Medieval Monastic Customaries on Minuti and Infirmi", p. 175-194. In *The Medieval Hospital and Medical Practice*, edited by Barbara S. Bowers. Aldershot: Ashgate, 2007.

Ziegler, Joseph. "Practitioners and Saints: Medical Men in Canonization Processes in the Thirteenth to Fifteenth Centuries." *Social History of Medicine* 12, no. 2 (1999): 191-225.

Zutshi, Patrick N. R. "The Office of Notary in the Papal Chancery in the Mid-fourteenth Century." In *Forschungen zur Reichs-, Papst- und Landesgeschichte*, edited by Enno Bünz, Karl Borchhardt and Peter Herd, vol. 2, 665–83. Stuttgart: Hiersemann, 1998.

———. "The Political and Administrative Correspondence of the Avignon Popes, 1305–1378: A Contribution to Papal Diplomatic." In *Aux origines de l'État moderne. Le fonctionnement administratif de la papauté d'Avignon*, 371–84. Rome: École française de Rome, 1991.

10 Compensatory Damages and the Construction of Injury in Prenatal Torts

Luke I. Haqq

This chapter suggests how an arena of civil litigation contributed to creating new incentives for parents and society to construct present and future children as injurious. It specifically focuses on the emergence of actions in which the plaintiffs are parents of a child whose existence they had sought to avoid. The defendants are usually physicians specializing in reproductive care, actors whom plaintiffs allege inhibited their abilities to make fully informed reproductive decisions.

Beyond the Supreme Court's reproductive policy jurisprudence and its impacts on state laws, the emergence of these types of legal claims in the United States reflected broader social changes in the twentieth century like the transition of childbirth from homes to hospitals, growing activism over women's health and equality in education and employment, as well as the development and routinization of prenatal technologies. This litigation also contributed to changes in law, medicine, and society. As healthcare transitioned away from an era of medical paternalism, for example, new forms of liability for malpractice in reproductive and prenatal care helped sift out bad actors from a medical profession that had been slow to do so itself.

In addition, these actions provided venues for plaintiffs to recover for numerous harms they could suffer as a consequence of malpractice in reproductive care. Palpable harms can befall parents when a child is born with a genetic disease, from the costs of accommodations to the obligations of a conservatorship that might require parents to give up personal or professional plans. In many jurisdictions, plaintiffs can also request general damages for pain and suffering, whether for the pain and suffering of pregnancy, labor, and delivery, or for loss of consortium of a spouse or parent.

The nature of these cases, however, has also brought many jurisdictions to permit plaintiffs to seek general damages for the alleged pain and suffering of their child's existence, rather than nonexistence. Other jurisdictions have described these damages as "inherently distasteful",[1] a key reason why this litigation came to be circumscribed in many jurisdictions,

DOI: 10.4324/9781003452324-14

either by judicial decision or by legislative acts. Some jurisdictions only allow requests for these damages if the child is not born healthy, and many deny requests for them altogether.

Where these damages are permitted, these actions provide motivations for parents and their legal counsel to co-construct, create, and imagine their children and future children as injuries. This is not to impugn the character of plaintiffs or lawyers who bring such claims but rather highlights an expressive function of damages in a particular legal context. These cases first emerged as society was reimagining the value or lack thereof of future children. This type of litigation uniquely came to define and reinforce notions of future children as injuries to their parents.

From *Dietrich to Zepeda:* The Common Law of Prenatal Injury

One could trace back to antiquity numerous ways in which parents and societies have constructed future children as pathological or injurious. Medievalists and early modernists, for example, have shown the pervasive influence of beliefs that birth anomalies were divine punishments for the sins of parents or entire communities.[2] Future children could be also constructed as injurious for a variety of reasons even in the absence of congenital disease or anomalies, whether because of the timing of childbirth, such as birth outside of marriage, or because of the child's sex.

For centuries, the law participated in constructing children and future children as injurious in these contexts. Not only were children born outside of wedlock, for example, stigmatized and denied privileges and rights, such a legal and cultural milieu also subject their parents to stigmatization. Still, the law had done little in terms of recognizing the existence of children or future children as injuries for which parents could seek compensation through litigation. Several factors facilitated the common law development of such legal injuries, as plaintiffs raised novel claims in courts. The legal concept of negligence—that is, a neglectful act or omission that reflects a lack of due care—had played a minor role in lawsuits for centuries, but as plaintiffs relied more heavily on it, this shifted attention away from the type of harm done to the plaintiff and placed greater scrutiny of the defendant's acts.[3] This perspective provided a vantage point from which new legal injuries could be created by plaintiffs and recognized by courts.

In addition, many judges became persuaded that it was necessary for courts to recognize certain new injuries in order for the law to keep pace with the times. Legal historian G. Edward White, for example, notes that urbanization brought Americans more frequently into contact with strangers, social and cultural conditions in which people more often stood to be injured by people with whom they had no prior relationship, contractual or otherwise.[4] Negligence doctrine, by focusing on whether a defendant's acts or omissions reflected a lack of due care, provided a legal standard for ascertaining culpability in such situations. Finally, facilitated by the new pedagogical approach of Christopher Columbus Langdell's case method, legal scholars like Oliver Wendell Holmes began to systematize and categorize the numerous and cumbersome types of actions that had built up within the writ system into a contained body of tort law.

A "tort" refers to a wrong or injury. Criminal law deals with wrongs by individuals against the state, and contract law revolves around wrongs judged primarily with reference to what parties agreed to in words or conduct, rather than more generalized conceptions of wrongfulness, as in the case of tort law. The precedent of earlier courts could often provide guidance in how to rule in a given case, but judges also encountered cases of first impression. This situation provided incentives for plaintiffs to perform, for their counsel to convince, a need for persuasion that was especially strong if judges interpreted plaintiffs to be requesting the court to recognize a new cause of action. Among other reasons that courts were reluctant to do so were the separation of powers considerations, that judges ought to leave it to legislatures to recognize or deny new causes of action.

Nevertheless, judges occasionally found it necessary to fashion new forms of legal actions, especially in situations that legislatures had not addressed. One reason that motivated Holmes to do so while serving as a judge on the Massachusetts Supreme Court was an increase in sources of injury from industrialization and urbanization that could affect people prior to birth, coupled with a lack of legal precedent on whether people could recover for such injuries. Holmes proffered what he described as the legal doctrine of "conditional prospective liability" for prenatal injuries; that is, he recognized that a defendant could be liable for injuries inflicted on an unborn individual if that person is then born.[5] This both accommodated the view that legal personhood did not begin in many ways until after birth, while also making it possible to bring personal injury claims for harms that one sustained prior to birth.

Though Holmes and judges in several other states over the early twentieth century were willing to entertain claims alleging prenatal injuries as valid causes of action in theory, in practice all of these cases were dismissed until 1946, when the first federal court found a defendant liable in a prenatal injury claim.[6] Up to that point, courts had either refused to recognize this type of liability in cases of first impression or, like Holmes, recognized it in a case that was ultimately dismissed for lack of standing because the plaintiff had died soon after birth from the prenatal injury. Several states began recognizing the right to sue for prenatal injuries soon after the first federal court did. Tort scholar William Prosser concluded in 1955 that the trend toward recognizing a right to sue for prenatal injuries was "so definite and marked as to leave no doubt that this will be the law of the future in the United States".[7]

Five years later, a state appellate court faced what it understood to be a distinct type of claim for prenatal injury. In all of the precedent on prenatal injuries up to that point, whether arising from sources like a fall, a car accident, or the use of forceps during delivery, the prenatally injured plaintiff still might have existed without the injury. Consequently, it was not difficult to justify allowing damages in these cases with respect to the purposes of tort law and damages—namely, if a defendant is found liable, damages are to make the plaintiff whole. More specifically, wholeness is usually understood in a comparative, counterfactual sense, where damages seek to make plaintiffs as close as possible to the state they were in if the wrongful act had never happened.

In *Zepeda v. Zepeda* (1960), a court was faced with a plaintiff alleging that he was prenatally injured by being conceived out of wedlock. Among other harms he alleged that these conditions of his conception caused him, the plaintiff claimed that he had been deprived of a "normal home", including a "natural right to be wanted, loved and cared for".[8] The prenatal injury he alleged, therefore, was one that he would not have existed without; his parents might have changed their circumstances and married each other, but any child in this counterfactual situation would not be the plaintiff but rather an entirely different person. In this alternative, the plaintiff would never have existed. It was thus not immediately clear that tort law offered a route for seeking compensation for this particular type of allegation, since there was no comparative reference other than nonexistence in terms of the position the plaintiff would have been in if it had not been for the defendant's act.

The court found that the case before it "seems to be the natural result of the present course of the law permitting actions for physical injury ever closer to the moment of conception".[9] It provided several hypotheticals in which it seemed intuitive to extend prenatal personal injury law to include situations in which the plaintiff counterfactually would not have existed. The first hypothetical it offered was a child injured after birth by a defective space heater, purchased before the child had been conceived. The court wondered, "Would there not be a right of action against the manufacturer despite the fact the negligence took place before the child was conceived?" It also considered a drug manufacturer that had failed to test a drug adequately for teratogenic risks.

Finally, it noted that "[p]hysicists and geneticists declare that thermonuclear radiation can so affect the reproductive cells of future parents that their offspring may be born with physical and mental defects".[10]

Such hypotheticals provided some support for the court to affirm the "creation of a new tort: a cause of action for wrongful life". And the court provided some legitimation to the specific congenital harm of illegitimacy that the plaintiff alleged, noting that "it would be pure fiction to say that the plaintiff suffers no injury. The lot of a child born out of wedlock, who is not adopted or legitimized, is a hard one".[11] Succinctly put, the court recognized that "[a]n illegitimate's very birth places him under a disability".[12]

At the same time, the law by the time of *Zepeda* had already enacted some reforms to reduce the disabling aspects of illegitimacy. The court took note that "an evolution has been taking place and illegitimate children are now being treated with more consideration".[13] It was not this, however, that the court took to be the major counterbalance to the harms alleged by the plaintiff but rather "[l]ove of life", what it explained was a "natural instinct to preserve life" that would impel the plaintiff "to cherish his existence". This core aspect of the plaintiff's claim was the court's primary motivation for determining that there were "overriding legal, social, judicial or other considerations which should preclude recognition of a cause of action".[14]

The appellate court ultimately affirmed the trial court's dismissal of the complaint. It concluded that the "legal implications of such a tort are vast, the social impact could be staggering".[15] Among other reasons, it feared a floodgate of litigation if it recognized that illegitimate birth in particular was a legally compensable prenatal injury. It did not fully reject the new tort but concluded that "[i]f we are to have a legal action for such a radical concept as wrongful life, it should come after thorough study of the consequences". It saw this task to be best suited for the state's general assembly, reflecting the court's "belief that lawmaking, while inherent in the judicial process, should not be indulged in where the result could be as sweeping as here".[16]

The Emergence of Wrongful Birth and Wrongful Conception

The abilities of plaintiffs to recover any damages, including damages for pain and suffering, in cases of first impression depended on convincing courts of the need to recognize a new action. Even if this hurdle had been overcome, success in recovering damages also often depended on eliciting sympathy for one's alleged injuries, such as from judges and juries. Legal historians have noted, for instance, how it was often easier for courts and legislatures to be sympathetic to injury claims involving women and children, facilitated in part by a greater willingness of women vis-à-vis men as plaintiffs to express their feelings and broader impacts of their injuries in court.[17] This precedent operated as a wedge that opened possibilities of recovery for subsequent plaintiffs.

Sometimes, as in *Zepeda*, courts took recognizing a right of recovery to be consequential enough that they were not willing to do so, leaving it to legislatures to determine public policy and what the law ought to be. When *Zepeda* and a second wrongful life case in the 1960s first raised a new inflection of prenatal injury, birth defects were gaining greater social visibility as problems that the law, science, and medicine could remedy. Among other causes and responses that brought them into attention were the molecular revolution, spikes in births affected by German measles and thalidomide, the Food and Drug Administration's addition of teratogenic effects to its drug-labeling requirements, and reforms in a dozen states following a model law of the American Legal Institute to decriminalize abortion in cases of fetal anomalies.

In the 1960s into the 1970s, the fate of the wrongful life claim remained indeterminate. *Zepeda* had set a precedent indicating concern that the type of harm it alleged failed to reflect an appropriate "love of life". Yet as diagnostic and screening reproductive technologies came to be routinized or otherwise became major factors that shaped reproductive decisions, many courts and legislatures saw public policy as supporting recognition of the birth of children with congenital diseases or anomalies as injuries to parents, rather than as injuries to the children born with such diseases, as would have been the case under the wrongful life claim. Instead, wrongful life came to be banned in nearly every jurisdiction that has entertained it, while two new torts—the actions for wrongful conception and wrongful birth—came to be far more widely accepted. In the United States, nearly every state has recognized wrongful conception and half recognize wrongful birth, though a dozen ban the latter.

The Supreme Court's reproductive rights jurisprudence transformed litigation over congenital injuries. Several parents whose children were born with congenital rubella syndrome (CRS) in the late 1950s into the 1960s filed lawsuits, alleging that they would have avoided the birth of their children if they had known about the risks of transmitting German measles. These lawsuits were the first "wrongful birth" cases, cases in which the plaintiffs are not the children born but rather their parents. More specifically, wrongful birth cases involve parents who claim that they would have aborted if it had not been for the defendant's alleged negligence. Special damages in a wrongful birth claim might cover the same damages that could have been recovered under wrongful life, namely, the costs of accommodations, but general damages under the parental claims were distinct: These compensated parents for their alleged harms because of their child's existence rather than nonexistence.

Early wrongful birth cases like *Gleitman v. Cosgrove* (1967) included wrongful life actions. Thus they built on *Zepeda*'s concept of wrongful life, but rather than alleging illegitimate birth as the congenital injury, the injury was instead CRS, which was imputed to medical malpractice. Key issues to *Gleitman* arose on April 20, 1959, when one of Mrs. Gleitman's physicians "told her that the German measles" that she had contracted earlier in the year "would have no effect at all on her [unborn] child". Mrs. and Mr. Gleitman sought to recover for their own harms in their wrongful birth actions, and they also brought an *ad litem* wrongful life action on behalf of their eight-year-old son with CRS. The New Jersey Supreme Court rejected the wrongful life claim. "This Court cannot weigh the value of life with impairments against the nonexistence of life itself". It reasoned that by "asserting that he should not have been born, the . . . plaintiff makes it logically impossible for a court to measure his alleged damages because of the impossibility of making the comparison required by compensatory remedies". The court therefore concluded that even if the conduct complained of were true, they do "not give rise to damages cognizable at law" for the wrongful life plaintiff.[18]

Turning to the wrongful birth claim, the court took note of Mrs. Gleitman's allegation that "an abortion would have freed her of the emotional problems caused by the raising of a child with birth defects", but it determined that wrongful birth damages also required the court "to evaluate the denial . . . of the intangible, unmeasurable, and complex human benefits of motherhood and fatherhood and weigh these against the alleged emotional and money injuries".[19] It consequently found that the wrongful birth action, much like wrongful life, ultimately sought damages that were "impossible for a court to measure".[20]

The holding of the case was not based only on an objection to the impossibility of damages, however. Rather, the court emphasized a need to avoid awarding damages that failed to reflect an appreciation for the "preciousness" of life. As it explained:

> The sanctity of the single human life is the decisive factor in this suit in tort. It may have been easier for the mother and less expensive for the father to have terminated the life of their child while he was an embryo, but these alleged detriments cannot stand against the preciousness of the single human life to support a remedy in tort.

The majority thus held wrongful birth and wrongful life to be "precluded by the countervailing public policy supporting the preciousness of human life".[21] Years later, after the Supreme Court's landmark decisions on reproductive policy, the New Jersey Supreme Court saw public policy as having changed, motivating it to recognize wrongful birth as well as wrongful life, though only for special damages in the latter action.[22]

Another case reaching a state's supreme court in 1967 overcame comparable concerns with devaluing or failing to appreciate the preciousness of human life. *Custodio v. Bauer* (1967), on the one hand, was similar to

Gleitman in that parents alleged that they were harmed by being denied an opportunity to have prevented their child's existence, but by avoiding conception, rather than relying on abortion; this is what characterized it as an action for "wrongful conception". On the other hand, it was different from *Gleitman* and the first wrongful life cases because the child at issue in *Custodio* was born without congenital injury, yet his parents still alleged that his birth was injurious to them. When such a fact pattern had reached another state's supreme court in the 1930s as a breach-of-contract action against a surgeon over unsuccessful sterilization, the court was dismissive of a plaintiff seeking the costs of raising a child to adulthood in such circumstances. For this earlier court, such damages were odious to public policy.[23] *Custodio*, the first time wrongful conception was brought as a tort, reflected a change in attitudes toward contraception.

The case involved a healthy rather than prenatally injured child, whose parents brought the action because "Mrs. Custodio [alleged] 'that she had more than sufficient children'" and had sought to prevent the existence of the latest child by obtaining a tubal ligation.[24] *Custodio* included seven causes of action. More historically significant than their breach-of-contract claims was their allegation of malpractice based on negligence. Among other damages, the plaintiffs sought $1,500 in medical expenses associated with labor, delivery, prenatal and postnatal care, $250,000 for Mrs. Custodio's emotional distress, and $500,000 in punitive damages.[25] They further sought damages for the harm that they alleged their additional, healthy child brought them. Mrs. Custodio requested $50,000 in damages for the cost of caring for and raising her child to maturity.

Mr. Custodio sought separate special damages of "$50,000 to care for and raise" their child, and general damages on the grounds that his "emotional and nervous system will be affected by said pregnancy and subsequent birth of said child".[26]

In order to establish that the defendant's actions had left them harmed, the plaintiffs needed to conceptualize their complaint "in terms of a child being unwanted and a burden".[27] Among the other burdens they alleged were new strains on "the family exchequer [by] the new arrival [that may] deprive the other members of the family of what was planned as their just share of the family income".[28] The court considered that it might be "repugnant to social ethics with respect to the family establishment" to permit plaintiffs to recover such damages, but it was ultimately more persuaded by "some trend of change in social ethics with respect to the family establishment".[29]

Since the court did not find the novel wrongful conception tort to be contrary to public policy but rather took it to be supported by changing social attitudes, the appellate court reversed the trial court's dismissal of the case. Though it clarified issues of law, the appellate court found that in "the present state of the record", the matters of whether a duty of care had been breached and the scope of damages "cannot be ascertained". If the plaintiffs provided adequate facts to establish liability, the trial court was directed to apply the California Civil Code on tortious conduct, which provided that "[f]or the breach of an obligation not arising from contract, the measure of damages . . . is the amount which will compensate for all the detriment proximately caused thereby, whether it could have been anticipated or not".[30]

The greater willingness of the *Custodio* court to permit the action before it in comparison with *Gleitman* can be explained in part by the latter being an action for wrongful birth. *Gleitman* involved parents would have aborted, whereas *Custodio* involved parents who alleged they never would have conceived their child. But some courts were not persuaded that this difference overcame concerns about the public policy reflected by permitting damages. Another state's supreme court rejected a wrongful conception claim before it in 1975, for example, one involving the birth of a sixth child after unsuccessful sterilization. Not only did parents allege that their healthy child was a harm to them, the case included loss of consortium claims by their other five children as well for being deprived of parental affection. The court determined that "the value of a human life outweighs any 'damage' which might be said to follow from the fact of birth, and recovery on any such thesis would violate both our public policy and the law governing provable damages".[31] The court summarized that, at the time, "[m]ost courts have decided that the addition of a normal child to the family is a gift of great benefit to the recipients, rather than a cause of damage to them".[32] *Custodio* was the exception.

Nevertheless, wrongful birth and wrongful conception claims soon bore the imprimatur of the Supreme Court's reproductive rights jurisprudence. *Dumer v. St. Michael's Hospital* (1975) reflects this impact on state courts. *Gleitman*, brought before *Roe*, was dismissed on public policy grounds, while *Dumer* appeared after that landmark decision and indicated that public policy might be changing. The fact pattern in *Dumer* straddled both sides of *Roe*. The alleged malpractice underlying *Dumer* occurred on March 18, 1972—less than a year before *Roe*—though the case only reached the Wisconsin Supreme Court in 1975. Like *Gleitman*, *Dumer* involved a child affected by CRS and also included wrongful birth and wrongful life actions. Rather than physicians specializing in obstetrics and gynecology, however, Mrs. Dumer had sought treatment for a skin rash with the personnel of an emergency department.[33]

Part of the negligence claim alleged that the nurses and doctors she saw on this visit failed to diagnose that she had contracted German measles.[34]

Mrs. Dumer was one month into pregnancy at this visit, though the complaint did not allege that she had conveyed this to any nurses or doctors at the time.[35] Nevertheless, the complaint further alleged that the doctor and hospital staff were negligent for failing to inquire as to whether she was pregnant, failing to warn her about the risks that she could transmit rubella to a fetus, and failing to provide her information about where she could obtain a lawful abortion in 1972.[36]

The Wisconsin Supreme Court in *Dumer* affirmed the dismissal of claims against the hospital and its staff, explaining that "[n]urses and attendants, under these facts, are not required to make a temporary diagnosis nor advise the patient as to a course of treatment".[37] It also affirmed the dismissal of the child's wrongful life action. Within a year of *Roe*, the court had already heard wrongful life and wrongful birth cases of first impression, but these involved healthy children. One of these, *Slawek v. Stroh* in 1974, was like *Zepeda* in that a plaintiff complained of being "born an adulterine bastard" because of false promises of marriage to her mother, resulting in her "suffer[ing] mental pain and anguish [from] public humiliation and embarrassment".[38] The court raised the impossibility of calculating damages in that case and affirmed this in *Dumer* as its primary reason for finding that the child had not stated a valid cause of action in alleging a wrongful life injury, citing favorably to *Gleitman*.[39]

The second case mentioned by the *Dumer* court, *Rieck v. Medical Protective Co.* (1974), involved the birth of a healthy yet "unwanted addition to the family circle" and was a wrongful birth rather than a wrongful conception action. "What is demanded" in damages, the court explained in *Rieck*, "is that the costs of rearing the child be transferred to the obstetrician, the clinic and their insurer".[40] The Wisconsin Supreme Court rejected such damages as contrary to public policy, especially because the child was healthy.

Unlike *Rieck*, the child in *Dumer* was not healthy but rather born with numerous impairments, including "cataracts and heart malfunctions".[41] The court recognized that her condition required and "will continue to incur additional extensive hospital, medical and supportive expenses".[42] If the facts alleged in the complaint were true, the court concluded that the defendant should be found negligent for failing to diagnose the German measles, failing to ask whether Mrs. Dumer was pregnant, and failing to inform her of risks of transmission to the fetus. However, since there was "no question as to the life or health of the mother", it reasoned that the defendant doctor had no duty to advise her about the availability of abortion. The court noted that this called for "a legal opinion, not a medical one", given that abortion was still criminalized when she had been pregnant.[43]

Constructing Injury in Wrongful Birth and Wrongful Conception Claims

Congenital disease like CRS or births shaped by the teratogenic effects of thalidomide impacted more than only the children born; they also transformed the lives of parents and other family members as well. But many other wrongful conception and wrongful birth cases over the late twentieth century did not involve any congenital pathological conditions but rather children born healthy. To be sure, litigation has also included cases in which there is no diagnosis or specific name for congenital conditions that are still manifestly grave or severe. Other cases have included parents suing for conditions that seem far less pathological, however, such as one involving a child whose parents would have chosen to abort because of the child's missing hand,[44] or another because the child had an alleged "emotional problem".[45]

Even cases involving congenital conditions with known etiologies have provided spaces for constructing children as injuries. As legal historian Leslie Reagan writes in describing an early wrongful birth case arising from CRS:

> Through [their child's] body, the [parents'] attorney invited the jury to feel and imagine parental and child emotions. The use of the person herself may offend—perhaps the child was exploited by her lawyer or by her parents. The display of the disabled child inevitably called upon both voyeuristic "freak shows" and the pity induced by March of Dimes "poster children" and Jerry Lewis's telethons for muscular dystrophy. This conscious display of the disabled body in court violated the rules of politeness that taught people to avoid looking at the . . . disabled by insisting that the jury look. The courtroom was a public space in which the rules of politeness and privacy were broken. Like science and like the freak show, the jury and the courtroom were invited and required to look and to stare. [46]

Reagan captures one way that congenital conditions could be constructed into injuries to parents in courtrooms, namely, as part of the process of persuading a jury that their child's existence brought them overall harm.

But cases like *Custodio* in which the children at issue were born healthy were more directly and necessarily sites at which parents constructed their children into injuries. Whether healthy or not, a child whose existence parents would have avoided can contribute to a range of harms to parents, whether as a source of discord within their relationship or as an impediment to personal plans or goals. Yet many courts and legislatures have been reluctant to permit general damages allocated to these purposes, most often for reasons rooted in what these damages express about the value of existence, future children, and people with disabilities. Over a dozen states outright ban the wrongful birth action for these reasons, and in jurisdictions that do allow the action, most often they do not allow general damages for the purposes of compensating parents for their child's existence rather than nonexistence.

Reluctance to award these damages has been especially strong for wrongful birth actions. Yet courts have also espoused the same sentiments in wrongful conception claims. A court considering the "plaintiffs' claim that the surgeon should be compelled to assume financial responsibility for raising and educating the child", for example, affirmed the lower court's determination "that such damages may not be recovered in a court of law because they proceed on the premise that the life involved is 'wrongful'. [This] was clearly correct . . . as a statement of public policy".[47] Another court that recognized the wrongful conception tort while also limiting damages found that "to rule that a plaintiff may recover the cost of rearing her healthy but unplanned child" seemed to imply "that a child is not worth what it costs to raise it", and was thus "something inherently distasteful" that "is a matter best left to measured legislative action rather than to judicial fiat".[48]

Jurisdictions that do permit parents to seek general damages for their claimed pain and suffering because of their child's existence have often underscored that costs like the expenses of raising a child to adulthood were foreseeable consequences for defendants like sterilization surgeons. Of course, plaintiffs in these cases still carry the burden of demonstrating that they have been injured and are entitled to compensation for it. As one state's supreme court explained in permitting the wrongful conception action, for the plaintiffs to recover any damages:

> requires that the parents demonstrate not only that they did not want the child but that the child has been of minimal value or benefit to them. They will have to show that the child remains an uncherished, an unwanted burden so as to minimize the offset which the defendant is entitled (i.e., an offset to signify the value of the child's existence).[49]

They must construct their child into a problem, into an injury to themselves.

Some jurisdictions, as mentioned, do not allow them the opportunity to do so. A state's supreme court summarized some of the reasons why the "majority of courts of other jurisdictions have held that no damages may be recovered for the costs of rearing and educating a healthy, normal child born as a result of malpractice":

> (1) A parent cannot be said to have been damaged by the birth and rearing of a normal and healthy child. (2) Benefits of joy, companionship, and affection which a healthy child can provide outweigh the costs of rearing that child. (3) The recovery of rearing costs would be a windfall to the parents and an unreasonable burden on the negligent health

care provider, wholly out of proportion to the culpability of the physician. (4) Recovery should be denied to protect the mental and emotional health of the child . . . who will one day learn that he or she not only was not wanted by his or her parents, but was reared by funds supplied by another person. (5) Other reasons include the speculative nature of damages and the possibility of fraudulent claims. . . . Many other reasons for the adoption of the majority rule are stated in the cited cases, but we need not base our opinion upon them. We hold simply that under the public policy of this state, a parent cannot be said to be damaged by the birth of a normal, healthy child, and the parent may not recover damages because of the birth of such a child.[50]

By contrast, courts permitting more extensive recovery in wrongful birth and wrongful conception claims downplay their expressive impact. One court thought that:

[t]he once unwanted child's knowledge that someone other than the parents had been obliged to pay for the cost of rearing him or her may in fact alleviate the child's distress at the knowledge of having been once unwanted.[51]

In another case in which a state's supreme court recognized wrongful birth for the first time, the court assured that "given [the child's] severe cognitive disabilities" in the case before it, "there is nothing in the record to indicate that he will someday understand his parents sued over their lost opportunity to avoid his birth".[52]

In other contexts outside of an adversarial legal process, there may be less of an inherent tendency to disvalue or construct children as injurious. In her book on clinical dysmorphology, for example, sociologist Joanna Latimer underscores how many of the congenital conditions that people now avoid through contraception and abortion were just being discovered at the molecular level as prenatal technologies like amniocentesis were starting to be incorporated into clinical practice. Consequently, many conditions were not just clinical disease entities that were diagnosed by physicians but rather were co-constructed by parents, who often provided physicians with intimate information about their children, reports which then reciprocally informed how physicians understand the pathological aspects of these conditions.[53]

But when placed within an adversarial process, there is an inherent tendency for any plaintiff seeking the largest possible recovery in a wrongful conception or wrongful birth claim to construct children into problems and injuries. How courts and legislatures have responded to wrongful birth and wrongful conception litigation has reflected their understandings of public policy with respect to matters like reproductive rights, the value of unplanned children, and what these lawsuits might convey about the value of people with disabilities. In the United States, by the end of the twentieth century, published awards reached into the millions in general damages allocated solely to pain and suffering because of a child's existence rather than nonexistence. In the twenty-first century, some general damages in these cases have reached eight-figure awards.

The scope of recovery in other countries contrasts sharply with the United States. The vast majority of countries allowing wrongful birth or wrongful conception only permit special damages and potentially limited general damages. For those countries that permit childrearing expenses for healthy children, damages are rarely above five or six figures. In the precedential British case on recovery for childrearing damages for a healthy child after unsuccessful sterilization, for example, the court envisioned using a "conventional figure of £15,000".[54] More recently, a court in India spent considerable time deliberating over whether the plaintiff's request of 75,000 rupees for childrearing expenses after a negligently performed tubal ligation was excessive.[55] This was not a request for millions, but rather just over a thousand dollars.

Conclusion

This chapter has highlighted reasons why the actions for wrongful conception and wrongful birth provide incentives for parents to construct their children into legal injuries. These actions gained traction as social and legal attitudes toward unplanned or unanticipated children were undergoing thorough transformations. Their availability has created spaces in which plaintiffs seeking the fullest damages are thereby incentivized to devalue their children, to construct them into burdens and injuries, as impediments to their personal plans, relationships, or careers. This domain of litigation largely reached settled law in most states as each reflected its own public policy after *Roe*, but with *Dobbs v. Jackson* (2022), many states are revisiting the extent to which children and future children have been imagined and created as injuries.

Notes

1 Flowers v. D.C., 478 A.2d 1073, 1076 (D.C. 1984).
2 Mary Fissell, *Vernacular Bodies: The Politics of Reproduction in Early Modern England* (New York: Oxford University Press, 2007); Marie-Hélène Huet, *Monstrous Imaginations* (Cambridge, MA: Harvard University Press, 1993).
3 J. H. Baker, *An Introduction to English Legal History*, 3rd ed. (London: Butterworths, 1990), 455.
4 G. Edward White, *Tort Law in America: An Intellectual History* (New York: Oxford University Press, 1980), 16.
5 Dietrich v. Inhabitants of Northampton, 138 Mass. 14, 16 (Mass. 1884).
6 Bonbrest v. Kotz, 65 F. Supp. 138 (D.D.C. 1946).
7 William Prosser, *Handbook of the Law of Torts*, 2nd ed. (St. Paul: West Publishing, 1955), § 36.

8 Zepeda v. Zepeda, 41 Ill.App.2d 240, 249 (Ill. Ct. App. 1963).
9 *Zepeda*, 41 Ill.App.2d at 249.
10 *Zepeda*, 41 Ill.App.2d at 250.
11 *Zepeda*, 41 Ill.App.2d at 259.
12 *Zepeda*, 41 Ill.App.2d at 258.
13 *Zepeda*, 41 Ill.App.2d at 255.
14 *Zepeda*, 41 Ill.App.2d at 258.
15 *Zepeda*, 41 Ill.App.2d at 259.
16 *Zepeda*, 41 Ill.App.2d at 262.
17 Nancy Woloch, *Muller v. Oregon: A Brief History with Documents* (Boston: Bedford, 1996), 3; Barbara Welke, *Recasting American Liberty: Gender, Race, Law, and the Railroad Revolution, 1865–1920* (New York: Cambridge University Press, 2001), 171–202.
18 Gleitman v. Cosgrove, 227 A.2d 689, 692 (N.J. 1967).
19 *Gleitman*, 227 A.2d at 693.
20 *Gleitman*, 227 A.2d at 692.
21 Ibid (citations omitted).
22 Procanik v. Cillo, 478 A.2d 755 (N.J. 1984); Schroeder v. Perkel, 432 A.2d 834 (N.J. 1981).
23 Christensen v. Thornby, 255 N.W. 620 (Minn. 1934).
24 Custodio v. Bauer, 251 Cal.App.2d 303, 307 (Cal. Ct. App. 1967).
25 *Custodio*, 251 Cal.App.2d at 308–9.
26 *Custodio*, 251 Cal.App.2d at 309.
27 *Custodio*, 251 Cal.App.2d at 324.
28 *Custodio*, 251 Cal.App.2d at 323.
29 *Custodio*, 251 Cal.App.2d at 325.
30 *Custodio*, 251 Cal.App.2d at 326.
31 *Custodio*, 251 Cal.App.2d at 326–27.
32 Coleman v. Garrison, 327 A.2d 757, 771 (Del. Super. Ct. 1974).
33 Dumer v. St. Michael's Hospital, 233 N.W.2d 372, 373 (Wisc. 1975).
34 *Dumer*, 233 N.W.2d at 374.
35 *Dumer*, 233 N.W.2d at 373.
36 *Dumer*, 233 N.W.2d at 374.
37 Ibid.
38 Slawek v. Stroh, 215 N.W.2d 9, 32 (Wisc. 1974).
39 *Dumer*, 233 N.W.2d at 376.
40 Rieck v. Medical Protective Co., 219 N.W.2d 242, 245 (Wisc. 1974).
41 *Dumer*, 233 N.W.2d at 373–74.
42 *Dumer*, 233 N.W.2d at 376.
43 *Dumer*, 233 N.W.2d at 377.
44 Charlie Schwalm, Sarah Pierce and Tyler Schwalm v. Janna Doherty, Jury Verdicts LEXIS n.p. (Cal. Super. Ct. 2013).
45 Stellhorn v. Victory Medical Group, Jury Verdicts LEXIS n.p. (Cal. Super. Ct. 1990).
46 Leslie J. Reagan, "Rashes, Rights, and Wrongs in the Hospital and in the Courtroom: German Measles, Abortion, and Malpractice Before *Roe* and *Doe*," *Law and History Review* 27, no. 2 (2009): 267.
47 Coleman v. Garrison, 349 A.2d 8, 12–13 (Del. 1975).
48 Flowers v. D.C., 478 A.2d 1073, 1076–78 (D.C. 1984).
49 Cockrum v. Baumgartner, 447 N.E.2d 385, 393–94 (Ill. 1983).
50 Byrd v. Wesley Medical Center, 699 P.2d 459, 465–70 (Kan. 1985).
51 Burke v. Rivo, 551 N.E.2d 1, 8–9 (Mass. 1990).
52 Plowman v. Fort Madison Community Hospital, 896 N.W.2d 393, 407 (Iowa 2017).

53 Joanna Latimer, *The Gene, the Clinic, and the Family: Diagnosing Dysmorphology, Reviving Medical Dominance* (London: Routledge, 2014).
54 Rees v. Darlington Memorial Hospital NHS Trust, [2003] UKHL 52, at 8; *cf.* McFarlane v. Tayside Health Board, [2000] 2 A.C. 59, at 114.
55 State of Kerala v. P.G. Kumari Amma, I.L.R. 2011 (Kerala) 1.

Reference List

Baker, J. H. *An Introduction to English Legal History.* 3rd ed. London: Butterworths, 1990.
Bonbrest v. Kotz, 65 F. Supp. 138 (D.D.C. 1946).
Burke v. Rivo, 551 N.E.2d 1 (Mass. 1990).
Byrd v. Wesley Medical Center, 699 P.2d 459 (Kan. 1985).
Charlie Schwalm, Sarah Pierce and Tyler Schwalm v. Janna Doherty, Jury Verdicts LEXIS n.p. (Cal. Super. Ct. 2013).
Christensen v. Thornby, 255 N.W.2d 620 (Minn. 1934).
Cockrum v. Baumgartner, 447 N.E.2d 385 (Ill. 1983).
Coleman v. Garrison, 327 A.2d 757 (Del. Super. Ct. 1974).
Coleman v. Garrison, 349 A.2d 8 (Del. 1975).
Custodio v. Bauer, 251 Cal.App.2d 303 (Cal. Ct. App. 1967).
De Ville, K. A. *Medical Malpractice in Nineteenth-Century America.* New York: NYU Press, 1990.
Dietrich v. Inhabitants of Northampton, 138 Mass. 14 (Mass. 1884).
Dumer v. St. Michael's Hospital, 233 N.W.2d 372 (Wisc. 1975).
Flowers v. D.C., 478 A.2d 1073 (D.C. 1984).
Fissell, M. *Vernacular Bodies: The Politics of Reproduction in Early Modern England.* New York: Oxford University Press, 2007.
Gleitman v. Cosgrove, 227 A.2d 689 (N.J. 1967).
Huet, M-H. *Monstrous Imaginations.* Cambridge, MA: Harvard University Press, 1993.
Latimer, J. *The Gene, the Clinic, and the Family: Diagnosing Dysmorphology, Reviving Medical Dominance.* London: Routledge, 2014.
Procanik v. Cillo, 478 A.2d 755 (N.J. 1984).
Prosser, W. *Handbook of the Law of Torts.* 2nd ed. St. Paul: West Publishing, 1955.
Plowman v. Fort Madison Community Hospital, 896 N.W.2d 393 (Iowa 2017).
Reagan, L. J. "Rashes, Rights, and Wrongs in the Hospital and in the Courtroom: German Measles, Abortion, and Malpractice before Roe and Doe." *Law and History Review* 27, no. 2 (2009): 267–79.
Rees v. Darlington Memorial Hospital NHS Trust, [2003] UKHL 52.
Rieck v. Medical Protective Co., 219 N.W.2d 242 (Wisc. 1974).
Schroeder v. Perkel, 432 A.2d 834 (N.J. 1981).
Slawek v. Stroh, 215 N.W.2d 9 (Wisc. 1974).
State of Kerala v. P.G. Kumari Amma, I.L.R. 2011 (Kerala) 1.
Stellhorn v. Victory Medical Group, Jury Verdicts LEXIS n.p. (Cal. Super. Ct. 1990).
Welke, B. *Recasting American Liberty: Gender, Race, Law, and the Railroad Revolution, 1865–1920.* New York: Cambridge University Press, 2001.
White, G. E. *Tort Law in America: An Intellectual History.* New York: Oxford University Press, 1980.
Woloch, N. *Muller v. Oregon: A Brief History With Documents.* Boston: Bedford, 1996.
Zepeda v. Zepeda, 41 Ill.App.2d 240, 249 (Ill. Ct. App. 1963).

Afterword

Eliza Buhrer

As I read through the historical accounts of malingering explored in this volume, I was struck by how the subjectivity of pain and the fact that people's symptoms do not always align with recognized medical disorders makes it difficult to determine whether an illness or impairment is real, imagined, or feigned. This is illustrated by essays in which the veracity of people's claims of illness remain ambiguous, such as Caroline A. Day's exploration of a princess whose nervous fits defied belief, Wendy J. Turner's investigation of an early modern schoolteacher who possibly feigned madness, Emma Trivett's study of medieval queens alleged to have faked their pregnancies, and Herb Leventer's discussion of patients' struggles to get doctors to take their unexplained symptoms seriously. However, I have also been thinking about this due to my own family's recent experience with injury and chronic pain.

In February, my husband fell down the stairs and broke his spine after a sleepless night of caring for our infant son who had been hospitalized for dehydration a few days earlier (he is fine and healthy now). In the hospital and at appointments afterward, doctors remarked on how improbable my husband's injury was, not because it was caused by something so mundane—stairs account for a surprisingly high percentage of vertebral fractures—but because he suffered a burst fracture of his T9 vertebra and his spinal cord remained intact. In contrast to less severe compression fractures, a burst fracture shatters the vertebra in all directions and bone fragments frequently splinter into the spinal cord. As a result, most burst fractures cause neurological deficits, including muscle weakness, loss of bowel and bladder control, and paraplegia. Rather than splintering into the spinal cord, though, my husband's vertebra crumpled in on itself, leaving his spinal cord unscathed, so he was told that he could expect to fully recover without surgery. Six months after his injury, however, he still experiences debilitating pain, but because X-rays and CT scans show that his spine has healed, there is technically no medical explanation for this. His

DOI: 10.4324/9781003452324-15

pain then is a medically unexplained symptom, like those discussed by Herb Leventer in this volume.

Locating Pain, Real and Imagined

As absurd as this may seem, his experience is not atypical. Doctors are frequently unable to identify the source of chronic back pain, which can have numerous causes—anatomical changes to bones, muscles, ligaments, and joints, nerves sending abnormal signals to the brain, and the vicious feedback loop between these conditions and psychosocial conditions like depression and anxiety.[1] For these reasons, insurance companies are reluctant to cover diagnostic tests that are expensive and often inconclusive. Further, since pain is subjective, patients are often unable to communicate their pain in a way that aligns with physicians' expectations for how pain should be present. For these reasons, many people with chronic back pain suffer for months or years without a diagnosis.

This can pose seemingly insurmountable challenges to people seeking treatment and support. In the United States, insurance companies generally will not cover procedures to manage pain unless the source of the pain is identified. Moreover, while it is widely recognized that chronic back pain can leave people whose livelihoods depend upon physical labor unable to work, Americans cannot receive social security disability insurance (SSDI) or social security supplemental income (SSI) unless their pain is the result of a "medically determinable impairment".[2] Thus, although chronic back pain is one of the leading causes of disability among adults, SSDI/SSI claims for chronic back pain are denied more often than they are approved, and applicants for these benefits are frequently suspected of malingering. SSDI/SSI fraud is not unheard of; indeed, as Courtney A. Krolikoski's investigation of responses to feigned leprosy in thirteenth-century Bologna shows, medical fraud has been a perennial concern for those who want to "ensure that their hard earned-money [is] going to people and institutions who [are] truly deserving".[3] However, it is less common today, than generally assumed.[4] Instead, the struggles endured by those who suffer from chronic back pain without a known cause illustrate a point that Charles Rosenberg made in his seminal essay on framing disease; that "in some ways, disease does not exist until we have agreed it does—by perceiving, naming, and responding to it".[5]

For these reasons, as my husband has sought treatment, he has learned that he must perform illness in a way that communicates that his pain is severe enough to require medical intervention. He has learned how to translate the sensations of his body to a ten-point pain scale—not rating his pain 1–3 if he wants it to be taken seriously, but not rating it 9–10 either lest he be suspected of exaggeration or malingering. While his instinct is to be stoic about the ways pain has limited his activities, he has also learned that he must exhaustively detail the ways that pain has altered his life.[6] Fortunately, my husband's medical providers have taken his pain seriously. He was recently referred to a pain clinic, and after some back-and-forth with our insurance company, he has a treatment plan that will involve using radiowaves transmitted through a needle to cauterize the nerves around his fracture to prevent them from sending pain signals to his brain. In many respects, this is a good outcome. There are some 19.6 million Americans who experience chronic pain that interferes with their daily life or work activities. Yet, due to the difficulty of getting referrals from primary care doctors, inadequate insurance coverage, the widespread assumption that pain is a normal part of aging, and a national shortage of pain management specialists, most never receive treatment.

My husband's efforts to get his pain treated speak to many of the same issues brought into focus by this collection. Whether focused on malingering, physicians' and quacks' attempts to gain legitimacy, or patients' struggles to get doctors to recognize and treat symptoms that do not fit into known diagnostic categories, the essays in this collection demonstrate that patients must perform and narrate illness in conformity with contemporary medical ideas about illness, disease, and health, to have their claims accepted. When they are unable to do so—either because medical understandings of the body and its debilities are in flux, the framework physicians rely upon for understanding illness is inadequate to make sense of reported symptoms, physicians and the public view illness and disease through different interpretive lenses, or simply because pain is so subjective and our experiences of embodiment so varied, that two people can have radically different experiences the same biological phenomenon—they will struggle to have their accounts believed.

Explaining That Which Was Thought Malingering

We are increasingly familiar with modern examples that illustrate this point. Beyond the medically unexplained symptoms or "factitious" disorders that Herb Leventer discusses, for many years physicians and researchers dismissed fibromyalgia and chronic fatigue syndrome as psychosomatic because they were unable to identify organic causes or biomarkers for either disorder. As a result, people with fibromyalgia and CFS were often suspected of malingering or told that their symptoms were purely psychological.[7] However, the medical community's understanding of both disorders has evolved over the past decade.[8] Researchers have recently identified biomarkers for CFS and suspect that it may be triggered by Epstein–Barr virus, human herpesvirus 6, or varicella-zoster virus.[9] Similarly, after studies revealed that people with fibromyalgia have evidence of neuroinflammation and abnormalities in the region of their brain that processes pain, scientists now believe that fibromyalgia may be a disorder of the nervous system.[10] Ultimately, the histories of CFS and fibromyalgia highlight how much the modern biomedical model of illness struggles to make sense of symptoms that do not fit into recognized diagnostic categories, one of the central points of Herb Leventer's chapter in this volume. Further illustrating this, sufferers of long COVID are now confronted by many of the same challenges people with CFS and fibromyalgia have faced.[11]

One of the primary reasons that people with CFS and fibromyalgia struggled to get the medical community to accept that they were afflicted with organic rather than psychosomatic disorders is that since the mid-nineteenth century, physicians have understood disease through clinical-pathological correlations. It was only when these correlations were discovered for CFS and fibromyalgia that they were able to fit into the framework through which physicians understand the disease. I believe that one of the values of this collection is that it demonstrates that these problems are not unique to modern medicine. While most of the chapters focus on malingering rather than patients' inability to get physicians to recognize "real" conditions, they nevertheless show that long before physicians thought about illness in terms of discrete disease categories, people had to translate their subjective experiences of illness into narratives that aligned with contemporary medical understandings to have their claims accepted, regardless of whether those claims were truthful or fictitious.

Wendy J. Turner illustrates this when she suggests that the sixteenth-century teacher William Hawkyns may have successfully feigned madness to avoid trial for treason because he was familiar with medicolegal concepts of and terms for mental illness. So does Ninon Dubourg when she shows that infirm petitioners seeking exemptions from religious obligations from the Avignon Papacy succeeded when physicians revised their petitions using medical terms, and often offering "detailed diagnoses, including the name of the condition from which the supplicants suffered". On the other hand, Lisa LeBlanc's and Carolyn A. Day's essays speak to what happens when patients' performances of illness fail to meet physician expectations. In her study of malingering in antiquity, LeBlanc recounts how Galen accused a slave of malingering when his swollen knee did not respond to medicine as expected. In Day's discussion of Princess Sophia's "fitts", Sophia's relations, physicians, and attendants ceased to believe she was "afflicted" with a "violent nervous disorder" when her "hysterical faintings" did not follow expected patterns, sometimes occurring too frequently, and other times, not occurring enough.

Moving Beyond the Foucauldian Narrative

This is not to say that the essays in this collection support a Foucauldian narrative, in which physicians are "articulators and agents of a broader hegemonic enterprise—the medicalization of society, one aspect of an oppressive ideological system".[12] However, when read together they show that medical paradigms—whatever people and physicians considered "disease", "illness", and "medicine" in a given time period—exercised discursive power over how people described, and perhaps even understood, pain, illness, and infirmity, well before the advent of modern medicine. In doing so, they make an interesting historiographical intervention.

Influenced by Foucault's argument in *The Birth of the Clinic*, contemporary authors writing on the history of medicine hold that prior to the rise of teaching hospitals in the eighteenth century, the relationship between doctors and their patients was one of collaboration between near equals. Before medical technologies, like X-rays, blood tests, and even stethoscopes, could reveal the secrets of patients' bodies, physicians had to rely upon their patients' accounts of how they had fallen ill and how their symptoms had progressed to diagnose and treat them. According to Mary Fissell, this coupled with the fact that "medical knowledge was part of popular culture [so] patients had a wealth of concepts and remedies upon which to draw", meant that "doctors lacked control over the production or consumption of such knowledge and had to tailor their diagnoses and treatment accordingly".[13] In other words, prior to the mid-eighteenth century, physicians' diagnoses had to reflect patients' expectations of medicine, as much as patient narratives had to conform to physicians' understandings of disease and illness. The trial of the fourteenth-century quack Roger le Clerk, which Chelsea Silva discusses in her broader exploration of pre-modern quackery, exemplifies this. Silva argues that le Clerk's credibility, and the credibility of premodern medical practitioners more broadly, depended not upon the efficacy of their cures, but on their ability "to look, speak, and act in accordance with popular expectations about who a physician was, and what a physician did".[14] The treatment le Clerk prescribed was absurd—he promised to cure a woman of her fever if she wore a parchment inscribed with a prayer around her neck—and yet it was not the treatment's inefficacy that revealed his status as a quack, but rather the discovery that he was illiterate and the parchment blank.

It is generally assumed that this changed with the rise of hospital medicine in the eighteenth and nineteenth centuries.[15] Physicians had previously been concerned with treating the whole person, guided by the belief that, since each person had a unique humoral balance, treatments needed to be tailored to the individual. In contrast, hospital medicine focused on discovering clinical–pathological correlations between symptoms and diseases. To establish these correlations, physicians observed and collected data on the people who received treatment in the hospital and conducted postmortem dissections to discover how external symptoms corresponded to internal pathologies. As this new empiricism came to define how medicine was practiced and how illness and disease were understood, the relationship between physicians and patients became more hierarchical. Patients' accounts of their symptoms now mattered less than what their bodies could reveal during a physical examination, and if their reported symptoms did not correspond to a recognized diagnostic category or align with expectations for how disease should present and progress then, their narratives were discounted.

The essays in this collection do not fully refute this narrative, but they do make an argument for nuance. Several chapters that focus on earlier periods support the idea that physicians placed more trust in patient narratives prior to the nineteenth century. For instance, in Dubourg's study of medical petitions to the Avignon papacy, the fact that the physicians tasked with evaluating petitioners' claims of incapacity were willing to translate their accounts of illness into the language of learned medicine suggests that they did not doubt the veracity of the petitioners' claims, even though the petitioners emphasized their functional limitations rather than the medical causes of their limitations. Likewise, in Caroline Day's essay, Princess Sophia's physicians seem to have taken her accounts of nervous fits at face value for much longer than most modern physicians would, given how significantly they diverged from contemporary understandings of nervous disorders.

These examples suggest that physicians might have assigned greater importance to patient narratives prior to the nineteenth century. Yet, they also show that the relationship between doctors and patients was hierarchical long before the rise of hospital medicine. The fact that the petitioners Dubourg discusses needed to have their accounts of illness rewritten in the first place demonstrates that physicians were already beginning to act as gatekeepers by the fourteenth century. We see similar evidence of gatekeeping in Galen's insistence that patients must be malingering if they did not respond to treatment as expected or refused to take a medicine he prescribed. Similarly, Princess Sophia's physicians, friends, and relations began to suspect she was malingering as her actions became increasingly disconnected from medical expectations, suggesting that medicine's discursive power limited the trust physicians and laypeople placed in patient narratives before the birth of the clinic.

Nevertheless, people with "real" conditions and malingerers alike accepted medicine's authority by seeking out physicians' opinions and allowing their experiences to be translated into the language of medicine, long before efficacious treatments existed for most diseases and disorders. This is somewhat surprising. Medicalization, the process by which normal human conditions are reimagined as medical disorders in need of treatment, is often portrayed in a negative light, as an instrument of social control, or a tool of pharmaceutical companies that profit from pathologizing human difference. We can see some of the reasons for this in Irina Metzler's fascinating examination of medieval Dansomnia and the 1996 Berlin Love Parade. Metzler argues that observers in both instances interpreted dancing through medical lenses; medieval chroniclers suggested dancers were suffering from demonic possession or epilepsy, while journalists used medical language and contagion metaphors to describe the ecstatic revelry of the Love Parade. In doing so commentators, both medieval and modern, obscured the fact that the dancing they witnessed contained undercurrents of social protest. Metzler suggests that this was advantageous—for by pathologizing dance, authorities were able to restore the social order the dancers had subverted.

Yet, aside from Metzler's chapter, and Leventer's suggestion that modern medicine's emphasis on pathologic–clinical correlations has led doctors to treat disorders rather than people to the detriment of those with unexplained symptoms, there is little resistance to interpreting ailments through a medical lens in the stories told in this volume. Instead, most chapters focus on people who welcomed or actively sought medical labels for their conditions. This undoubtedly reflects the fact that most of the chapters focus on malingering, and to succeed at malingering one must convince others that they are ill enough to require treatment or accommodation. In some cases, such as the stories of William Hawkyns or the "false" lepers in medieval Bologna, people to sought to convince others that they were afflicted with medical conditions for reasons similar to those associated with malingering today; they wished to avoid criminal prosecution or work. Yet, I think there is another way to read these stories.

Reading Past Malingering for a Real Cause or Crisis

Malingering is often imagined as something people do in pursuit of unjust advantages, or to escape from their duties or work. Yet, many of the people identified as malingerers in the essays in this volume experienced significant hardships that their societies either ignored or stigmatized. I want to suggest they may have readily translated their experiences into the language of medicine, because doing so enabled them to communicate what was otherwise incommunicable. In other words, they used medical concepts to describe real problems, just not the problems they were devised to describe. For example, the petitioners Dubourg discusses emphasized their functional limitations when requesting exemptions or dispensations from the Avignon papacy. By using precise medical terminology to describe these limitations, however, the physicians who rewrote their petitions did so with "words that would be understood by other medieval elites". Medicine thus served as a tool for communicating the subjective experience of disability, which might otherwise remain unrecognized and unaccommodated. By acknowledging petitioners' suffering, even when their descriptions did not reference or map perfectly onto recognized medical conditions, medieval physicians seem to have done what Herb Leventer argues modern physicians fail to do when they do not take medically unexplained symptoms seriously: They treated people rather than diseases.

Similarly, recent scholarship on the history of "hysteria" in the eighteenth and nineteenth centuries might help us better understand Princess Sophia's "hysteric faintings". While late twentieth-century scholarship interpreted hysteria as a patriarchal diagnosis, Heather Meek has recently suggested that during the long eighteenth century it might better be understood as "a malleable term that, in the hands of doctors, sometimes implies female inferiority or inherent unruliness, but in the hands of its sufferers can emerge as a distinctly female articulation of discontentment".[16] Sophia's attendants came to view her spells and spasms as attention seeking when they ceased to conform to medical understandings of nervous disorders. However, when her "nervous disorder" began in 1793, Sophia had many reasons for discontentment. Her father, King George III, to whom she had been close, had begun his descent into madness in 1788, and at the same time, her mother, Queen Charlotte, had withdrawn her attention from her daughters to focus on her husband's health. After this, Sophia and her sisters were discouraged from bringing up their futures to avoid upsetting the king, who had expressed reluctance to see them marry. Sophia was 16 years old in 1793, an age at which marriage would have been on the horizon. However, her father's madness forestalled seeking a match, and Sophia was instead forced to live as Queen Charlotte's companion, constantly chaperoned, and so secluded that she and her sisters complained of living in a nunnery.[17]

As one of 12 royal offspring, far removed from the line of succession, Sophia's circumstances would have been of little consequence to anyone but herself, so she undoubtedly would have had few opportunities to express her misery and no ability to gain control over her life. Indeed, in 1804, she complained in a letter to a friend that her father's affection and "over kindness" greatly alarmed her, which some modern scholars have interpreted as a reference to sexual advances.[18] Within this context, it is easy to imagine that by feigning a nervous disorder, Sophia was not basely seeking attention, but expressing despair that could otherwise not be expressed. While her distressing circumstances could be ignored, her nervous fits and "hysteric faintings" could not. Perhaps for Sophia, illness and the freedoms it afforded became a refuge.

It could similarly be argued that the plaintiffs in the wrongful conception and birth lawsuits that Luke I. Haqq examines used the language of pathology to describe "unwanted children", to bring to light suffering that society would otherwise fail to acknowledge. Haqq argues that parents pathologize "unwanted children" when they sue doctors for failed sterilization procedures or for withholding medical information about a developing fetus that might have led them to terminate their pregnancy. Haqq suggests that since damages in these cases are limited to those that redress the ways an unwanted child's existence harms their parents, plaintiffs not only "have incentives to overemphasize and even fabricate" any medical problems their child may have, but also to "construct, create, imagine, or feign injuries to themselves" from the birth of healthy unwanted children who may nevertheless bring them "irreplaceable joy".[19]

It is not difficult to understand why some may find it morally repugnant for parents to argue that they were harmed by the birth of a child they love. Yet, this overlooks the profound harm that comes from having one's reproductive autonomy violated. Damages in prenatal torts are limited. When a child is healthy, parents can seek damages for the costs of raising the child; although, these are sometimes reduced by the "value of the benefits conferred by having and raising the child".[20] Some jurisdictions also allow parents to seek damages associated with pregnancy, including medical expenses, emotional distress, and the pain and suffering of pregnancy and childbirth. In cases where a child is unhealthy or disabled, parents can also seek damages for the extra costs associated with the child's condition and sometimes, "the emotional distress or mental distress of birthing and raising a disabled child".[21] As a result, wrongful conception and birth torts focus on the ways a living child's existence harms their parents, which Haqq argues incentivizes parents to exaggerate the burdens of raising children.

If plaintiffs make arguments that "construe their actual children as pathological", perhaps this reflects society's failure to fully recognize the importance of reproductive autonomy since the Roe era. In the majority opinion in *Planned Parenthood of Southeastern Pa. v. Casey*, Justice Kennedy described the decision to "bear or beget a child", as among "the most intimate and personal choices a person may make in a lifetime". In Kennedy's reading, these choices are so "central to personal dignity and autonomy", that they are "central to the liberty protected by the fourteenth amendment".[22] While *Planned Parenthood v. Casey* focused on whether states could limit the right to abortion, if American society had broadly accepted these ideas about why reproductive autonomy matters, then parents in wrongful conception and birth suits may not need to argue that they are harmed by the existence of a child they love. Instead, they could seek damages for the gross violation of their dignity and autonomy that occurred when the choice of whether to become pregnant or carry a pregnancy to term was made for them by someone else. If parents are malingering by overemphasizing the costs and burdens created by an "unwanted child", then perhaps it is because the law provides no way to redress this grievous wrong.

Emma Trivett's study of medieval queens who allegedly feigned pregnancy similarly suggests that what at first appears to be malingering may reflect a more complex reality. Trivett suggests that there are multiple ways to interpret accounts of feigned royal pregnancies. Since infertility was seen as a sign of female failure in the Middle Ages, medieval chroniclers may have fabricated these accounts to malign queens and cast doubt on their legitimacy. Alternatively, Trivett suggests that the queens could have been pregnant but miscarried before their pregnancies were detectable by others. For while there was no surefire way to detect early pregnancy prior to the invention of pregnancy tests and ultrasounds, numerous symptoms can reveal to a woman that she is pregnant: a missed period, swollen breasts, nausea, and fatigue, along with many others.[23] Thus, what society and chroniclers considered to be feigned pregnancy, could have simply been a pregnancy that society failed to recognize. Finally, Trivett notes that some scholars have argued that faking pregnancy might also have been a way that "a woman could harness some authority or control over her (usually dire) circumstances using her reproductive role".[24]

In these instances of historical malingering, it seems plausible that if people intentionally feigned illness, they did so in response to desperate circumstances that they had no other way to address due to the limitations imposed upon them by their societies. In other words, they feigned illness to adapt to hardship. The idea that malingering may be an adaptive response to adversity or unmet needs is well established in modern medical literature.[25] For example, one study of malingering in emergency settings found that more than 50% of patients who malingered did so because they needed food or shelter.[26] This way of explaining malingering, which is known as the adaptational model, may not have seemed unfamiliar to some of the people discussed in this volume.[27] For instance, Lisa LeBlanc argues that ancient literary texts were relatively sympathetic to malingering, "often presenting the situation as the only or best solution available".[28]

Conclusion

The point of these re-readings is ultimately to suggest that the line between malingering and illness is more fluid than commonly assumed. For if disease is to some extent socially constructed, then should not the same be true of malingering? Except in obvious cases of fraud, assuming certainty about malingering also requires assuming that the diagnostic categories recognized at a given time are adequate for describing any "real" symptoms a person might have. Yet, the map is not territory. Since the beginning of the nineteenth century, numerous diseases and disorders have been added to our medical lexicon, while others that were once understood as medical disorders are no longer viewed through a medical lens.[29] As the history of fibromyalgia and chronic fatigue syndrome shows, moreover, new medical discoveries can fundamentally change the way we understand existing disorders.

If illness, real or feigned, involves performance, then we must acknowledge that some people's performances are more likely to be believed than others. Just as Galen suspected the slave whose knee he examined was malingering because slaves were "prone to lie", people marked by stigma are more likely to be suspected of malingering when they seek medical attention for real problems. It is well documented, for instance, that Black people are undertreated for pain due to doctors' racial biases and the disturbing persistence of ideas about how people of different races tolerate pain that originated in the antebellum era.[30] Similarly, many doctors take women's reports of pain less seriously than men's. In emergency settings, doctors often misattribute women's pain to anxiety and offer them sedatives or anti-anxiety medication rather than analgesics. Women also wait longer than men for treatment during medical emergencies.[31] In outpatient settings, women with conditions that cause chronic pain are frequently told that their pain is psychosomatic and offered anti-depressants rather than treatment.[32] The convergence of these two biases can lead to devastating outcomes. Black women in the United States are two to three times more likely to die of complications related to pregnancy and childbirth than white women, and this is in part because doctors do not take their reported symptoms seriously.[33]

The essays in this volume suggest that these problems have a long history. They further provide insight into how illness was performed and imagined in the past, how medical expertise was once defined, and how doctor–patient relations and medical paradigms shaped the way people understood, described, and experienced illness. However, they also raise questions about the nature of malingering that puts the past into dialogue with contemporary questions. Concern about malingering seems to have both been a historical constant and a reflection of culturally specific biases, and beliefs about disease and illness. Ultimately, the accounts of illness we trust and the accounts we view with suspicion say as much about our own values as the motives of alleged malingerers.

Notes

1 Adaku Nwachuku, "4 Big Reasons Why Back Pain Is Hard to Diagnose," *Spine-health*, last updated February 28, 2020, https://www.spine-health.com/blog/4-big-reasons-why-back-pain-hard-diagnose. Low Back Pain Fact Sheet,

National Institute of Neurological Disorders and Stroke, last updated July 25, 2022, https://www.ninds.nih.gov/low-back-pain-fact-sheet.

2 "How We Evaluate Symptoms Including Pain," Code of Federal Regulations 404.1529, Social Security Administration, last updated January 18, 2017, https://www.ssa.gov/OP_Home/cfr20/404/404–1529.htm.

3 Courtney A. Krolikoski's article in this volume, 183–206.

4 The Office of the Inspector General estimates the fraud incidence rate among recipients of SSDI to be "less than a fraction of one percent." https://www.ssa.gov/disabilityfacts/facts.html.

5 Charles E. Rosenberg, "Disease in History: Frames and Framers," *The Milbank Quarterly* 67. Supplement 1. Framing Disease: The Negotiation of Explanatory Schemes (1989): 1–15.

6 Numerous online resources that advise patients with chronic pain on how to communicate with doctors. See for instance: https://health.clevelandclinic.org/how-to-talk-to-your-doctor-about-pain/, https://uspainfoundation.org/blog/how-to-talk-about-pain-so-your-doctor-will-listen/, https://www.npr.org/sections/health-shots/2018/07/23/626202281/words-matter-when-talking-about-pain-with-your-doctor. The fact that such resources exist is indicative of how difficult it is for chronic pain patients to get adequate treatment.

7 "What Is ME/CFS?" U.S. ME/CFS Clinician Coalition, last updated 2021, https://mecfscliniciancoalition.org/about-mecfs/.

8 Committee on the Diagnostic Criteria for Myalgic Encephalomyelitis/Chronic Fatigue Syndrome: Board on the Health of Select Populations, Institute of Medicine, "Beyond Myalgic Encephalomyelitis/Chronic Fatigue Syndrome: Redefining an Illness," *National Academies Press*, February 10, 2015, https://nap.nationalacademies.org/catalog/19012/beyond-myalgic-encephalomyelitischronic-fatigue-syndrome-redefining-an-illness.

9 See for instance, R. Esfandyarpour, A. Kashi, M. Nemat-Gorgani, J. Wilhelmy, and R. W. Davis, "A nanoelectronics-blood-based diagnostic biomarker for myalgic encephalomyelitis/chronic fatigue syndrome (ME/CFS)," *PNAS* 116, no. 21 (April 2019): 10250–57.

10 "What Causes Fibromyalgia?: Signs Point to Changes in the Brain," Cleveland Clinic, last modified October 4, 2019, https://health.clevelandclinic.org/what-causes-fibromyalgia/.

11 For the first year of the COVID-19 pandemic, physicians and researchers often dismissed long COVID symptoms as psychosomatic. As a result, much of our initial knowledge about long COVID comes not from scientific studies, but from information compiled by online support groups, like https://www.reddit.com/r/Longhaulers/, where people afflicted with lingering sequelae gathered to compare symptoms, discuss potential treatments, and seek support. Due in part to the efforts of these groups, the medical community eventually recognized long COVID as a legitimate disorder; in the first half of 2022 researchers finally identified its biomarkers, began to understand its physiological causes, and identified factors that might predispose people to developing it. Nevertheless, people with long COVID are still frequently suspected of malingering. Exemplifying this, Senator Richard Burr recently rejected the Biden administration's request for funding to study and treat long COVID on the grounds that since "no one can even diagnose long COVID, people would certainly lie in order to receive disability payments."

12 Rosenberg, "Disease in History," 4.

13 Mary Fissell, "The Disappearance of the Patient's Narrative and the Invention of Hospital Medicine," in *British Medicine in the Age of Reform*, eds. Roger French and Andrew Wear (New York: Routledge: 1991), 93.

14 Chelsea Silva's article in this volume, 25–54, quote at 26.

15 Herb Leventer discusses this transition in his chapter, although he associates these changes with the publication of the Flexner Report in 1911 due to his focus on American medicine.

16 Heather Meek, "Medical Discourse, Women's Writing, and the 'Perplexing Form' of Eighteenth-Century Hysteria," in *Early Modern Women* 11 (2016): 186.

17 Jeremy Black, *George III: America's Last King* (New Haven: Yale University Press, 2006): 156.

18 Janice Hadlow, *A Royal Experiment: The Private Life of King George III* (New York: Henry Holt and Company, 2014), 508; Flora Frasier, *Princesses: The Six Daughters of George III* (New York: Anchor Books, 2006), 207.

19 Luke I. Haqq's article in this volume, 245–262.

20 "Prenatal Torts," Legal Information Institute, last modified July 2020, https://www.law.cornell.edu/wex/prenatal_tort.

21 "Prenatal Torts," Legal Information Institute, last modified July 2020, https://www.law.cornell.edu/wex/prenatal_tort.

22 Planned Parenthood v. Casey, 505 U.S. 833, 112 S. Ct. 2791 (1992).

23 "Getting Pregnant," Mayo Clinic, last modified December 3, 2021, https://www.mayoclinic.org/healthy-lifestyle/getting-pregnant/in-depth/symptoms-of-pregnancy/art-20043853.

24 Emma Trivett's article in this volume, 115–137.

25 Richard Rogers, "Development of a New Classificatory Model of Malingering," *Bulletin of the American Academy of Psychiatric Law* 18 (1990): 323–33.

26 B. D. Yates, C. R. Nordquist, and R. A. Schultz-Ross, "Feigned Psychiatric Symptoms in the Emergency Room," *Psychiatric Services* 47 (1996): 998–1000.

27 Shortly after the adaptational model was introduced by the forensic psychologist Richard Rogers, psychologists began to recognize it as more useful than other explanatory models which attributed malingering to mental illness or criminal motivations. See R. Rogers, K. W. Sewell, and A. M. Goldstein, "Explanatory Models of Malingering: A Prototypical Analysis," *Law and Human Behavior* 18 (1994): 543–52.

28 Lisa LeBlanc's article in this volume, 11–24.

29 See, for example, Bert Hansen, "American Physicians' Earliest Writings About Homosexuals, 1880–1900," *The Milbank Quarterly* 67, Supplement 1. Framing Disease: The Creation and Negotiation of Explanatory Schemes (1989): 92–108.

30 Kelly M. Hoffman et al., "Racial Bias in Pain Assessment and Treatment Recommendations, and False Beliefs About Biological Differences Between Blacks and Whites," *Proceedings of the National Academy of Sciences of the United States of America* 13 (2016): 4296–301.

31 J. Crook and E. Tunks, "Women with Pain," in *Chronic Pain: Psychosocial Factors in Rehabilitation*, eds. E. Tunks, A. Bellissimo, and R. Roy (Malabar, FL: R. E. Krieger Publishing Company, 1990), 37–48.

32 Diane E. Hoffman and Anita J. Tarzian, "The Girl Who Cried Pain: A Bias Against Women in the Treatment of Pain," *Journal of Law and Medical Ethics* 29 (2001): 13–27. Also see Joe Fassler, "How Doctors Take Women's Pain Less Seriously," *The Atlantic Monthly*, October 15, 2015, https://www.theatlantic.com/health/archive/2015/10/emergency-room-wait-times-sexism/410515/.

33 Nina Martin and Renee Montagne, "Nothing Protects Black Women from Dying in Pregnancy and Childbirth," *ProPublica*, last modified December 7, 2017, https://www.propublica.org/article/nothing-protects-black-women-from-dying-in-pregnancy-and-childbirth.

Reference List

Black, Jeremy. *George III: America's Last King*. New Haven: Yale University Press, 2006.

Committee on the Diagnostic Criteria for Myalgic Encephalomyelitis/Chronic Fatigue Syndrome, Board on the Health of Select Populations, Institute of Medicine. "Beyond Myalgic Encephalomyelitis/Chronic Fatigue Syndrome: Redefining an Illness." *National Academies Press*, February 10, 2015, "How We Evaluate Symptoms Including Pain." Code of Federal Regulations 404.1529, Social Security Administration, last updated January 18, 2017. https://www.ssa.gov/OP_Home/cfr20/404/404-1529.htm.

Crook, J., and E. Tunks. "Women With Pain." In *Chronic Pain: Psychosocial Factors in Rehabilitation*, edited by E. Tunks, A. Bellissimo, and R. Roy. Malabar, FL: R.E. Krieger Publishing Company, 1990.

Esfandyarpour, R., A. Kashi, M. Nemat-Gorgani, J. Wilhelmy, and R. W. Davis. "A Nanoelectronics-Blood-Based Diagnostic Biomarker for Myalgic Encephalomyelitis/Chronic Fatigue Syndrome (ME/CFS)." *PNAS* 116, no. 21 (April 2019): 10250–57.

Fassler, Joe. "How Doctors Take Women's Pain Less Seriously." *The Atlantic Monthly*, October 15, 2015. https://www.theatlantic.com/health/archive/2015/10/emergency-room-wait-times-sexism/410515/.

Fissell, Mary. "The Disappearance of the Patient's Narrative and the Invention of Hospital Medicine." In *British Medicine in the Age of Reform*, edited by Roger French and Andrew Wear. New York: Routledge, 1991.

Frasier, Flora. *Princesses: The Six Daughters of George III*. New York: Anchor Books, 2006.

"Getting Pregnant." Mayo Clinic. Accessed December 3, 2021. https://www.mayoclinic.org/healthy-lifestyle/getting-pregnant/in-depth/symptoms-of-pregnancy/art-20043853.

Hadlow, Janice. *A Royal Experiment: The Private Life of King George III*. New York: Henry Holt and Company, 2014.

Hansen, Bert. "American Physicians' Earliest Writings About Homosexuals, 1880–1900." *The Milbank Quarterly*, 67, Supplement 1. Framing Disease: The Creation and Negotiation of Explanatory Schemes (1989): 92–108.

Hoffman, Diane E., and Anita J. Tarzian. "The Girl Who Cried Pain: A Bias Against Women in the Treatment of Pain." *Journal of Law and Medical Ethics* 29 (2001): 13–27.

Hoffman, Kelly M., et al. "Racial Bias in Pain Assessment and Treatment Recommendations, and False Beliefs About Biological Differences Between Blacks and Whites." *Proceedings of the National Academy of Sciences of the United States of America* 13 (2016): 4296–301.

Low Back Pain Fact Sheet. *National Institute of Neurological Disorders and Stroke,* last updated July 25, 2022. https://www.ninds.nih.gov/low-back-pain-fact-sheet.

Martin, Nina, and Renee Montagne. "Nothing Protects Black Women From Dying in Pregnancy and Childbirth." *ProPublica,* last modified December 7, 2017. https://www.propublica.org/article/nothing-protects-black-women-from-dying-in-pregnancy-and-childbirth.

Meek, Heather. "Medical Discourse, Women's Writing, and the 'Perplexing Form' of Eighteenth-Century Hysteria." *Early Modern Women* 11 (2016): 186.

Nwachuku, Adaku. "4 Big Reasons Why Back Pain Is Hard to Diagnose." *Spine-health,* last updated February 28, 2020. https://www.spine-health.com/blog/4-big-reasons-why-back-pain-hard-diagnose.

Planned Parenthood v. Casey, 505 U.S. 833, 112 S. Ct. 2791 (1992).

"Prenatal Torts." Legal Information Institute, last modified July 2020. https://www.law.cornell.edu/wex/prenatal_tort.

Rogers, R. "Development of a New Classificatory Model of Malingering." *Bulletin of the American Academy of Psychiatric Law* 18 (1990): 323–33.

Rogers, R., K. W. Sewell, and A. M. Goldstein. "Explanatory Models of Malingering: A Prototypical Analysis." *Law and Human Behavior* 18 (1994): 543–52.

Rosenberg, Charles E. "Disease in History: Frames and Framers." *The Milbank Quarterly* 67. Supplement 1. *Framing Disease: The Negotiation of Explanatory Schemes* (1989): 1–15.

"What Causes Fibromyalgia?: Signs Point to Changes in the Brain." Cleveland Clinic, last modified October 4, 2019. https://health.clevelandclinic.org/what-causes-fibromyalgia/.

"What Is ME/CFS?" U.S. ME/CFS Clinician Coalition, last updated 2021. https://mecfscliniciancoalition.org/about-mecfs/.

Yates, B. D., C. R. Nordquist, and R. A. Schultz-Ross. "Feigned Psychiatric Symptoms in the Emergency Room." *Psychiatric Services* 47 (1996): 998–1000.

Contributors

Eliza Buhrer, PhD, is Teaching Associate Professor in the Department of Humanities, Arts and Social Sciences at Colorado School of Mines. Her research and publications focus on the relationship between medicine, law, and disability in premodern Europe, and the early histories of mental disorder and intellectual disability. She has also published on poverty and charity in premodern Europe, and she is the editor of the Bloomsbury Cultural History of Poverty in the Middle Ages.

Carolyn A. Day, PhD, is Associate Professor of History at Furman University. Day studied microbiology before becoming a full-time historian of science and medicine in British history. She is the author of *Consumptive Chic: A History of Beauty, Fashion and Disease* (Bloomsbury, 2017), which focuses on material culture and the social space occupied by tuberculosis in the late eighteenth and first half of the nineteenth century. Her current research focuses on the individual experience of illness in eighteenth- and nineteenth-century Britain.

Ninon Dubourg, PhD, studied at the University of Paris, France, and she is currently working as a postdoctoral scholar at the University of Liège, Belgium. Already an accomplished scholar with many publications, editorial work, and service to the medical history community, her research includes medieval people with physical and mental disabilities among both laypeople and clerical from the twelfth to the fifteenth centuries. Her work highlights the medieval Church's comprehension of the social experience of disability.

Luke I. Haqq, JD, is an attorney in the Public Health Law Center of the Mitchell Hamline School of Law. His research, which focuses on intersections of law, medicine, religion, and reproductive policy, has received several awards and appeared in numerous law journals.

Courtney A. Krolikoski, PhD, is Assistant Professor of History in the Department of History at Jacksonville University. Her research concentrates on the intersection of the social, medical, and religious history of leprosy in High Medieval Bologna, Italy. She also works on issues of gender, religion, sexuality, science, and digital history as it applies to humanistic and social scientific studies.

Lisa LeBlanc, PhD, is Associate Professor in the Department of English at Anna Maria College, and she has a degree in medieval literature. She also recently completed a License in Mental Health Counseling, and her current research focuses on the intersection of mental illness and ancient through early modern literatures.

Herb Leventer, PhD, is adjunct Assistant Professor in the Department of Philosophy at Yeshiva University and Affiliate Instructor in the Division of Medical Ethics of the Department of Population Health at the NYU School of Medicine. He teaches medical ethics, environmental ethics, philosophy of art, and epidemiology. His research has focused on ethical issues of infectious diseases, and philosophical problems in clinical diagnosis raised by new discoveries of the multifactorial causes of most maladies.

Irina Metzler, PhD, is Fellow of the Royal Historical Society. She is the author of numerous publications, and she is most well known for her monograph, *A Social History of Disability in the Middle Ages: Cultural Considerations of Physical Impairment* (Routledge, 2013). She has been the recipient of many grants and awards, including a research fellowship in Medical Humanities and History from the Wellcome Trust.

Walton O. Schalick, III, MD/PhD, is on faculty in the Department of Orthopedics and Rehabilitation, the Waisman Center, and Medieval Studies. He works with and for pediatric patients as a physiatrist and pediatrician at the University of Wisconsin. He co-edits Amsterdam University Press' *Premodern Health, Disease, and Disability* with Wendy J. Turner and Christina Lee, and Manchester University Press' *Disability History* with Julie Anderson. His published research ranges from pediatric clinical studies to research ethics to the history of modern disabilities. The core of his medieval research is focused on the intersections between medicine, pharmacology, and wider society.

Chelsea Silva, PhD, is Assistant Professor of English at Oklahoma State University. She works on disability studies, medical humanities, and Middle English literature. Her in-progress monograph, *Bedwritten: Middle English Medicine and the Ailing Author*, explores the intersection of healthcare and literary production in late medieval England. Her work has been supported by fellowships from the ACLS, the Huntington Library, and the University of Wisconsin–Madison, among others.

Emma Trivett, PhD, is an independent scholar in Dundee, UK. She recently finished her doctoral thesis on royal infertility in medieval England and Scotland at the University of Edinburgh. Already an accomplished author and scholar, Trivett is interested in the social and political significance of (in)fertility for medieval kingship and queenship.

Wendy J. Turner, PhD, is Professor of History and holds affiliate professorships in The Graduate School and the Center for Bioethics and Health Policy in the Institute of Public and Preventative Health at Augusta University. Her research interests lie at the intersection between law and medicine in medieval England, primarily on the history of disabilities, mental health, and intellectual disabilities. Her works include *Care and Custody of the Mentally Ill, Incompetent, and Disabled in Medieval England* (Brepols, 2013) along with numerous articles. She has edited four other books and sits on four editorial boards. She is currently researching pandemic history and the history of old age in medieval England.

Index

For Product Safety Concerns and Information please contact our EU
representative GPSR@taylorandfrancis.com
Taylor & Francis Verlag GmbH, Kaufingerstraße 24, 80331 München, Germany

www.ingramcontent.com/pod-product-compliance
Lightning Source LLC
Chambersburg PA
CBHW061626220326
41598CB00026BA/3900

9 78103 2 589626